INTEGRATING NARRATIVE MEDICINE AND EVIDENCE-BASED MEDICINE

T0321408

Integrating Narrative Medicine and Evidence-based Medicine

The everyday social practice of healing

JAMES P MEZA MD

and

DANIEL S PASSERMAN DO

Forewords by
PETER WYER and RITA CHARON
and
MARK H EBELL

Radcliffe Publishing
London • New York

Radcliffe Publishing Ltd
33–41 Dallington Street
London
EC1V 0BB
United Kingdom

www.radcliffepublishing.com

Electronic catalogue and worldwide online ordering facility.

British Library Cataloguing in Publication Data

A catalogue record for this book is available from the British Library.

ISBN-13: 978 184619 350 7

The paper used for the text pages of this book
is FSC® certified. FSC (The Forest Stewardship
Council®) is an international network to promote
responsible management of the world's forests.

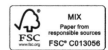

Typeset by Phoenix Photosetting, Chatham, Kent, UK
Printed and bound by TJI Digital, Padstow, Cornwall, UK

Contents

Part IV: Epilogue

Afterword

Part V: Appendices

Index

Dedication

Dedicated to our loving wives Carol and Tracy

The Social Practice of Healing

When doctors listen to patients' stories, they merge the individual's narrative with the cultural power of the medical profession and produce a co-constructed narrative within the context of an institutionalized social framework, creating coherence between the 'inner experience' of the individual and the socially authorized version of the same story. This practice harmonizes two stories, creating personal meaning and reinforcing social norms.

Foreword

We appreciate the appearance of this book as evidence of the emergence into the clinical mainstream of a stereoscopic way of knowing in clinical medicine. In 2008, our group at Columbia University coined the name 'Narrative Evidence Based Medicine', being careful to not insert hyphens between the words. We tried thereby to keep in play the concepts of 'narrative evidence' as well as 'evidence based medicine' and, by the long view, 'narrative medicine' as the encompassing or embracing concept. Evidence – of all kinds – sits at the center of what the overarching effort reaches for, that is, a scientifically informed narrative medicine.

Dr Meza and Dr Passerman do a great service to clinical trainees and practitioners in this serious yet welcoming review of the practice of evidence based medicine along with the conceptual hints of the relational, social, and political aspects of narrative medicine. This young book helps us all to envision a time in clinical practice when doctors know how to listen to their patients' narratives of illness while partnering with their patients to accurately answer the questions they ask.

We take heart from a book like this one, for its appearance now signals that the field of narrative medicine, which was inaugurated at Columbia in 2000, has had an impact on the mainstream practice of medicine, not only among the literary types but also among the 'in-the-trenches' doctors in practice. That two family medicine residencies in the Midwest teach narrative evidence based medicine grounds our own impression that mainstream clinical medicine *needs* the fruits of our work in narrative medicine and endorses our joining of narrative ways of thinking in medicine with the search, always, for the firmest and 'truest' thinking in the scientific foundations of clinical practice.

Peter Wyer and Rita Charon
Columbia University, New York, NY
March 2011

Foreword

Let me tell you a story.

Got your attention, didn't I? Human beings are hard-wired to hear and tell stories, and to use the story to communicate complex ideas, emotions, and experiences. Stories teach us values, they emphasize connections and connectedness, and help us build community. Learning to truly listen to our patients' stories is the essence of narrative medicine.

The area under the receiver operating characteristic curve was 0.89.

Still there? Receiver what? The language of evidence-based medicine is too often complex and opaque, and almost always lacks poetry. In short, it lacks the narrative elements that tell a story. No wonder so many physicians and learners quickly lose interest in evidence-based medicine, and have so much difficulty applying it in their practice.

In fact, narrative medicine and evidence-based medicine have often been thought of as non-overlapping magisteria, much in the way Stephen Jay Gould described the domains of religion and science.[1] To paraphrase his thoughtful and influential essay, religion asks *why* questions, while science asks *how* questions. But are they truly non-overlapping? Are we biologically predisposed toward altruism, xenophobia, and even spirituality?

Similarly, are the magisteria of narrative and evidence-based medicine truly non-overlapping? In this important book, Meza and Passerman argue that the domains of narrative and evidence-based medicine can and must be integrated to provide the best possible care for our patients.

Many years ago, as a college freshman, I read CP Snow's *The Two Cultures*.[2] Snow described a chasm between the humanities and sciences, with members of each camp ignorant of the achievements of the other. Too many physicists could not quote Shakespeare, and too many literary critics could not describe the second law of thermodynamics. But just as Snow saw a way forward toward a 'third culture' that mediated the cultural chasm, Meza and Passerman have proposed a way forward for medicine.

They are not alone in their vision for a more integrated approach to the care of patients that learns from both the patient's story and the best available scientific evidence. It is noteworthy that so much of their book addresses concepts like POEMs (Patient Oriented Evidence that Matters), DOEs (Disease Oriented Evidence), and the SORT rating (Strength of Recommendation Taxonomy, based on the POEMs concept). This transformative framework was first proposed by Allen Shaughnessy and David Slawson in 1994 and was an important first step in linking narrative and evidence-based medicine.[3]

Shaughnessy and Slawson argued convincingly that we must listen to our patients, so we can learn the outcomes that they care about most. Those patient-oriented outcomes address how long and how well they live, not just how high or low their numbers are. Only by keeping our focus on POEMs can we decide which evidence is most important to our patients.

Ultimately, our success as a profession, as healers, depends on our ability to integrate our patients' stories with the evidence. Otherwise, we become slaves to technology. As CP Snow famously said: 'Technology is . . . a queer thing. It brings you gifts with one hand, and stabs you in the back with the other.'[2] We perform more CT scans per capita than almost any country in the world, and there is no doubt that some patients benefit from this technology some of the time. But we are sickening tens of thousands with unnecessary radiation exposure, overdiagnosing and then overtreating disease and predisease, and bankrupting our society with the cost of unthinking and careless use of these technologies.

Meza and Passerman have written a groundbreaking work that successfully teaches physicians how to practice both narrative medicine and evidence-based medicine. Both are intimidating to the uninitiated, but in this pragmatic book we can see how both can be successfully integrated into our daily care of patients.

Only by forging a partnership with patients, built on listening to their stories, truly understanding their questions, and informed by the best available evidence, can we hope to provide the most efficient, effective and compassionate care possible.

Mark H Ebell, MD, MS
Associate Professor, Dept of Epidemiology and Biostatistics
College of Public Health, University of Georgia, Athens
March 2011

REFERENCES

1 Gould SJ. Nonoverlapping magisteria. *Natural History.* 1997; **106**: 16–22.
2 Snow CP. *The Two Cultures.* Cambridge: Cambridge University Press; 1959.
3 Shaughnessy AF, Slawson DC, Bennett JH. Becoming an information master: a guidebook to the medical information jungle. *J Fam Pract.* 1994; **39**: 489–99.

Preface

A NEW TYPE OF MEDICAL KNOWLEDGE

Good medical care is delivered within the context of a healthy doctor–patient relationship and incorporates the best scientific evidence available at the time. These two ingredients are the recipe for making good decisions. The inescapable fact that decisions must be made in the course of providing medical care highlights the need for us to understand how those decisions are made. Both a healthy relationship and science are necessary, but each is insufficient without the other. Too often, this fact is overlooked and cloaked in the mysteries of 'professional opinion' and 'bedside manner.'

Although there has been an explosion of technology and medical science in the past 20 years, what we describe here is a totally different type of medical knowledge, one that is contingent, emergent, and situated within a social context. This type of medical knowledge is completely different than a purely biomedical model. It is uniquely conceptualized for practicing physicians.

OUR CHANGING WORLD

The only constant in our world is constant change. This book is written at a specific point in time. Technologies will certainly continue to change, but there are parts of medicine that are timeless and enduring. By necessity, if we want to describe the timeless and enduring process of providing medical care, we have to use contemporary (outdated) examples. So, you will see some of both in this book. We remember attending a Society of Teachers of Family Medicine (STFM) Annual Spring Conference about ten years ago. One of the presenters talked about his several years of experience with evidence-based medicine and, at the conclusion of the presentation stated that the topic was 'dead' because of how difficult it was to access the evidence and create knowledge. At the time, he had a convincing argument. Times have certainly changed. All of us are wired and connected to the internet in so many different ways it is hard to imagine what life was like just a few short years ago. All of us have the technology to access information at a frighteningly rapid pace – but do we know what it means? Even more importantly, what does it mean for our patients?

During the same period of time, advances in medical knowledge have progressed as rapidly. Whatever is true today has a half-life measured in months. 'Specialists' used to claim authority because they knew everything there was to know about a particular topic. Because of the proliferation of knowledge, specialists these days have to claim authority in a smaller and smaller scope of practice. In cardiology, we have nuclear medicine cardiology, congestive heart failure specialists, interventional cardiology, electrophysiology cardiology, transplant cardiologists, etc. Nobody is just a plain old cardiologist. The same phenomenon is true across specialties. Neurologists have movement disorder specialists, stroke specialists, seizure specialists, etc.

A MEDICAL PRACTICE THAT IS TIMELESS AND ENDURING

With all the changes, we asked ourselves, 'What will be constant in health care no matter what changes occur in the next decade or two?' It seemed there were two answers to that question. The first will be the enduring value of the doctor–patient relationship. No matter what type of stress that relationship encounters, patients look to doctors (providers) who provide caring and compassion. Ideally, it will be someone that they know and trust, someone who accepts them with all their imperfections, someone who can help them understand the unfamiliar or distressing sensations that they experience, making sense out of symptoms and explain what the symptoms mean. This type of relationship is best described in the context of 'Relationship Centered Care.' In order to provide that type of care, doctors need to be self reflective. They need to know how they themselves affect the process of care.

The second attribute that will remain constant despite any change in health care is that patients will always want a doctor who really knows their stuff ... someone who is up to date on the latest advances and knowledgeable about current treatments. It is impossible for any doctor to know everything, so we can't define ourselves by a specific body of knowledge – in order to 'know our stuff' we need to know how to find the information at the point of care, evaluate the quality of the information, and apply the information to the specific situation that brought the patient to our office to begin with. What this really means is that we need to be experts in critical thinking and analysis. It is a more adaptable approach to 'medical information' than memorizing a specific body of specialized knowledge. So 'Information Mastery' is a new skill that needs to be added to knowing the patient and having clinical experience.

A STUMBLING BLOCK TO INTEGRATING NARRATIVE AND EVIDENCE

It is the combination of these attributes – relationship skills and critical thinking with analytic skills – that will prepare physicians to re-claim their role in the health care of the future. This type of doctor is what one of our friends calls 'a complete physician.' Unfortunately, those skills are not often found in equal proportions in any one individual. Again, at an STFM Annual Spring Conference we attended a session of a working group that had spent a year trying to integrate evidence-based medicine with 'communication skills.' The working group's conclusion was that 'The two concepts couldn't be combined in a consistent way.' We vividly remember breaking into small discussion groups and having a pre-eminent patient communication expert who led one of the small groups start with the statement, 'I don't know what to say because I don't know anything about evidence-based medicine.' Sitting there, we wondered, 'Why is this so difficult? This seems like what we do every day in the clinic.' Articulating exactly what we do took several years and resulted in this book.

DIFFERING EPISTEMOLOGIES (DIFFERING 'WAYS OF KNOWING')

Before we proceed, it is worth taking a moment to understand why narrative medicine and evidence based medicine have been so difficult to integrate into a single process of care. Understanding this difficulty requires concepts borrowed from the philosophy of science. For simplicity, we will discuss four basic philosophical perspectives rather than specific philosophical arguments; those four are empiricism, positivism, relativism, and realism. *Empiricism* (seeing is believing) was popularized during the Enlightenment, a time when Western medicine began to develop its current structure. Diseases were observable in the form of abnormal organs discovered at autopsy. Empiricism was followed by logical positivism. *Positivism* holds that there is a single truth and science discovers that truth. Truth exists apart from human endeavors and what we do is seek to discover truth through science. Empiricism and positivism are the legacy that medicine inherited and what many doctors take for granted, forming the philosophical basis of biomedicine.

The form of knowledge in narrative is something we call *relativism*. Relativism means that all truth is only as true as it is perceived. There can be many truths depending on one's perspective. This sticks out as 'unscientific' (otherwise known as the 'marked category' – different than 'normal'). For this reason, Narrative medicine has to always be making an argument that it belongs in what we otherwise consider the scientific endeavor of medicine (biomedicine). In order to accomplish the feat of integration, we reject both of those philosophies of science in favor of 'realism.' *Realism* implies that there is a truth, even if we can never know it fully. What we can do is continuously approximate it more closely. You will hear us talk about the science in narrative and the narrative in science. What we are doing is mixing these two different ways of knowing (epistemologies) so that they can be integrated into a single 'way of knowing.'

Consider the following quotation. It implies that the patient's way of knowing is different than the doctor's way of knowing:

> My wife's recent illness taught me that patients are not only texts read by their physicians but also the authors of their bodies and stories. As 'reader-response' theorists point out, each reading is necessarily a reconstitution of the text. By rewriting in medical terminology, physicians, like literary critics, put patients' texts into more abstract terms, transforming patients into cases and their illnesses into diseases. Physicians can thus discuss, understand, and treat disease, although the stories may become unrecognizable to their original authors. Unlike critics, however, physicians are responsible for the well-being of their patients. They must, therefore, retranslate medical cases back into individual narratives using the patient's language. Thus, patients can retake control of their illnesses and become again the primary authors of their lives. (Paul C Sorum. Patient as author, physician as critic. *Arch Fam Med* 1994; **3**: 549–6)

What this quotation illustrates is a give and take, a journey traveled together by patient and doctor, a process that acknowledges both the full humanity of the patient and provides the best of medical science. It is a collaboration – a relationship with moral dimensions. It is a way to recapture the essence of what it means for physicians to serve patients. To truly integrate narrative and 'evidence,' we take this process one step further, inviting the doctor to enter the patient's world and way of knowing an illness narrative and inviting the patient to enter the doctor's world and way of knowing scientific evidence. *Both doctor and patient can claim 'knowing' in both these domains, enabling a conversation that results in a co-constructed narrative.* Others concluded that it can't be done, but we do it, and in this book we hope to show how you too can do it.

THE INTERDEPENDENCE OF NARRATIVE MEDICINE AND EVIDENCED-BASED MEDICINE: T1, T2, T3, AND BEYOND

In a way, this practical guide of 'how to' presages the theoretical work that integrates two separate movements in medicine that are currently being pursued in a parallel fashion. There are hints that these two movements will converge: see comments by one of Narrative medicine's champions, Rita Charon:

> He [evidence based medicine practitioner] came to us to say, 'Evidence based medicine lacks what you in narrative medicine know.' I was able to say to him 'Narrative medicine lacks what you in evidence based medicine know.' So we have formed a joint intensive study seminar. We call it narrative-evidence-based medicine, realizing that there is evidence to be had in narrative ... So, to dichotomize those two seems a mistake to me, and seems to relinquish a lot of what I

> believe is salient to clinical practice, which is to say narrative based medicine, by definition, is not meant to point to medicine that does not have evidence ... We're at a point in this field already of high complexity. (Rita Charon, cited in John D Engle *et al. Narrative in Health Care: healing patients, practitioners, profession and community.* Radcliffe Publishing: Oxford, 2008)

Rita Charon is saying exactly what we hope to reinforce – the integration of narrative and evidence based medicine is necessary if we are to face the challenges of medicine as it is practiced today. Indeed, the Narrative Evidence-based Medicine Working Group at Columbia University have expressed this in the language of the National Institute of Health's (NIH)Translational Research roadmap. The NIH characterizes the challenges as T1, getting knowledge from the bench sciences into clinical research, and T2, getting clinical research into clinical practice. The critical flaw in the NIH roadmap is the assumption that 'knowledge' is positivist knowledge, true in and of itself and when clinicians know it they will use it; both clinician and patients will recognize (positivist) truth and behave accordingly. The NEBM Working Group has critiqued the term T3 and its many variations (shared decision making, implementation science, knowledge translation, practice based research, etc.), pointing out:

> Most published versions of the translational research pipeline stop at the cusp of the individual patient, whose final decision to adopt or not adopt a therapeutic recommendation will determine the success or failure of the whole biomedical enterprise. The complexity of the issues that determine whether patients actually adopt and benefit from healthcare recommendations qualifies this domain as independent and translational in a fashion not true of the other proposed ('T3') extensions we have reviewed. (R Goyal, R Charon, H Lekas, *et al.*, 'A local habitation and a name': how narrative evidence-based medicine transforms the translational research paradigm. *Journal of Evaluation in Clinical Practice* 2008; **14:** 732–41)

They have recognized what we know to be true: the NIH stopped short of including the patient in their 'translational research paradigm.' We argue that the real translational challenge for clinicians is to translate knowledge into a social setting. Instead of the term T3, we use the term 'translational practice' because of socio-cultural overtones of the word 'practice.' This knowledge is no longer 'positivist' truth, but a new type of knowledge that we will continuously emphasize as contingent, emergent, situated, and contextual. This type of knowledge can be incorporated by scientific realism when it is recognized as a social practice.

We agree with everything implied by NEBM, but attempt to extend it further. Narrative evidenced-based medicine is a *method*. We believe that it is a particularly good method that holds promise to lead us toward improved health outcomes. However, we extend the argument to a broader social *theory* of healing. This book has two messages to tell. The first is a practical primer on Narrative evidence-based medicine and the second uses that method as an example to explain the theory and why the method works. We think both are important. Although these two messages are juxtaposed in Parts I and II compared to Part III, we hope this format gives the reader a deeper understanding of the process of care. It is the articulation of both the theory and the method that allow us to move forward to scientifically research *the practice of healing*.

Also in Part III of this book, we will describe the context of health care and how it has changed. Large organizations driving a 'commodification' of services with well meaning administrators espousing chronic disease management, pay for performance, proliferation of guidelines, patient satisfaction scores, and measures for many things, whether or not it is related to the vital mission of medicine. Doctors often feel stressed, frustrated, and disheartened because they can't practice the way they think is good or right for the patient. This puts a strain on professionalism. The accepted definition of professionalism as a 'social contract' is insufficient in today's world where medicine is a commodity, a service and a moral practice all at the same time. It seems our country is forever in a 'health care crisis.' *We suggest that a reasonable response for doctors is to re-connect with the timeless roots of medicine as a social practice of healing.*

THE LEARNING PLAN TO MOVE FROM NOVICE TO MASTER

To be expert in the actual skills required to use the process we describe requires practice and continuous learning. Although there is deep scholarship within the fields of narrative medicine and evidence-based medicine, this book is written at a beginner level and provides only the most essential tools to be able to start using this method of care in your own practice. There are resources elsewhere in the literature to guide your further learning in each of the components. We have tried to include some of the standard readings as references. We did not invent narrative medicine or evidence-based medicine; there are others far more expert in those fields. We try to reinforce the interdependence of these two highly developed concepts and we hope by the end of the book you will realize that they truly are part of each other and cannot be practiced independently of each other. What is unique about this book is our assertion that NEBM fulfils a necessary social role of healing.

We will, however, include our 'practical wisdom' based on our experiences of how to go through the process. This will primarily be in the form of how to use Google Scholar efficiently to address the requirements of evidence-based medicine structure. Since we are sharing practical wisdom based on experience, we quite naturally include our opinions. Feel free to disagree or experiment on your own. No two practitioners will interpret the evidence the same way. We have always acknowledged legitimate differences in opinion. That is what keeps medicine fascinating and fun. Rather, we strived to develop a common language so that informed clinical discussions can occur among a group of experienced clinicians. We use the word 'doctor' instead of the more politically correct 'practitioner'; we do that intentionally because, in Part III, we will be making a cultural argument and 'doctors' have been around longer than nurse practitioners, physician assistants, and other types of mid-level providers. We use the word 'doctor' to refer to anyone in the medical field entering into a therapeutic relationship with patients. Likewise, all examples are dramatized or fictionalized and do not refer to any real patient. The case that we follow throughout the book was completely confabulated for illustrative purposes. Believe us when we say that every day in the office has equally dramatic stories if you care to listen.

We believe that any physician can follow this process. We provide a practical textbook or learning plan for young and young-at-heart physicians to discover something besides the standard medical school or residency curriculum. Later in the book, we will provide some theoretical reflections; they can be read as merely reflective essays or as theoretical grounding for the science of healing. For now, simply try the process we describe. Just like learning a musical instrument or a new language, it takes practice, practice and more practice. We recommend using the patients in your own clinical environment for case examples. When introducing this process as a curriculum to our colleagues, we simply chose a case from the past one or two days that seemed workable; cases are easy to find. When first learning, avoid rare and strange cases that are unlikely to have any medical literature. When you have more experience, you can still use the process, but telling a story about '... we don't know anything about ...' is not going to help you learn the process. Don't be afraid of failure, use parts of the process when you are able, but keep in mind that the sequence of events is critical to success. Eventually, you will develop a 'cognitive schema' for the process of care as described and that is when it becomes seemingly effortless because you will achieve that 'it's just the way it is' type of thinking that makes things effortless. Changing your thinking changes your practice.

THE LEARNING ENVIRONMENT

As learners, this process addresses the mandated competencies from the American Council on Graduate Medical Education (ACGME) related to Practice-Based Learning, Communication, Medical Knowledge, and Patient Care. We will emphasize repeatedly that we are describing a process and that in order for the process to work correctly, the steps have to be done in the correct order.

However, if you are practicing in a teaching program, you should not necessarily learn them in the order you do them. Like any academic course, there are prerequisites. In this case, we suggest focusing on: (1) Journal Club and learning to critique research methodology; and (2) reflective practitioner skills. Historically, our family medicine residency has had reflective writing sessions, 20-minute unstructured listening sessions with patients, book reviews, essays, cinema learning, oil painting and Balint Group. Rita Charon also describes skill-building exercises for narrative medicine as part of a medical school curriculum. Our local medical school teaches the skills of clinical epidemiology and critical appraisal of research methods beginning in the first year of medical school. If a first year medical student can do it, so can you! All you need to do is practice, practice and more practice.

NARRATIVE COMPETENCE

Rita Charon suggests many narrative competency exercises in her writings. Although telling stories is a normal part of our culture, medical practitioners are trained to think predominately with the biomedical disease-oriented story. Doctors seem to have lost their ability to listen to illness stories. Learning how stories are constructed and the internal relationships within the story to *discover the meaning* is referred to as narrative competence. Although developing narrative competence is a life-long pursuit, we only assume a beginner level skill set – one that a person in our culture can understand. The challenge is to for practitioners to be open or willing to listen before having the biomedical story close the door to understanding. Later, we will discuss Balint Groups as a way to learn narrative competence. There are many other learning and skill-building programs that we don't have the time to incorporate here; just realize their importance. Whatever method is used to achieve narrative competence, it can only occur when physicians embrace the pathos of clinical practice. This is not easy, as physicians need to become vulnerable to begin to understand suffering. Far too often we rigidly protect ourselves from painful emotions. A healthier way to deal with the emotional labor of medical practice is to work on it in small, safe amounts. Whatever exercise or skill development exercise you choose, keep working at expanding those skills. These efforts are so important because *one simply cannot practice narrative medicine without being a self-reflective physician.*

HOW THE BOOK IS ORGANIZED

We would like to say a few words about how this book is organized. The entire book is structured around two office visits. The first office visit (Part I) emphasizes diagnosis and the second office visit (Part II) emphasizes therapy. In both parts, the individual chapter title begins with an 'A' so we refer to the process as, 'The six "A"s.' Subsequent chapters continue sequentially through the list to the next 'A,' which all together describe the complete process. They are:

1 **Acquire** enough information to understand the patient's concern.
2 **Ask** a clinically relevant question.
3 **Access** information to answer the clinically relevant question.
4 **Assess** the quality of the information.
5 **Apply** the information to the clinical question.
6 **Assist** the patient to make a decision.

Each chapter begins with *key concepts to remember* and then has didactic material related to the topic emphasized within that chapter identified by the heading *Learning About* ... . We include examples occasionally, but also include a feature called *Story Time*, a demonstration within the book about the book's theme. We next highlight *The Narrative Aspects of* ... 'the science.' We chose to emphasize this because we hope to overcome the (unmarked) assumption that science discovers reality. This is actually our attempt to blend the interface of these two ways of knowing (epistemologies) we discussed earlier. Next follows a section heading called *Application to Our Case Scenario*, which always refers to our single case study that is used as an example throughout the entire book. We finish each chapter with a reflection of how this part of the process of care created *contingent, emergent, situated, and contextualized medical knowledge*.

This book is a careful explanation of two office visits and one doctor–patient relationship. We painstakingly explain it as a *process of care*. It must always be remembered that it is a process of care. Doing things in the correct order is paramount in order to have a good outcome. It becomes easier once you understand the whole process. It is particularly helpful if you have prior knowledge of evaluating the quality of the research methodology (it helps when searching for information) but it is not necessary for you to have a comprehensive background since we explain things at a basic level. Again, our purpose is to demonstrate that integrating narrative medicine and evidence based medicine can be done; this is a demonstration project. Our target audience is beginners at all stages of their careers who want to be healers. Our goal is to explain the process sufficiently well that the reader can begin using the process with the next patient they see.

Part III changes from practical methods to theory development. We attempt to show how narrative and evidence are both cultural tools used in medical care. We believe Western medicine can be improved by using narrative evidenced-based medicine, but that method is only what works for us here and now, a subset of the globally available types of healing, which we perceive to be a social function. In this social context, it is vital to distinguish 'healing' from 'cure.' People are healed, not diseases. Similarly, people can be healed without being cured, cured without being healed, both, or neither. Clinical medicine includes all of these under the broader term 'sickness.' Other small scale societies can accomplish 'healing' with witchcraft and shamanism. Although we strongly adhere to narrative evidence-based medicine, we acknowledge that other methods may be efficacious to accomplish the social function of healing.

REMEMBER: PRACTICE, PRACTICE, PRACTICE ... YOU TOO CAN DO IT

In this book, we set out to show you one example of *how* it is done to demonstrate that *it can be done*. In fact, once you learn this process of care, it becomes second nature and makes the practice of medicine more efficient (and easier to deal with all the complex, insolvable problems we face on a day-to-day basis). Every office visit contains an opportunity to add to the co-constructed narrative.

About the authors

JAMES P MEZA, MD

Dr Meza received his Bachelor of Science degree in biomedical sciences from the University of Michigan, followed by his Doctor of Medicine degree from the University of Michigan Medical School. He subsequently completed his Family Medicine residency at the same institution. Since that time, he maintained a primary care medical practice for over twenty years, a time when his patients taught him much about how to practice medicine. In the interim, he received a Master of Science of Administration degree in healthcare administration from Central Michigan University and received a Certificate of Added Qualifications in Geriatrics from the American Board of Family Medicine. His interest in the psychological dimensions of clinical practice resulted in pursuing additional training, which led to becoming a Credentialed Balint Leader from the American Balint Society. He is currently finishing a Doctor of Philosophy degree in Anthropology, with special interests in Narrative Theory, Cognitive Anthropology, and Medical Anthropology. He works with Oakwood-Annapolis Family Medicine Residency as Associate Residency Program Director and Director of Research. Oakwood Health System is affiliated with Wayne State University School of Medicine, where Dr Meza is an Assistant Professor in the Department of Family Medicine and Public Health Science. He is the Course Director for Translational Medicine and Evidence-based Practice, part of the longitudinal curriculum at the Medical School.

DANIEL S PASSERMAN, DO

Dr Passerman received his bachelor of Science in Engineering from the University of Michigan. He worked in the private corporate sector for two years before returning to Michigan State University College of Osteopathic Medicine. He completed his Family Medicine post-graduate training at Henry Ford Hospital in Detroit Michigan. He is currently practicing medicine with the Henry Ford Health System in Detroit, Michigan where he teaches evidence-based medicine in the departments of Family Medicine and at Henry Ford Wyandotte Hospital's department of medical education. He is the Program Director of the osteopathic family medicine residency at Henry Ford Wyandotte Hospital. He is also a Clinical Assistant Professor at AT Still University Kirksville College of Osteopathic Medicine. Special areas of interest include teaching evidence-based medicine as described in this book.

Introduction

In this book, we will be presenting a different way of understanding the social world in medicine and how sickness is embodied and negotiated within that context. We will be drawing on two established domains of knowledge that at first glance seem like oil and water. The conceptual path to a new form of knowledge will be demonstrated by integrating narrative medicine and evidence based medicine. Once integrated, it transforms into something different than what we typically understand our usual practice to be.

The National Institute of Health (NIH) has spent billions of dollars supporting basic science research. The expectation from this investment of time and treasure was that the health of the population would improve. Disappointingly, there remain intractable problems with health disparities and translating basic science into practice. Currently, the NIH is emphasizing 'translational research,' to close this gap. We believe that neither 'science' nor 'management' will solve the problem. Rather, we perceive the problem as integrating scientific knowledge into social practices. Unless we understand this source of complexity and difficulty in making this 'translation,' we won't be able to address the perceived need by the NIH to actualize the benefit of our investment.

We will be taking the viewpoint that both narrative medicine and evidence based medicine are social practices, which creates the opportunity for true integration. In our society science has a status almost equivalent to truth. Having spent years critiquing the medical literature (evidence-based medicine) it has become apparent to us that scientific research papers are actually a form of narrative. They have a speaker (author), a specific audience, a specific context, a persuasive viewpoint and an underlying structure to support claims of 'truth.' Like any other story, after reading the article we ask ourselves and others, 'Do you believe it?'

Similarly, narrative medicine stakes a claim to understanding the world our patients live in. It is well accepted that psychological and social aspects of life impact health outcomes. The patient's narrative thus becomes one of the unrecognized independent variables when we measure health outcomes. Unfortunately, since narrative cannot be quantified, the psychosocial input to biomedical outcomes is infrequently incorporated into biomedical research agenda.

By integrating these two forms of knowledge (two different epistemologies), we create a blended form of medical knowledge that is contingent, emergent, situated, and contextual. This type of medical knowledge is not reified as truth that can be tested with multiple-choice exams. It is a form of knowledge that is embodied in practice. The contingent aspect of this new type of medical knowledge reflects the unknown future capable of holding multiple possibilities simultaneously throughout the process of care. The emergent aspect reflects recognition of the chronological or time sequence of clinical care patterns and clinical decisions. The situated nature of this knowledge reflects the uniqueness of how both narrative and biomedical research are applied to individual patients and individual concerns within the doctor–patient relationship. The contextual nature of this knowledge recognizes that neither the patient nor the doctor are independent actors, rather they both draw on vast and differing forms of knowledge as well as a shared cultural framework.

At this point, we have practical experience that shows this can be done and later in the book we will suggest a theoretical framework within which this contingent, emergent, situated, and contextual medical knowledge can become the object of scientific research. Practicing medicine is a social act, affecting not only the patient, but also society. What we provide in Part I and Part II is simply a methodology for this style of clinical practice. Recognizing the advantages and disadvantages of the process we describe, we are confident that this method better meets the needs of our patients and society than continuing on our present course. In Part III we present a theoretical argument about why we believe this method better meets the needs of our patients.

We are going to begin this journey together by initially focusing on narrative (Chapter 1); subsequent chapters will describe our perspective on evidence based medicine. Throughout the book however, we will try to emphasize the *science in narrative* and the *narrative in science* so that the reader can come to understand this process of care as an integrated, unified, unique form of medical knowledge. We start with the following definitions from the *American Heritage College Dictionary*:

> **Contingent**: Liable to occur but not certain; possible. Dependent on conditions or occurrences not yet established; conditional.
> **Emergent**: Coming into view, existence, or notice ... Arising or occurring unexpectedly ... Occurring as a consequence.
> **Situated** (situate): Having a place or location; located. To place under particular circumstances or in a given condition.
> **Contextual** (context): Of, involving, or depending on a context ... the part of a text or statement that surrounds a particular word or passage and determines its meaning ... The circumstances in which an event occurs; a setting.

PART I
The Process of Care for a Diagnostic Narrative Dilemma

CHAPTER 1

Acquire Enough Information to Understand the Patient's Concern

KEY CONCEPTS TO REMEMBER

➤ Storytelling is a natural form of human interaction.
➤ We assimilate the meaning of a story naturally, without analyzing it.
➤ Stories that are analyzed for meaning are called 'narratives.'
➤ Medical narratives have an essential scientific role – to make sure we answer the correct question in the clinical interview.
➤ Narrative competence is more than mastering communication skills – practitioners need to understand the structure of narratives.
➤ Narratives allow doctors to engage with the patient's illness experience.

LEARNING ABOUT HOW TO UNDERSTAND THE PATIENT'S CONCERN

Stories are Everywhere

People tell stories every day. They tell stories at work, at parties, and commonly when arriving home. 'How was your day?' is an invitation to reflect and select the meaningful experiences and organize them into a summary of the events since the last gathering of the family. Stories are a form of sharing. They create a social fabric and a web of meaning. Stories are told and re-told, both by the same individual and also passed along to others. 'Did you hear what happened to Sally last week?'

Storytelling is natural – small children haltingly tell stories and adults patiently listen, even if the point of the story is missing or the story is about childish things that adults have long since disregarded as not important. The facts that adults wait patiently while listening to young children and parents who might know the meaning of the child's verbalizations will intercede and say something like, 'Now tell Uncle Joe what the teacher said when the frog jumped out of its bowl ...' indicate that learning to tell a story is an essential skill in functioning in an adult social environment.

Everybody tells stories. These stories surround us. As a cultural form, we simply assume and assimilate the information in a story. Most stories are not consciously analyzed; this is because human cognition includes something called a narrative schema.[1] For the moment, we will equate story with narrative and look closer at the idea of schema. A schema is cognitive scaffolding that relates each part to the others and to the whole. When we hear a story, we simply insert details in a framework and understand the meaning without consciously, laboriously analyzing what we have just heard (or read). We think with schemata which are often nested from very small relationships in our world and social world to combinations of very complex schemata that result in larger, comprehensive narrative schemata.

Stories Have Meaning

Sometimes, however, we actually examine a story for meaning. This is often in the form of a parable or fable where there is a specific moral tale or meaning and we take the extra time to understand the meaning explicitly, even going to the point of discussing, sharing, or explaining the lesson. Bible stories are used repetitively, often extrapolated to current day situations with an attempt to apply the lessons embedded in the story to our own lives. With expensive stories such as cinema or theater, there may even be an argument or alternative meanings or lessons discussed among the audience, an interpretation.

The Structure of Narrative

A story becomes a narrative when the listener examines the structure, content, context, format, frame, plot, dramatic moments, purpose or desire, and the temporality of the story as a means of understanding the specific social role of the story.[2, 3] We examine the story for plot lines, core metaphors, and rhetorical devices, all in the hope of interpreting the story to uncover its meaning. 'Meaning' assumes that we can represent the 'inner life' of another person and bring that into a social interaction. Uncovering the 'meaning' is an interpretive act.

Literary Terms and Narrative

Most of these descriptors are literary terms; a few deserve further discussion here. Let us take *suspense* first. What could be more suspenseful than waiting for a biopsy report? Suspense is a mixture of the unknown and the possibility of multiple different outcomes, or twists in the plot. The *plot* is the causal sequence that takes you from episode A to episode B, and then from episode B to episode C, etc. Although not necessarily lived in 'narrative time' human experience is understood that way. One of the purported functions of narrative is to give order to the inchoate experiences of life – it is a way of knowing and understanding. *Metaphors* summarize incredibly complex ideas and convey them succinctly. In our example which follows, we talk about the heart. Culturally, 'the heart' is portrayed as courage, sadness, strength, love, tenderness, etc. The list goes on. Medical metaphors often incorporate elements of symptoms, diseases, and illness experiences.

Another key literary component is *drama*. Drama is heightened when emotions are heightened. Any skillful story-listener has to understand emotions.

From a social perspective, emotions are cognitions (the result of neurological activity) for an individual and a social signal between people. The simplest example is the flight or fright response. When confronted by an angry patient, we interpret the social setting in any number of ways. Most commonly, we try appeasement. The patient is using anger to control the social setting. At other times, the physician refuses to interact if the patient is too angry, and simply says something like, 'I'll come back later when you're less upset and maybe we can discuss your care then.' In this second example of anger, the doctor is controlling the social setting and likely the medical care that follows. Emotions are part of clinical care and they are part of the story. Listening (to the story) and responding defines the co-creation of that story that follows. That is what narrative medicine is all about.

The Narrative Dilemma is Part of the Scientific Enterprise

For most physicians, this all seems quite wishy-washy; could we please just stick to the facts? *In fact*, examining stories our patients tell, i.e. medical narratives, has an essential scientific role. Any good scientist will tell you that the most important process is to ask the correct question; answering questions, particularly ones we already know the answers to, is less illuminating. Every clinical case is filled with hundreds of questions. We know that most health care is actually self care. We suspect that only when our patients can no longer deal with the difficulty, complexity or risk of their life story – those times when they experience a narrative dilemma – do they seek professional advice. The question that the patient wants answered is embedded in their story, their medical narrative. It is this question that we have to find before we begin the process of diagnosis and treatment. If doctors assume they know the question, they risk answering the wrong question. It is poor scientific practice to answer the wrong question or answer a question not worth asking (Type III and Type IV statistical errors).[4] It also leads to poor patient care. We recognize that doctors can also add legitimate questions to the process of care, but we should never ignore or devalue the patient's narrative dilemma.

Patients' Stories, Doctors' Cases

Once again, the reader may be wondering if the doctor as scientist got lost. We recognize the inherent paradox, but have learned to embrace it. One day when struggling how to integrate narrative medicine and evidence based medicine, we looked up at the diploma hanging on the wall and there it was, 'Doctor in the Arts and Science of Medicine.' Doctors have to be able to keep multiple different narrative interpretations in mind simultaneously, exactly in the same way they maintain a differential diagnosis, and work through the emergent experience, all the while evaluating how the story needs to unfold to best care for this particular patient. Usually the story gets told as a co-constructed narrative, the work of both the doctor and patient. Realizing both you and the patient are in it together is exactly how narrative and evidence become integrated – it is a share and share-alike adventure called clinical medicine. All we are doing is making explicit what typically goes unnoticed and is taken for granted.

In order to participate in this realm of medicine with some degree of understanding of what is actually happening, the doctor must develop skills of mindfulness and self reflection. Without mindfulness and self reflection, we operate on auto-pilot using cultural scripts that may or may not be appropriate to the clinical case at hand. We confuse our story with the patient's story. Doctors need to acknowledge that in each clinical encounter they have to listen to an illness narrative before they create the diagnostic or therapeutic story using the classical medical syntax of a 'history and physical.'

Does the Shoe Fit? Is Narrative a Part of Medicine?

It is important to recognize the tension and the ambiguity in the very term 'narrative medicine.' To do that, we have to look back at the history of medicine. What we call medicine today originated in the time of the Enlightenment of Europe in the 1700s. At that time, the naturalists and empiricists dominated epistemology (the branch of philosophy that studies the nature of knowledge)[5] and medicine's foundation was built upon this philosophy. For the first time, we organized medicine by anatomical structures and medical knowledge derived from empirical 'experiments' and observations. Medicine was an objective science. With the modernist trend in the 1950s, technology and science became ascendant and reinforced these cultural realities. We call this pinnacle of accomplishment 'biomedicine.' Indeed biomedicine is so strong a cultural force that it survived almost unscathed by the Postmodernism of the 1980s, which questioned the order, structure, and unity of epistemology in many other disciplines. At this point in time, there was literally an explosion of narrative studies in many disciplines. Narrative became a theory and a method in philosophy, literary studies, psychology, anthropology, history, linguistics, social sciences, law, etc.[2, 6] Simultaneously, medicine was criticized for becoming too impersonal, technology driven, and abandoning the humanism of the core values of professionalism in medicine.[7,8,9,10] George Engel coined the phrase 'biopsychosocial' as a specific response to this criticism.[11, 12] Scholars interested in the doctor–patient relationship started to look at a broader definition of medicine and that led to eventually developing the role of narrative in medicine. Today, there is a well-developed argument that narrative actually does have merit and is legitimately part of the grand enterprise we call medicine.

Hierarchy of Knowledge Systems

Unfortunately, narrative medicine practitioners are still considered 'alternative' because narrative is simply not scientific enough to compete with biomedicine.

On the other hand, others argue that a purely biomedical approach to medicine is inadequate because it leaves too many human needs unmet. The body of literature on narrative and narrative medicine has several consistent and recurrent themes: the therapeutic nature of telling stories while someone listens, the creation of coherence by re-ordering of experiences into meaningful accounts, the embodied nature of narrative in medicine, the cultural communication aspects of narrative, and the creation of relationship with self and other.[3, 9, 11, 13–32] Narrative is often used as a critique of biomedicine.[33] To a much lesser extent there is recognition of the fact that they may be related endeavors. Rarely is there any practical advice about how to integrate these two systems of knowledge.[29]

The thought of integrating an interpretive enterprise such as narrative with the positivist epistemology of biomedicine is enough to make most physicians turn green. It is difficult to acknowledge the epistemological contradiction openly, so we euphemistically say that a doctor has 'good bedside manner.' To develop bedside manner, we teach 'communication skills.' We will argue that communication skills facilitate 'narrative competence,' a term coined by Rita Charon and her colleagues,[34] and that communication skills are important, but fall short of *narrative competence*.

Indeed, you have to be able to listen if you want to hear a story. One of the most fundamental aspects of narrative medicine is to allow the patient to tell their story. Incredibly, doctors do not seem to be able to do this consistently.[35, 36] When doctors interrupt, they irrevocably disrupt the narrative thread of the story, the embedded meaning coded in the sequencing, the content, and the intended meanings of the patient when telling the 'history of present illness' story. *If you get nothing else out of this entire book, try to remember to ask open-ended questions, listen without interruption, and organize the clinical interview using the patient's narrative thread. Only when you understand the patient's narrative dilemma should you start 'to think like a doctor.'*

Narrative Competence

We mentioned many of the skill development exercises in the preface, which can be found in the published literature. While reflective writing sessions, 20-minute unstructured listening sessions with patients, book reviews, essays, cinema learning, oil painting and other activities can develop narrative competence, we believe Balint Group sessions as structured by the American Balint Society are among the best reflective practitioner experiences. Clive Brock, MD once said, 'the patients have the best stories to learn with.' He was referring to the multi-faceted, multi-dimensional approach to exploring stories within stories and being able to keep many different possibilities in mind while caring for patients.

Balint Groups are not as popular as some of the easier, less time consuming activities that require less of a commitment of precious curricular time to develop narrative skills, but Balint Groups have the advantage of exploring the patient, the doctor, and the patient–doctor relationship in an intensely self reflective way. Michael Balint himself compared the doctor to a drug, with beneficial effects and adverse side effects. Unless the doctor can be self reflective, he/she cannot listen to the patient's story without distinguishing self from the patient. These groups are time and resource intensive. They also require quite a bit of courage to acknowledge the personal foibles we as physicians typically prefer not to demonstrate in public under the guise of professionalism. Essentially, Balint Groups are small group, case-based presentations where the presenter gives a short history of a patient case that is 'difficult' in some way, but also requires an ongoing relationship. After the presentation, the other group members 'take' the case and begin to speculate. In this way, multiple different, even contradictory interpretations or feelings emerge. The practitioners explore what it must be like to be the physician, what it must be like to be the patient, and what type of relationship between the two is best for patient care. There is explicitly no 'answer,' but only an exploration of all the hitherto hidden dimensions of the social interaction embedded in the doctor–patient relationship. Metaphor is explored, as well as transference and counter-transference. It requires experienced leaders and absolute confidentiality to maintain the safety of the group members. It is, however, a wonderfully rich way to develop as an individual and as a narrative practitioner. Our advice is to participate in a Balint Group if available, but use all the other narrative skill building techniques described in the literature.

We also recognize that narrative competence is more than a sum of the parts – mastering communication skills will not result in narrative competence. Stories have structures. Stories have context. There is the story of why the patient is in the clinic that day and there is the story of how that episode fits into broad themes of the patient's life. There is the life story and the meaning of a person's existence.

Narrative Power

Stories have a speaker and a listener and the story has an intended consequence or intended impact by the storyteller for the story-listener. Sometimes stories are used to provoke a special social action.[37] Cheryl Mattingly is an anthropologist who has worked extensively with narrative theory. While working with the World Bank in Calcutta, she noted:

> I recognized that stories were not just told after experience but were constructed while people were still very much in the midst of action. This active storytelling played a critical role in team strategizing about how to turn project implementation in a more desirable direction. Thus, I began to examine narrative as an aesthetic form with rhetorical powers, one which could become a persuasive tool for convincing others to see the world in a certain way.[6]

Patients can also tell stories that have persuasive effects and change social interactions. Since we live in the northern hemisphere, it gets cold in the winter and we all know homeless patients that can recite a chest pain story well enough to secure a warm bed for 24 hours. The narrative is not really about coronary artery disease, but unmet physical needs.

Mattingly also describes the 'co-constructed narrative' – inherent in taking turns being the listener or storyteller:

> Narrative meaning is not something which belongs to the narrator so much as something which is co-constructed in a social interaction (for example, an interview) between speaker and listener – 'For it is clear ... that stories or narrative are somehow jointly produced, and not by the patient alone ...'[6]

In order to use this process of care, it is vital for the clinician to acknowledge, monitor, and share the inherent power distribution in the doctor–patient relationship.[37, 38] The default is biomedical doctor-talk dominates and controls the social interaction. In a hospital setting, Arthur Frank describes his own cancer treatment experience as 'a circulation of stories.' If the Illness Story was trumped by Biomedical Story, Frank called this *narrative surrender* and *biomedical colonization*. The paternalistic medicine of the 1950s gave way to the Patient Centered care; the current standard is the Relationship Centered Care described by Beach and Inui.[39] This awareness of reciprocal influence is essential to acquire the patient's narrative, but even more essential in working with the patient to create a co-constructed narrative, a preferable outcome to narrative surrender or biomedical colonization. It turns out that the doctor has to translate between the two cultures of the patient's world and the world of biomedicine to facilitate the creation of this co-constructed narrative; that's what most of this book is about.[40]

There is a Difference between Narrative Interpretation and Narrative Analysis

Before we proceed, we need to make certain our readers understand the difference between *narrative interpretation* and *narrative analysis*. Remember that we mentioned that narrative has been embraced by a wide range of disciplines within academia. What we have been describing and will demonstrate shortly is narrative interpretation. Like singing, anyone can do it, even if some of us can only do it in the shower. Narrative interpretation is done daily by all of us simply to negotiate our daily lives. People tell stories all the time. We understand these stories intuitively. *Narrative interpretation* is simply saying out loud what we think the story was about or attempted to communicate. The skill building we referred to is developing the ability to enrich the interpretation.

Narrative analysis, on the other hand, is a scientific methodology for qualitative researchers and requires special training. The best review of narrative analysis we have read is by Catherine Riessman.[41] In general, there are four types of narrative analysis. The first is *thematic analysis*, where the text is examined in societal context and emphasis is directed toward understanding big issues in the particular research setting. The second type of analysis is *structural analysis*, which examines how parts of the narrative are related to the whole and how each part functions within the text. Special emphasis is given to the local context. The third type of analysis is *dialogic* or *performative analysis* which examines the roles played by the narrator and its particular effects within a social context. It explores the social actions of the narrator and the emphasis is both on the local context and society level. The last method is *visual analysis*, which is a bit beyond the brief description we offer here. Likewise, discourse analysis is an analytic tool that incorporates all the para-linguistic information, such as pauses, interruptions, duplicate meanings, sequencing of words or phrases, etc. This is done with a line-by-line, word-by-word perspective. For our purposes, it is important to know it exists, but is not taught in this book. The reader must understand that nothing in this book pretends to achieve the scientific method of narrative analysis. Rather, we focus rather on practical, everyday thought processes and behaviors that doctors and patients use when they interact with each other.

The Narrative Aspects of Science

By exploring the realms of evidence based medicine and clinical epidemiology, physicians become more aware of uncertainty in medicine and more critical of how medical knowledge is socially constructed through the research enterprise. Indeed, scientific research is a highly structured form of storytelling amongst a highly selected group. 'Research as storytelling' is most apparent when the 'discussion' comes to a conclusion not supported by the 'results.' Analyzing how the 'research story' is constructed with its strengths, weaknesses, and bias is another way to describe evidence based medicine. The paucity of high quality scientifically valid studies demonstrating causal effect still only answers questions at the population level; our patients are primarily concerned about what those research studies mean for them. Although this might be an uncomfortable migration toward rapprochement of narrative and scientific enterprises for some physicians, we find that not only is it possible, but it is also a more satisfying way to practice medicine. We would go so far as to say that the integration of the two approaches has more truth value than either alone.

Narrative and Medicine

Narrative interviewing is a skill unto itself. It requires that the clinician track the patient's logic and find what the connections are from the patient's point of view. As doctors, we have a hard time and little patience for this endeavor because we want to construct our own story of a disease. In many ways, narrative interviewing in clinical practice is like ethnographic interviewing in anthropology. You have to start by assuming you know absolutely nothing about what the patient is attempting to describe and facilitate the patient to reveal to you how he/she makes sense of the story elements. You have to be patient to even discover what the story elements are! John Launer's *Narrative-based Primary Care – a practical guide* is a good source to 'retrain' your brain to this new style of interviewing.[42, 43] If successful, you can uncover what Arthur Kleinman, MD calls the patient's 'explanatory model.'[40, 44] Hidden in this explanatory model is a clinical question that dare not be ignored.

Listening

By incorporating narrative into the practice of medicine, doctors are able to deal not only with the disease, but also to engage more fully with the illness experience, allowing them to reclaim their social role as 'healers.'[20, 45] Diagnosing and treating disease is a totally different endeavor than 'diagnosing and treating illness experiences.' We suggest doctors as healers must do both. The fundamental role of doctors is to relieve suffering. Using biomedicine, we can cure disease and prevent the suffering that disease would have caused. But there are others forms of suffering embedded in the illness story that can only be relieved by 'bearing witness' to the patient's story of suffering.[46, 47] Because listening is embedded in a therapeutic relationship, it often provides relief in and of itself. We have many experiences of patients saying 'thank you' for simply listening – we turn to the residents and ask, 'What was that patient thanking us for?' We believe it comes from the universal 'need to be known,'[6] understood, accepted; we have a need to be in a relationship, connected in the social world. What better way to get to know someone than to listen to their life story? Remember, there is all the difference in the world between, 'taking a medical history,' and 'listening to an illness narrative.'

A Practical, Doable Daily Practice

Although there is scholarly, theoretically driven work to support the concepts presented, we focus mostly on the learning or practicing physician that is looking for a new way to engage his/her patients. It is important to realize that we present a process of care. That means that sequence is important – it will not work if you do not do things in the correct order. The first two parts of this book are mostly a practical 'how to' book, with only enough theory to make the process of care we describe plausible. We recognize that narrative medicine or evidence based medicine may not have been taught in medical school or post graduate training, so we will do some teaching along the way. Primarily, however, we will be sharing practical methods worked out locally to meet the demands of two different frames of reference: narrative and EBM/clinical epidemiology. We encourage our readers to explore and learn both narrative and EBM/clinical epidemiology – we hope to only demonstrate enough of each to show how they work together. The only evidence of effectiveness we can present is that it works in our busy everyday primary care practices and that our patient satisfaction scores are excellent. We have been able to maintain stable patient panels when others have melted under the stress of changes in the health care system.

What is a Narrative Dilemma?

Patients 'write their own life story.' As we mentioned before, we suspect that only when they can no longer deal with the difficulty, complexity or risk of their life story they experience what we are calling a *Narrative Dilemma*. That is when they seek professional advice and embark on the process of the co-constructed narrative. The question that the patient wants answered is embedded in their story; doctors help them discover that question by listening attentively. Often answering one question provokes another so that there are stories within stories. This is how the doctor–patient relationship is built over time. The doctor can ask, 'What part of this story is missing?' as a way to identify the narrative dilemma. Stories are complex. Often the doctor and the patient are working on multiple different parts of the story simultaneously. Clinical care, like storytelling, has to take place one episode at a time, however. For each visit or encounter, it is the narrative dilemma of the day that we have to find and confirm with the patient before we begin the process of diagnosis and treatment. It is the narrative dilemma that structures and organizes the process of care. It is the ongoing relationship with its ongoing narrative that facilitates healing.

STORY TIME

A resident physician presented a case on rounds about an elderly man. She began, 'The patient was noncompliant and stopped taking his diabetic medicines,' Implying that non-compliance was the cause of all subsequent medical complications. The patient developed polyuria (increased volume of urine) so severe that he went into acute renal failure from dehydration, causing hyperkalemia severe enough to require emergency dialysis. In addition, he was found to have an extensive deep vein thrombosis affecting his entire left leg. Although the presentation was excellent (according to the medical cultural script), we explained that *non-compliance* does not exist and that *non-adherence* is a behavior that can be understood by listening for the patient's perceptions and reasoning. We said, 'What you really need to know is what he was thinking when he made that decision.' The next day, the resident updated the management and all the complexities of the medical case, then fell silent. Eventually she said, 'I talked to him about why he stopped his medicines ...' He said that he went to his doctor and the doctor told him he had to start insulin. The doctor said his blood sugars were not controlled and unless he started insulin, there would be damage to his organs. The patient was terrified of needles and objected. At that point, the doctor became more insistent about starting him on insulin. When the patient said he would prefer to take the pills even if his blood sugar wasn't perfect, the doctor said, 'Those medicines can damage your kidneys, too.' The patient said he got home and was so scared of everything, including his pills, that he simply *stopped* taking them!

The point of this story is – by ignoring the patient's narrative and pursuing his own story of diabetic control, the doctor caused a negative outcome.

CLINICAL CASE SCENARIO

1	*Doctor:*	Good morning Mrs Smith. How are you today?
2	*Patient:*	I am fine doctor.
3	*Doctor:*	Let me just wash my hands and we can get started. (wash ...
4		wash ... sit)
5		So, how have things been going since the last time we talked?
6	*Patient:*	Fine doctor.
7		Pause
8		Pause
9		I have had some trouble with my son. Jason's ex-wife took
10		him to court again about child support. You know I love
11		those kids to death and I just wish Jason would be a more
12		responsible father. I have practically raised his kids, but I
13		worry about how they are going to turn out because of all the
14		fighting in the family.
15	*Doctor:*	Fighting?
16	*Patient:*	I just wish things would run smoothly, you know, everyone
17		respectful and do their job. I think kids should have chores,
18		but all I hear is fighting and my son is too distracted to be a
19		consistent parent. I'm the one that has to make everything run
20		smoothly.

21	*Doctor:*	This has been a worry of yours for a long time now; I was
22		curious and wondering about whether or not you think that
23		this has affected your health.
24	*Patient:*	Sometimes I think my blood pressure medicine can't take
25		all the stress. I know I was reluctant to take them at first, but
26		now I am almost glad I take those pills. I do feel under a lot
27		of pressure and something has gotta keep me stable. I mostly
28		worry about what is going to happen in the future. I hope it's
29		nothin' like the past.
30	*Doctor:*	Tell me about Jason and the past ...
31	*Patient:*	Why did you ask me that? He was such a handful. I was a
32		single parent and I depended heavily on my father to watch
33		him and help while I was working, which is why I feel I need
34		to help Jason now. So why did you ask me that question?
35	*Doctor:*	I am just trying to understand what it has been like for you
36		from the beginning, what's going on now. You mentioned you
37		are worried about what is going to happen in the future, but it
38		seems to me the past is always connected to the future. That's
39		why we have these talks. We have known each other a long
40		time. I remember you telling me about when your Dad died ...
41	*Patient:*	That's when all of the trouble started. Everything was so
42		sudden. All I remember is my sister screaming on the phone
43		that I had to come to the hospital and when I got there
44		she kept saying, 'Daddy's gone, Daddy's gone.' It was a very
45		confusing time. Back then they didn't tell you much in the
46		hospital, but I do remember a nurse shaking her head and
47		saying, 'those blood clogs can be so cruel.' That is when my
48		life really got difficult and Jason started acting out.
49	*Doctor:*	So what helped you get through those difficult times?
50	*Patient:*	I am not sure I have ever recovered. Whenever things get
51		stressful, I still think about that day.
52	*Doctor:*	So what do you think happened to your father?
53	*Patient:*	He wasn't one to complain. But the whole week prior to the
54		day he died, he kept saying that he had this funny sensation
55		in his chest near his shoulder. I think that he probably had
56		a heart attack. Nowadays they probably would have done
57		one of those roto-rooter things and taken the clogs out of his
58		arteries. If only they had some of the technology we have now,
59		I think he would still be here today.
60	*Doctor:*	It sounds like you still miss him.
61	*Patient:*	I miss him so bad ... my heart aches.
62		Pause

63		Pause
64		Pause
65		That's one of the reasons why I am here today.
66	*Doctor:*	Can you tell me about that?
67	*Patient:*	I've been getting this funny feeling right here in front of my
68		shoulder. (Patient points to left chest, near her shoulder.) It's
69		sharp, sometimes enough to take my breath away. Of course
70		all that I can think about is what happened to Daddy and I
71		don't want to do that to Jason.
72	*Doctor:*	I can sense how unsettling this experience must be. It would
73		help me if you could go back to when that funny feeling first
74		started and share the whole story, including anything you felt
75		or thought since the beginning.
76	*Patient:*	I've had it now for three weeks. The first time was after a fight
77		with Jason when he stormed out of the house taking my
78		grandchild with him. I didn't think too much about it at the
79		time because it was just stress. But then the next day I got it
80		two more times and that was just on a Sunday when I didn't
81		have much to do. I was in church and I got that same pain,
82		but this time it was a little bit more achy. I got scared so I
83		had to sit down in the pew and stop singing. That lasted for a
84		couple of minutes, but after service was over, I felt fine. Later
85		that same day I was putzing in the garden and it happened
86		again. That's when I started worrying that it might be serious,
87		you know, my heart. I called for an appointment, but today
88		was the first time I could talk with you. The only other thing
89		I noticed in the meanwhile is it seems to happen more often
90		when I'm carrying groceries. I also get a bit winded at those
91		times. I'm glad I quit smoking when I did.
92	*Doctor:*	We have had this discussion before. I think that you have
93		been worried about your heart since the first day that I met
94		you. Two years ago, you were having similar problems and
95		we got that stress echocardiogram that didn't show any heart
96		problems.
97	*Patient:*	That's when you tricked me.
98	*Doctor:*	What's that?
99	*Patient:*	You heard me. You wanted me to take pills and I told you that
100		I don't want any foreign chemicals in my body ... so I had to
101		stop smoking after you asked me how many chemicals were
102		in the cigarettes.
103	*Doctor:*	And I'm very proud of the fact that you were able to do that.
104		Pause

105		Pause
106	*Patient:*	So here we are again, talking about my heart. I just have this
107		feeling that something is going to happen to me and it is
108		going to be sudden just like my daddy. He was too young
109		to die. My grandparents and mom all had heart problems,
110		but they passed when they were older ... It just seemed more
111		natural at that age.
112	*Doctor:*	It seems like there's two things that are bothering you at
113		this time. The first one is the turmoil with Jason and the
114		grandkids. The other one is ...
115		Pause
116		Pause
117		Pause
118	*Patient:*	I am worried that I have a clog in my heart.
119	*Doctor:*	What is a clog?
120	*Patient:*	You're the doctor ... you know, a clog. Just like when the drain
121		gets filled with all that junk and plugs up so that the water
122		can't get through. In your heart, it plugs the artery and kills
123		your heart. Don't you remember showing me that picture on
124		the computer with the clogged artery?
125	*Doctor:*	Is that what's bothering you the most right now?
126	*Patient:*	I wasn't thinking about it that way before this appointment,
127		but now that you mention it that is exactly what I am worried
128		about. I know it sounds silly, and you've done your best to
129		take good care of me. My blood pressure's good, the stress test
130		was OK, and I have been too afraid to take those cholesterol
131		pills, but I keep remembering that nurse saying that blood
132		clogs can be so cruel and I am afraid that it might happen
133		to me. (Patient opens purse) I brought you this article that I
134		clipped from the newspaper that says there is a new test which
135		is a fancy X-ray that can tell you if you have any blocked
136		arteries. Do you think that I should get one of those?
137	*Doctor:*	This newspaper article is describing a CAT scan that shows
138		the shape of your arteries on an X-ray film. I suppose our
139		job is to decide whether or not ordering such a test would
140		be helpful for you at this time. Correct me if I don't describe
141		your concern accurately, **you want to know if you have any**
142		**clogged or blocked arteries.**
143	*Patient:*	Yes, on some level that has always been on my mind.
144	*Doctor:*	We do have tests and treatments that can help those things,
145		but to tell you the truth, we think the real problem is only
146		those blockages that bust and cause a clog. Our problem is

147		that we can't tell which ones will bust and which blockages
148		won't ever affect your health.
149	*Patient:*	That's fine for you, but if I don't have any blockages I won't
150		have one that busts either. It doesn't matter to me if you can't
151		tell which ones bust or not, I just need to know that I don't
152		got any at all.

NARRATIVE INTERPRETATION OF CLINICAL CASE

For the purposes of discussion we are going to reflect upon the narrative components of the above conversation. This will help give the reader a sense of how a narrative oriented doctor would approach a clinical interview. Instead of trying to do a discourse analysis, which is analyzing the text line by line, we will discuss the interview as a whole unit, hoping to give a sense of the story telling elements of a brief clinical interview.

Lines 1–9: The first thing to notice is that this is a return visit between a patient and a doctor that have talked previously. From this perspective, we know that the 'frame' of the story extends beyond this single conversation and includes not only the continuity relationship of shared experiences but also the patient's life story. When the doctor washes his hands, he reinforces not only the germ theory of disease, but 'ritually' distinguishes clean from unclean. This is a powerful para-linguistic metaphor about creating a setting where life's messiness can be discussed. When the doctor asks 'How are you today?', the patient gives a polite response, 'Fine doctor.' Instead of directing the conversation by saying something like 'What's been bothering you,' which has a hidden assumption that the office visit is about a problem and that the problem should be a medical one, the doctor just simply sits with the patient. This serves to make sure that the patient has the opportunity to self define the topic of discussion.

Lines 10–23: Spontaneously, the patient starts talking about trouble with her son and raising his children. Although not necessarily a 'medical problem' this social context certainly affects the patient's health. One gets the sense that this patient bears a lot of responsibility. The drama is heightened by the hidden emotions in a phrase such as, 'I love those kids to death.' Obviously this has been an ongoing concern because the doctor recognizes it as 'a worry of yours for a long time now.' This demonstrates how the illness experience develops over multiple office visits and from a narrative perspective can be considered 'chapters' in the life story of the patient. This is a qualitative way for a subject to define the critical or most important landmarks or turning points of their life. For our patient, the narrative practitioner should start to search for how a stressful day with child care is related to the main characters, themes, and actions in this patient's life. In this case, the doctor asks the patient to reflect about these troubles and responsibilities and how they relate to the patient's health.

Lines 24–40: The patient responds by talking about blood pressure. Linguistically, pressure, stress, responsibility, and high blood are sloppy or overlapping categories in patients' speech. They often confuse social discomfort or psychological distress with the word pressure. 'I'm under a lot of pressure.' High stress becomes high pressure, which is a colloquial term for hypertension. Hypertension of course is a highly technical biomedical term.

Instead of talking about blood pressure, the doctor tries to follow the patient's narrative thread of difficulties with her son Jason and he does this by repeating one of the last words the patient spoke ('past') and the topic that the patient started the interview with – her son Jason. The doctor introduces the 'temporality' of the 'story' by trying to anchor the conversation into the beginning, a key element of the beginning–middle–end definition of narrative. A non-narrative inclined physician would have been more comfortable talking about blood pressure and could have easily directed the conversation towards blood pressure, missing the reason for the patient's visit.

Lines 41–71: The next interaction demonstrates the parallelism behind receiving help, raising Jason, and helping Jason raise his own child. The story is starting to develop a theme. There is an assumed narrative flow in the conversational gap when the doctor asks about the sudden death of the patient's father. The patient immediately closes the narrative gap by relating it to the 'start of the troubles.' One gets the sense that the story is being retold, which draws on the strength of narrative as an interpretive therapeutic endeavor between listener and storyteller. The patient identifies a narrative transition when life got difficult and Jason started acting out. This is defined as 'emplotment' – a change in the direction of the story. When the doctor asked the patient to reflect, the patient says, 'I am not sure that I have ever recovered. When things get stressful, I still think about that day.' This is a literary metaphor: a 'clogged artery' resembles our patient who has a 'clogged emotional flow' associated with this grief. Instead of attempting to give the patient an interpretation, the doctor allows the patient to self interpret by saying 'So what do you think happened to your father?' This self interpretation moves the narrative closer to the climax of this narrative episode, which revolves around the connection between troubles, blocked grief, and heartache. The action plays out when the patient begins to describe symptoms of blocked arteries. The drama unfolds as the patient positions herself in the middle generation between her father and her son, again developing a narrative thread or theme. The doctor recognizes this heightened sense of drama. The drama is created by large emotional content, possibly fear, anger, guilt, sadness. Earlier, we discussed how social interactions are choreographed by emotions. If the patient is fearful, many physicians respond with 'reassurance by medical testing.' If only dealt with on this level, it is poor medical practice and dangerous. Anger provokes appeasement, '... you have every right to be angry with your father for abandoning you that way.' Guilt provokes reassurance, 'You didn't do anything wrong.' Sadness provokes consolation, etc. This is where the doctor has to understand the difference between his/her emotions and the patient's experience and emotions.

Lines 75–105: The doctor labels it by saying, 'I can sense how unsettling this experience must be.' Unsettling is a neutral term – not an emotion – again allowing the patient to self define the emotion and hence the story. This empathetic statement is a way of saying, 'I'm listening ...' He then asks for a chronological telling of the chest pain story.

Again, the doctor reflects back to the patient the thematic content of their entire relationship 'since the first day I met you' and highlights a similar episode of chest pain. Reminding the patient about the stress echocardiogram allows the patient to continue the narration. The doctor uses the same method as before, phrasing it as, 'tell me again ...' By leaving the clinical interview open to story telling, there is a surprising narrative twist when the patient talks about smoking and medications. The next statement is a clear example of counter transference when the proud parent/doctor provides support to the patient.

Lines 106–142: This provokes a deeper patient reflection and the patient reveals the reason for today's visit, 'I just have this feeling that something is going to happen to me.' At this point, the doctor is starting to get a sense of this particular episode in the meta-narrative and the doctor invites the patient to state the reason for the visit out loud. The patient states 'I'm worried that I have a clog in my heart.' The doctor explores the patient's cognitive understanding of arthrosclerosis and the patient relates a newspaper clipping about CT coronary angiography to her underlying concerns. The patient had a newspaper clipping regarding new technology in her purse. The fact that the patient shared the clipping means the interview was successful. The patient was able to bring her current state of the narrative dilemma out of her purse, out into the open to be discussed between herself and her doctor.

Lines 143–152: Of course these narrative reflections on the dialogue is an interpretive endeavor, but remember, the doctor's job as a scientist is to discover the most important question. This section is clarifying the narrative dilemma. We strongly believe that the most important question is the one the patient wants answered. This particular office visit is part of an ongoing narrative where the major characters are suffering a complicated bereavement, arthrosclerosis, strained family relationships, and things yet to be discovered in the next chapter. In order for it to make sense to the patient, however, the doctor needs to track the story from the patient's perspective. The doctor asks and repeats the narrative dilemma trying to get the patient to confirm that it is correct.

The narrative is only the beginning of the process. Remember this is an interdependent process where narrative and clinical epidemiology/evidence based medicine become part of each other and so the doctor must connect this narrative to the domain of different diagnostic tests that would be reasonable in this situation. At the end of the interview, the patient alluded to CT coronary angiogram, which has been reported in the local press. As clinicians, we should respond to such inquiries with an evaluation of the medical literature and an assessment of what is known and what is not. It does not seem clinically appropriate to proceed to invasive cardiac testing at this time.

The doctor tries to impose the biomedical view of plaque rupture, but that does not fit the patient's understanding of the problem. She will only be able to 'rest assured' if her coronary arteries 'are clean' and 'clear of 'clogs.' The doctor has to determine whether it is medically reasonable to proceed with this understanding. We usually give our patients a large amount of latitude in defining what information they personally need. Remember though, the doctor has to agree with the overall treatment plan as well. In this case, the doctor agrees to explore the patient's narrative dilemma instead of the biomedical script of vulnerable plaque rupture and risk factor modification. By agreeing to enter the patient's world of experience and knowledge, we begin the healing journey.

A CONTINGENT, EMERGENT, SITUATED, AND CONTEXTUAL MEDICAL KNOWLEDGE

This office visit has *contingent* medical knowledge because the office visit could have been about stress management, musculoskeletal pain, bereavement, none of the above, or coronary artery disease. Patients do not live their life in an exam room, but the story that develops is a reflection of that life that is lived. It seems reasonable to say that neither the doctor nor the patient could have totally predicted at outset the way the interview went.

The *emergent* part of this interview is when the patient said, '... I wasn't thinking about it that way before this appointment ...' The narrative dilemma emerges during the process of listening.

The *situated* part of this case is that the conversation could only have happened with this patient and doctor because they share a common knowledge based on previous appointments. Had a sports medicine doctor interviewed the patient or a cardiologist interviewed the patient, we think the diagnosis would have been musculoskeletal pain.

The *contextual* part of the case is the historical nature of the patient's life story.

REFERENCES

1   D'Andrade RG. Schemas and motivation. In: D'Andrade R, Strauss C (eds). *Human Motives and Cultural Models*. Cambridge: Cambridge University Press; 1992.

2   Charon R. *Narrative Medicine Honoring the Stories of Illness*. Oxford: Oxford University Press; 2006.

3   Engel JD, Zarconi J, Pethtel LL, *et al. Narrative in Healthcare: healing patients, practitioners, profession and community*. Oxford: Radcliffe Publishing; 2008.

4   Crabtree BF, Miller W, editors. *Doing Qualitative Research*. 2nd ed. Thousand Oaks, CA: Sage Publications, Inc; 1999.

5   *The American Heritage College Dictionary*. 4th ed. Boston, MA: Houghton Mifflin Company; 2002.

6   Mattingly C. *Healing Dramas and Clinical Plots: the narrative structure of experience*. Cambridge: Cambridge University Press; 1998.

7   Lown B. *The Lost Art of Healing*. New York, NY: Ballantine Books; 1996.

8   Lown B. The commodification of health care. *Physicians for a National Health Program Newsletter*. Chicago, IL; 2007.

9   Greaves D. *'The Healing Tradition' Reviving the Soul of Western Medicine*. Oxford: Radcliffe Publishing; 2004.

10 Brock C, Salinsky J. Empathy: an essential skill for understanding the physician patient relationship in clinical practice. *Family Medicine*. 1993; **25**: 245–8.

11 Engel G. The need for a new medical model: a challenge for biomedicine. *Science*. 1977; **196**: 129–36.

12 Engel G. From biomedical to biopsychosocial: being scientific in the human domain. *Families, Systems & Health*. 1996; **14**(4): 425–33.

13 Cassell E. *The Healer's Art*. Cambridge, MA: MIT Press; 1985.

14 Borkan JM, Miller WL. Storytelling in medicine. In: Borkan J, Reis S, Steimetz D, Medalie JH (eds) *Patients and Doctors: Life-changing stories from primary care*. Madison: University of Wisconsin Press; 1999.

15 Divinsky M. Stories for life. *Canadian Family Physician*. 2007; **53**: 203–5.

16 Dossey L. *Healing Beyond the Body*. 1st ed. Boston: Shambhala Publications, Inc; 2001.

17 Elwyn GJ. So many precious stories: a reflective narrative of patient based medicine in general practice, *BMJ*. 1997; **315**(7123): 1659–63.

18 Frattaroli E. *Healing the Soul in the Age of the Brain*. New York, NY: Viking; 2001.

19 Galzigna M. *Aspects of medical practice: insight from Narrative Therapy. Psychoanalysis and Narrative Medicine*. 2004. Available at: www.english.ufl.edu/pnm/papers.html

20 Garro LC, Mattingly C. Narrative turns. In: Mattingly C, Garro LC (eds) *Narrative and the Cultural Construction of Illness and Healing*. Berkeley, CA: University of California Press; 2000. pp. 259–70.

21 Greenhalgh T. Narrative based medicine: narrative based medicine in an evidence based world. *BMJ*. 1999; **318**(7179): 323–5.

22 Greenhalgh T, Hurwitz B. Narrative based medicine: why study narrative? *BMJ*. 1999; **318**(7175): 48–50.

23 Hatem D, Rider EA. Sharing stories: narrative medicine in an evidence-based world. *Patient Education and Counseling*. 2004; **54**: 251–3.

24 Hunter K. *Doctors' Stories: The Narrative Structure of Medical Knowledge*. Princeton: Princeton University Press; 1991.

25 Kirmayer L. Broken narratives: clinical encounters and the poetics of illness experience. In: Mattingly C, Garro L (eds) *Narrative and the Cultural Construction of Illness and Healing.* Berkeley, CA: University of California Press; 2000.

26 Loxterkamp D. A vow of connectedness: views from the road to Beaver's Farm. *Family Medicine.* 2001; 33(4): 244–7.

27 Rapport F, Wainwright P, editors. *The Self in Health and Illness: patient, professionals and narrative identity.* Oxford: Radcliffe Publishing; 2006.

28 Smith R, Hoppe R. The patient's story: integrating the patient- and physician-centered approaches to interviewing. *Annals of Internal Medicine.* 1991; 115: 205–24.

29 Stewart M, Brown JB, Weston WW, *et al. Patient-Centered Medicine.* Thousand Oaks: Sage Publications, Inc; 1995.

30 Stuart M, *et al. The Fifteen Minute Hour: practical therapeutic interventions in primary care.* Philadelphia: Saunders; 2002.

31 Sulmasy DP. Is medicine a spiritual practice? *Academic Medicine.* 1999; 74(9): 1002–5.

32 Sparkes AC, Smith BM. When narratives matter: men, sport, and spine cord injury. In: Rapport F, Wainwright P (eds) *The Self in Health and Illness: patients, professionals and narrative identity.* Oxford: Radcliffe Publishing; 2006. pp. 53–68.

33 Adler HM. The history of the present illness as treatment: who's listening, and why does it matter? *Journal of the American Board of Family Practice.* 1997; 10(1): 28–35.

34 Charon R. Narrative and medicine. *New England Journal of Medicine.* 2004; 350(9): 862–4.

35 Realini T, Kalet A, Sparling J. Interruption in the medical interaction. *Archives of Family Medicine.* 1995; 4: 1028–33.

36 Beckman HB, Frankel RM. The effect of physician behavior on the collection of data. *Annals of Internal Medicine.* 1984; 101: 692–6.

37 Mattingly C. Emergent narratives. In: Mattingly C, Garro LC (eds) *Narrative and the Cultural Construction of Illness and Healing.* Berkeley, CA: University of California Press; 2000. pp. 181–211.

38 Frank AW. *The Wounded Storyteller: body, illness, and ethics.* Chicago, IL: University of Chicago Press; 1995.

39 Beach MC, Inui T. Relationship-centered care – a constructive reframing. *Journal of General Internal Medicine.* 2006; 21: S3–8.

40 Kleinman A. *The Illness Narratives: suffering, healing, and the human condition.* New York, NY: Basic Books; 1988.

41 Riessman CK. *Narrative Methods for the Human Sciences.* Los Angeles, CA: Sage Publications; 2008.

42 Launer J. *Narrative-based Primary Care: a practical guide.* Oxford: Radcliffe Publishing; 2002.

43 Launer J. Narrative based medicine: a narrative approach to mental health in general practice. *BMJ.* 1999; 318(7176): 117–19.

44 Kleinman A. *Patients and Healers in the Context of Culture.* Berkeley, CA: University of California Press; 1980.

45 Garro LC, Mattingly C. Narrative as construct and construction. In: Mattingly C, Garro LC (eds) *Narrative and the Cultural Construction of Illness and Healing.* Berkeley, CA: University of California Press; 2000, pp. 1–49.

46 Egnew TR. The meaning of healing: transcending suffering. *Annals of Family Medicine.* 2005; 3(3): 255–63.

47 Elwyn G, Gwyn R. Narrative based medicine: stories we hear and stories we tell: analysing talk in clinical practice. *BMJ.* 1999; 318(7177): 186–8.

Ask a Clinically Appropriate Question Based on the Patient's Concern

KEY CONCEPTS TO REMEMBER

➤ Transitioning from a narrative dilemma to a clinically relevant question requires the doctor to simultaneously think narratively and clinically so that nothing is 'lost in translation.'

➤ Maintaining a collaborative approach, explaining clinical terms to patients, and checking back with the patient to see if the transition to a clinical question was successful begins the 'co-constructed narrative.'

➤ Emphasize POEMs not DOEs when developing clinically relevant questions.

➤ Clinical questions about therapy use PICO structure.

➤ Clinical questions about diagnosis use test characteristics of a specific test for a specific disease (both are required).

LEARNING ABOUT ASKING CLINICAL QUESTIONS

The Transition from a Narrative Dilemma to a Clinically Relevant Question

We ended the last chapter by demonstrating how a narrative competent clinician overrides their impulses to seek a diagnosis by training themselves to listen to the patient's story. The story, or narrative, has a certain structure and is usually told for a specific purpose. This chapter begins by trying to find the question that will resolve the narrative dilemma for the patient. At each and every step of this care process it is important to get it right or subsequent efforts become inefficient, unhelpful, or wrong. So how do we turn the patient's narrative dilemma into an appropriate question that can be answered by using evidence?

While listening is the most important skill in narrative medicine, we have found that it is usually necessary to collaborate with a patient to rephrase the dilemma as a clinical question. This is a process of translation from the language of the Illness Narrative to the language of clinical medicine. We do not want anything to get lost in the translation. Most of us have heard funny stories of translations gone bad – well this step in the process requires the doctor to think in two 'languages' simultaneously, being very careful that the meaning of the narrative dilemma is not lost in translation. This co-operative, interactive process of speculating from a clinical perspective and checking with the patient to determine if the clinical question 'fits' the narrative is the beginning of the co-constructed narrative. Often, the patient will have a very narrow specific primary concern, not necessarily related to the 'clinical' facts of the case.

In the Preface we presented a quotation of the transition between the patient's illness narrative and the abstract language of diseases and medical jargon. This is a transition from one world of knowledge to a different world of knowledge. They are two different languages, but remember, there is only one patient. The quotation portrayed the process as a dichotomy – first the patient had an illness story, then the doctors used abstract language of medicine to provide an answer that was then translated back to the patient. We used the example to illustrate the general flow of the process, but it is incorrect to conceptualize these as independent activities with sharply demarcated boundaries of who does what. Rather, both the doctor and patient have to participate continuously, with recognizably different emphases. It is always a good rule of thumb to assume that the patient is listening and watching throughout the process. Do not leave them guessing – tell them what is going on. At this point, say something like, 'I'm trying to understand what you told me you needed to know and capture that in terms or words that doctors use.' It is with extreme caution, checking and double checking to ensure that the patient's narrative dilemma is captured in a clinically answerable question. When all else fails, ask the patient. This may require some patient education about specific tests or terms, but patients appreciate receiving the information that is being used to construct medical decisions[1] (aka emplotment of the narrative). All we can do is ask doctors to be cautious as they transition from a patient's concern to asking a clinical question.

During the discussion we say things like, 'Doctors like to use big words ... "cardiogenic shock." Shock means that the blood pressure is too low and the blood does not circulate or flow through the arteries enough to get oxygen to the tissues and organs. "Cardiogenic" means the root of the problem is the heart muscle is not pumping enough. So "cardiogenic shock" means the blood isn't getting oxygen to the organs because the heart isn't pumping hard enough. We use the word to distinguish it from other causes of problems with blood circulation.' At this point, the patient can recognize the language as an explanation and feels more comfortable asking about parts they do not understand. That is a big difference than just using the word embedded in a bigger explanation. When doctors use a lot of jargon, patients are easily intimidated and less likely to participate; doctors are also more likely to ask the wrong clinical question.

We need to check for meaning – not answers, at least not at this stage. 'Does the question capture the concern of the patient in a meaningful way?' This is vitally important because it means that the patient will be able to recognize the answer as relevant further along in the process.

Developing the Question

'Asking a clinically relevant question' is typically the first step in any evidence based medicine curriculum. In the following discussion, we hope to show that this 'evidence based medicine' skill is interdependent with the narrative process described above. This is not the responsibility of the doctor – it must remain a close collaboration with the patient. By refining the question, the doctor is inserting him/herself into the narrative, resulting in a co-constructed narrative.

Even though we have preserved the terms of orthodox evidence based medicine to help the reader correlate with that larger body of literature, we also hope the reader appreciates the subtle distinctions of meaning created by the blending and dual roles played by both the doctor and the patient that is unique to the process we describe.

Asking the correct question is vital to the process. The structure of the question will determine the structure of the search for evidence. This illustrates the need to do the process sequentially and avoid making errors early in the process. The first step is to acquire enough information to understand the patient's concern. If we do not understand the patient's concern, then how are we going to ask the correct clinical question? The next step after developing a clinical question related to the patient's concern is to access the information that will answer that specific question. Therefore, if we ask the wrong clinical question, we will access the wrong information and not be able to help the patient with their concern. Novices often want to breeze through this step. But remember, the goal of this process is to incorporate it directly into patient care to provide the patient with real-time answers.

Before we became proficient in being able to use this at the bedside, we would sometimes get lost searching for evidence. In retrospect, our mistake was not being careful enough in asking questions. Asking good questions improves the efficiency of steps further in the process. The importance of this step should not be underestimated.

CLINICAL EXAMPLE

A patient came in with the chief complaint of 'possible gallstones.' When listening to the story, it turns out that the patient had stomach pains and nausea. She was talking about it with the group of women with whom she plays golf and they all related the symptoms to their own experiences with gallstones. When trying to clarify the narrative dilemma, we asked, 'So really what you want to know is if this pain you had came from undiagnosed gallstones, right?' The patient said, '... yeah, sort of.' The non-narrative physician might have quickly decided that he/she knows how to check for gallstones and ordered an ultrasound, based on the clinical question, 'Does this patient have gallstones?' The narrative physician would have replied, '"Sort of" also means "Sort of, not ..." help me understand the other part of your concerns.' The patient went on to say that she was sure her friends were right, but that her husband's brother died five years ago from pancreatic cancer. She admitted it was 'silly' to worry about that, but it was there in the back of her mind. The true clinical dilemma was that the patient wanted to know if she had some terrible disease, so the narrative dilemma was really, 'Does this patient have an occult malignancy?' The doctor has to have some background knowledge that there are multiple ways to answer that question, based on what test is used. Options are ultrasound of the abdomen, CT scan of the abdomen, and Magnetic Resonance Cholangio-pancreatography. After relating the patient's narrative dilemma to the medical context, the doctor should re-state the narrative dilemma and review the pros and cons of each of the tests. In this particular case, the clinical question then became, 'What is the sensitivity and specificity of MRCP for gallstones versus malignancy?' For example, Magnetic Resonance Cholangio-Pancreatography (MRCP) has a different sensitivity and specificity for tumors verses choledocholithiasis.[2, 3] Notice how different the two clinical questions are, based on two minutes of conversation in the exam room. Notice also, the vast difference in the meaning of the two questions, not to mention the difference in evidence that should be used.

Only after the doctor is certain that he/she understands the patient's concern and has been able to ask a clinical question that relates to that concern, should the doctor consider other major risks or management issues for the patient. If the doctor prematurely jumps and steers the visit without understanding the patient's concern, then the doctor risks missing the patient's narrative dilemma and risks 'asking the wrong question.'

DOEs versus POEMs

Pathophysiology helps us understand disease and develop diagnostic and treatment modalities to help our patients. There are many pathophysiologic theories that lead to treatment modalities. Furthermore, the treatment modalities may demonstrate the lowering of a physiologic marker. For example, it was theorized that free radicals contribute to arthrosclerosis and coronary artery disease. Vitamin E reduces free radicals.[4] We would suspect that vitamin E is helpful to our patients as it should reduce coronary artery disease. However, studies have shown that vitamin E does not affect coronary artery disease. It is of no benefit.

Most of the medical literature includes articles that are classified as disease orientated evidence (DOE), such as the reduction of free radicals by vitamin E. Patients simply don't talk about or experience the levels of free radicals in their bloodstream. The reason for this is these proxy measures occur much earlier and are easier to measure than patient outcomes. For example, as a marker for diabetic control, hemoglobin A1C, is often used in studies to test the efficacy of diabetic pharmaceuticals. However, it is difficult to demonstrate that the particular drug improves outcomes that the patient really cares about, such as mortality, myocardial infarction, and renal dialysis. This latter category called patient oriented evidence that matters (POEMs), refers to outcomes that patient can notice and think the outcome is important. This vital concept was developed by Drs Allen Shaughnessy and David Slawson as part of an Information Mastery program dedicated to providing clinicians with the best possible information at the 'point of care' to assist their patients.[5]

A good example of patient oriented evidence that matters is the UK Prospective Diabetes Study (UKPDS trial). The researchers performed a large clinical trial that studied 'aggressive' diabetic care versus the 1980 diabetic standard of care, which was for the fasting blood sugar to be less than 280 mg/dl. The purpose of the UKPDS trial was to determine if improved glycemic control would also improve cardiovascular outcomes; less myocardial infarctions and less cardiovascular deaths.[6] Before and since this trial, there are numerous studies that clearly show poor glycemic control is associated with heart disease. In other words, the worse the patient's diabetes is, the worse the cardiovascular outcome will be. There are also numerous studies showing that insulin, sulfonylureas, and metformin lower the hemoglobin A1C (a disease oriented outcome). These are all surrogate markers and disease oriented markers – after all, people do not walk around saying their HgA1C is high this week. Interestingly, there has not been any study that showed lowering the hemoglobin A1C with these agents would actually improve cardiovascular outcomes. The UKPDS trial actually was unable to show this benefit. There was no cardiovascular difference between intense glycemic control and the standard of care (circa 1980). This is a real patient oriented outcome. Nonetheless, an entire ideology of diabetic care has evolved around the concept of lowering blood sugars in people with diabetes. Confirming the UKPDS trial results, the ACCORD[7] trial and the ADVANCE trial[8] were both published in 2008. Again, patient oriented evidence did not support the disease oriented research. These research trials should revolutionize the way we understand treating patients with diabetes (hopefully sometime soon).

Patients only care about the hemoglobin A1C because we tell them to. They come into the doctor's office and when motivated to manage their diabetes are often interested in lowering this number. They care about this because the medical community has taught them about the association between poor glycemic control and cardiovascular disease. We taught them this because we confused *association* with *cause and effect*. The patient believes that controlling their blood sugar will ultimately lower their risk of death. The patient really cares about dying, not about a number (blood sugar). That number is DOE, how well is the blood sugar controlled. But the patient really cares about death, which is POEM. Therefore, we only want to ask questions that our patient really cares about; we only want to ask questions that can be answered with POEMs.

Illness narratives are complex. There are usually multi-faceted web of concerns and behaviors. Using the above example of glycemic control, we actually re-frame the clinical questions about diabetic management to more closely align with the narrative dilemma (preserving good health) when working with our patients. Patients often respond with relief to not having to be perfect, simply by having us re-state their underlying concern (narrative dilemma) and changing the management questions.

Types of Questions

The medical literature is filled with editorials, health delivery research, epidemiology, etc. We tend to focus on diagnosis and treatment, since these are the bread and butter of practice. This limits the total body of literature that needs to be explored, making the process manageable. Other types of medical literature have other purposes, but we will not focus on that now.

We will next focus on how to structure questions for diagnosis and treatment. In Part I we are focusing on diagnosis, but here we will also say something about how to formulate treatment questions and then return to that subject in Part II. It should also be noted that the vast majority of narrative dilemmas and clinical questions do not require an expedition into the medical literature. Usually these questions can be answered simply with the doctor's fund of knowledge. The answer still needs to be translated back to the patient and we believe that the doctor must still verify that the knowledge is valid and not part of the unscientific, apprentice-type of 'knowledge.' If it is based on usual practice and not research literature, then the doctor has to declare that as well. This is all about being honest while in relationships with patients. We will be talking about conflict of interests and how it affects decision making later, but for now, let us look closer at how to formulate clinical questions for diagnosis and treatment.

Formatting a Clinical Question Using Test Characteristics

So then, how do we ask a clinically relevant question for a diagnostic test? All diagnostic tests can be described in terms of their sensitivity and specificity. Unfortunately, there is always a trade off between these two. For example, you can have a test with a very high sensitivity, but usually that diminishes the specificity and vice versa. Very technically to determine the maximization of both sensitivity and specificity we use receiver operator curves for different tests. Comparing the curves of different testing options is a reflection of the quality of the test. We are not going to go into that level of detail at this point.

Sensitivity and specificity together are referred to as the 'test characteristics.' Finding information about the test characteristics will help us format a clinically relevant question. The other piece of vital information that needs to be in the question is the target disease that we are testing for.

For a diagnostic test, we can simply combine the test with the test characteristics and the condition for which the test is being ordered to develop our question. For example, a patient presented to the hospital for a hip fracture. During her inpatient stay, she developed symptoms consistent with a pulmonary embolism. We discussed the purpose of the CT pulmonary angiogram on rounds and she was scared. She needed to know how good the test was. The clinical question then becomes: *What is the sensitivity and specificity of CT pulmonary angiogram for detecting pulmonary embolism?*

Formatting Therapeutic Questions

For therapeutic questions, we find that the most efficient method to connect the patient's clinical dilemma to the evidence is to use a process called PICO to structure the clinical question.[9, 10] PICO is an acronym that stands for Patient, Intervention, Control, and Outcome. In this case, we want to define the population that was studied to match our own practice demographics and our patient as closely as possible. The intervention is the therapy or management being considered. The control is the alternative standard of care. Consistent with our discussion with DOEs and POEMs, the outcome should be a patient orientated outcome that matters.

A patient came into the office and heard on TV that anti-anxiety drugs help with premature ejaculation. Even though we had seen this patient for several years, we had never discussed his sexual dysfunction before. This had been a chronic problem and had caused some marital problems for him. He was desperate for some help. He wanted to know if an anti-anxiety medicine would help. We thought he was referring to SSRIs as the anti-anxiety medication. The PICO question is as follows:

P = Patient Population: Patients that suffer from premature
     ejaculation
I = Intervention: Selective Serotonin Re-uptake Inhibitors (SSRIs)
C = Comparison: Placebo
O = Outcome: Premature ejaculation frequency reduction

PICO Question: In patients that have premature ejaculation, do SSRIs reduce the frequency of premature ejaculation compared to placebo?

STORY TIME

We were supervising a resident that asked and correctly answered a clinically important question, but missed the narrative dilemma and missed the second clinically relevant question that mattered most to the patient. The patient was well known to the resident and had a long standing history of menorrhagia and iron deficiency anemia. She was not very adherent to the iron because she suffered from iron induced constipation. Her chief complaint was fatigue. The resident, knowing the patient very well, quickly influenced the interview toward a discussion of menorrhagia by asking the patient about her heavy periods and her iron pill-taking habits. When he was precepting with us he labeled her as 'non-compliant' with her iron and that is why she was so tired. He answered the question, 'Will iron help my fatigue?' for the patient. However, that wasn't really the patient's concern/question. We re-interviewed the patient and elicited the patient's story, in which the patient was very worried about diabetes since she was obese and her friend, who has a normal body weight, was recently diagnosed with diabetes. She had read that fatigue could be a symptom of diabetes. The patient's narrative dilemma was 'Is diabetes causing my fatigue?' not 'Will iron help my fatigue?' It turns out that the patient did not have diabetes. After answering this question for her (her random blood sugar was less than 120 and a recent fasting blood sugar was 83), we were then able to move the office visit to address her anemia. The patient expects the physician to use his/her expertise. That is why the patient is there. The resident was correct; the patient had iron deficiency anemia and wasn't taking enough of her iron tablets – which is important, but insufficient from the patient's perspective. Notice that in this example, the 'evidence' is merely information already in the chart and available in the office visit. In other words, the evidence is our definition of diabetes. We do not need to proceed further in the Evidence based medicine process because we already have the evidence we need.

The point of the story is ... The doctor needs to collaborate with the patient, checking to make sure the clinical question is related to the narrative dilemma.

NARRATIVE ASPECTS OF ASKING A CLINICALLY RELEVANT QUESTION

We discussed above the importance of making the transition from a narrative dilemma to a clinical question. Howard Brody wrote an article with a wonderful title: 'Doctor, my story is broken, can you help me fix it?'[11] Another example is, 'Whose story am I in?' What we are essentially talking about is the fact that as the doctor starts to influence the co-constructed narrative, the patient needs to identify closely enough with the process to recognize it as a story that he/she can still relate to – something that has meaning for the patient. We highlight this point because all too often we have seen cases where the story gets 'abducted' by the doctor and there is no cohesiveness to the process of care, let alone within the life story of the patient. Whose story is it? At this point, both the patient and the doctor should begin to take ownership of the process and work together collaboratively.

APPLICATION TO OUR CLINICAL CASE SCENARIO

Let us apply the concepts and principles described above to the clinical vignette that was recorded in the previous chapter. First of all, we have to differentiate whether the question is about a diagnostic test or a treatment/therapy. Since the patient's concern is about the possibility of having undetected coronary artery disease, our job is to diminish the uncertainty related to that question. We need to demonstrate for her that the probability of having heart problems is so low that she is willing to stop worrying about it. We are not really talking about therapy, we are talking about diagnosis.

The patient brought in a newspaper clipping that alluded to Computed Tomography Angiogram (CT angiogram), but it is important for the clinician not to jump to conclusions. A good basis to continue the process of care would be to consider the available diagnostic tests that address the patient's underlying concern. Embedded in this example is the rather frequent scenario when the patient tries to provide the solution. All too often, the doctor takes the bait and focuses on 'the solution.' The wise physician focuses on the underlying question. Notice how the narrative drives the analysis, not the patient's suggestion or the doctor's predispositions. Available diagnostic tests include:

➤ Stress EKG.
➤ Stress (exercise or chemical) echocardiography.
➤ Stress (exercise or chemical) nuclear test (Thallium, etc).
➤ CT Coronary Angiography (16–64-slice, multi-detector).
➤ Magnetic Resonance Angiography.
➤ Coronary Catheterization.

In general we will start with less invasive testing. We also want to maximize the accuracy of the test and minimize the cost while still answering the patient's question to her satisfaction. So let us evaluate the patient's suggestion of CT angiography against those criteria. The patient already had a negative stress test. Her persistent symptoms are so concerning to her that the negative stress echocardiogram test is not enough to adequately address her concern. Based on her story, our concern as a physician is high enough to recommend further testing. However, it would be safer for the patient if we can avoid an invasive test, such as a coronary catheterization at this time.

Since the patient specifically mentioned CT coronary angiography, it seems appropriate from a narrative perspective to follow that thought process. This highlights the 'co-constructed' nature of the narrative. The doctor is using his/her medical authority to validate the appropriateness of the chosen diagnostic test. If there is disagreement, it needs to be discussed again with the patient about why that particular test was chosen. Let us explore how good CT coronary angiography is for this patient's specific problem, in the detection of coronary artery disease. Remember, we are trying to match a clinically relevant question to the patient's narrative dilemma.

We can ask, 'What is the sensitivity and specificity of CT coronary angiography to detect clinically significant coronary artery disease in patients with moderate risk for coronary artery disease?' This is our clinically appropriate question based on our patient's concern.

Let us go back and double check to see if this clinical question captures the narrative dilemma presented in the case scenario. The doctor stated and the patient confirmed that the narrative dilemma was, 'You want to know if you have any clogged or blocked arteries?' (end of line 141). This requires a judgment about the equivalence of 'clinically significant coronary artery disease' and 'clogged or blocked arteries.' It is best to check back with the patient to verify these definitions are truly equivalent to be relevant from the patient's perspective.

Only when we are sure that the clinical question matches the narrative dilemma do we proceed to the next step in the process. Remember, sequencing the steps in the process is vital. In this case, we feel ready to proceed.

A CONTINGENT, EMERGENT, SITUATED, AND CONTEXTUAL MEDICAL KNOWLEDGE

We hope to show that this process uses a different type of medical knowledge. Compared to 'science as truth,' we are looking to translate science into the social environment.

The *contingent* aspect of asking a clinically relevant question is demonstrated by the back and forth nature of translating the narrative dilemma into a clinical question. Multiple clinical questions have to be considered and measured against whether or not they describe the narrative dilemma. Eventually, questions will be considered and discarded, thus they were contingent until the social process progresses.

The *emergent* quality of asking a clinically relevant question is shown by the fact that one question (of many possible) is chosen and emerges as the link to the next narrative episode. It is a decision that defines the future. Notice also that it resets all the contingencies again. This is a reflection of a process in time.

The doctor has to *situate* the narrative dilemma within the body of research that addresses the question. At this point in the process that literature is known partially and discovered during the process of care as outlined in this book. As indicated, the co-constructed nature of the narrative is underway – asking a clinically relevant question is *situated* within the framework of that social interaction.

The *contextual* nature of our example that checks for gallstones versus identifying terrible intra-abdominal pathology reflects the patient's experience of having a brother-in-law who died of pancreatic cancer and the range of diagnostic tests available. Thus, context drives the clinical relevant question from both the patient's context and the doctor's context.

REFERENCES

1 Waitzkin H. Information giving in medical care. *Journal of Health and Social Behavior.* 1985; **26**(2): 81–101.
2 Adamek HE, Albert J, Breer H, *et al.* Pancreatic cancer detection with magnetic resonance cholangiopancreatography and endoscopic retrograde cholangiopancreatography: a prospective controlled study. *The Lancet.* 2000; **356**: 190–3.
3 Hochwald SN, Dobryansky M, Rofsky NM, *et al.* Magnetic resonance cholangiopancreatography accurately predicts the presence or absence of coledocholithiasis. *J Gastrointest Surg.* 1998; **2**: 573–9.
4 Ebell M. Information mastery. In: *FP Essentials, AAFP Home Study Edition No 318.* Leawood, KS: American Academy of Family Physicians; 2005.
5 Slawson DC, Shaughnessy AF. Becoming an information master: using POEMs to change practice with confidence. Patient-Oriented Evidence that Matters. *J Fam Pract.* 2000; **49**(1): 63–7.
6 UKPDS. Intensive blood-glucose control with sulphonylureas or insulin compared with conventional treatment and risk of complications in patients with type 2 diabetes (UKPDS 33). *The Lancet.* 1998; **352**: 837–53.
7 ACCORD SG. Effects of intensive glucose lowering in type 2 diabetes. *New England Journal of Medicine.* 2008; **358**(24): 2545–59.
8 ADVANCE SG. Intensive blood glucose control and vascular outcomes in patients with type 2 diabetes. *New England Journal of Medicine.* 2008; **358**(24): 2560–72.
9 www.cebm.net/index.aspx?o=1036
10 Sackett DL, Haynes RB, Guyatt GH, *et al. Clinical Epidemiology: a basic science for clinical medicine.* 2nd ed. Boston: Little Brown and Company; 1991.
11 Brody H. 'My story is broken; can you help me fix it?' Medical Ethics and the joint construction of narrative. *Literature and Medicine.* 1994; **33**(1): 79–92.

CHAPTER 3

Access Information Relevant to the Question

KEY CONCEPTS TO REMEMBER

➤ Technology is always changing, so lifelong learning is critical.

➤ Medline is a database driven search that is very sensitive; Google Scholar is an algorithmic search that is very specific. These two methods can be combined.

➤ We believe we are at a watershed moment in information technology when the clinician at the site of care is connected directly to the original scientific literature, cutting out the 'middle men' of EBM storehouses.

➤ Filters in Google Scholar, such as 'cited by #' and search from [date] to [recent date] allow you to determine how well you've accessed a complete body of literature.

➤ The patient participates in the searching/foraging process because we talk about what we are doing as we do it, thinking out loud.

LEARNING ABOUT ACCESSING INFORMATION

From Medline to Google

As discussed earlier, the approach described in this book is based on a practical experience. We would like to remind our readers that technological advances are progressing exponentially. The challenge of life long learning implies that clinicians must embrace these changes and adjust your medical practice accordingly. Some examples would be the recent addition of Google Scholar to selectively retrieve academic information. Another example would be the University of Michigan's project to create a digital image of their entire university library. We can only expect that such advances will continue into the future. What we present here is based on our current best practice.

Approximately eight years ago, we were working with a neurologist in the hospital setting caring for a patient with a rare neurological disorder (Fragile X Ataxia Syndrome). In the middle of the discussion, our colleague opened the internet browser and did a Google search with the name of the syndrome. We were astonished at the speed and relevance of the journal articles retrieved. This was the first crossing of the threshold away from Medline searches toward our current practice. Over the next several months we experimented with using Google as an entry for accessing information and were pleasantly surprised at the ease of use compared to Medline.

Our previous experience with Medline was a tedious process because we had to manually find the relevant articles through the hundreds of irrelevant articles that Medline queries displayed. In retrospect, Medline searches have an underlying structure of a database, and the query will result in all matches of the search terms using the MeSH to find original articles. At that time, individual physicians had to depend on reference librarians to narrow the search to a manageable number of articles. This process often took days or weeks. Meanwhile, the opportunity to use the evidence to help the patient make a medical decision was lost. Our patient is sitting in front of us worried about her heart. She needs a decision today, not at a follow-up appointment in a few weeks. A busy clinician cannot review the literature for patients if the process is tedious. The theme of this chapter is a description of how the task of reviewing relevant research evidence can be done quickly and efficiently.

In contrast, our experience with the neurologist showed us that the information search with the Google search engine resulted in information that was incorporated contemporaneously with our clinical discussion. Later, we came to understand that a Google search uses an algorithmic process that ranks orders by the relevance of the search. This shortened interval for retrieving relevant information changed the nature of applying medical literature to clinical cases.

Google Scholar

Subsequently, Google Scholar became available in November 2004, which is where we start today. Google Scholar is a web search engine that only focuses on scholarly literature, including books, peer-reviewed papers, and journal abstracts. It eliminates the commercial-based sites that are found on Google. Like Google, it sorts the search in order of relevance, with the most relevant articles near the top of the first page.[1] Since it is proprietary knowledge, the source content, indexing, or relevance algorithms are not publicly available. One of its strengths is scholarly literature in the discipline of medicine (compared to chemistry, for example). The algorithm uses a 'crawl' of full-text journal content from commercial and open source publishers, including PubMed. This relevance algorithm is a closely guarded proprietary secret.[2] Even though full text access is not available on the web, Google has agreements with publishers for access to such information. That is why you can often only get access to the abstract on Google Scholar. We prefer to have the complete article in PDF format for review and evaluation of the quality of the evidence. This gives us access to the data in the 'Results' section of the paper. The general public often may only be able to get the abstract of the article, depending on the journal. However, we work at academic institutions and are also associated with a medical school in a university setting. Both of these institutions have hundreds of subscriptions to online medical literature. For the community physician, we recommend pursuing an affiliation with a teaching institution because that provides access to electronic library services. Otherwise, individual subscriptions can be purchased.

The Usefulness Equation

The Usefulness Equation says that the 'usefulness' of medical information is equal to the (relevance of the information X validity)/the (work involved to retrieve the information).[3] We have demonstrated that the work of retrieval has plummeted with the advent of Google Scholar thereby increasing the usefulness. The relevance of the information goes up when put into the narrative frame of the patient's concerns and the validity is what we will review in this chapter. So, to summarize:

$$\downarrow \text{work}$$
$$\uparrow \text{relevance}$$
$$\updownarrow \text{validity}$$

This means that the information used in this process is a lot more useful than just a few years ago. It used to be said that primary care doctors relied mostly on colleagues, pharmaceutical representatives, review articles, and consultants for information. We believe those days are gone. We do not trust pharmaceutical representatives and after applying the principles in the next chapter during Journal Club or case conferences we are frequently asked, 'Why do the journal editors allow these articles to be published?' Yes, there is a bit of a learning curve, but it is well worth it. Your patients will thank you for demonstrating that you have access to the latest information and you know whether it is valid or not. It builds professional self esteem and improves your ability to communicate with consultants at a much more sophisticated level. Occasionally, you can protect one of your patients when a specialist can't fit the evidence into the patient's life story. Primary care physicians need to be guardians of their patients, assisting them to get every test that is helpful or useful, but protecting them against the harmful effects of being over tested and over treated.[4]

Google Scholar is Useful and Marks a New Era in Information Mastery

With this knowledge, a thorough and relevant literature search can be accomplished. Google Scholar searches 'came of age' when Mark Ebell, MD, MS included a screenshot of a Google search page in an article about how to find answers to clinical questions. We believe this is a 'watershed moment' transitioning from relying on others to pre-digest the medical literature for the practitioner to having the practitioner directly interact with the primary evidence itself – the original research articles. Most of what we teach is how to do that efficiently. We have to admit that after having practiced this way for several years, it was gratifying to have someone as pre-eminent as Mark Ebell give the technique legitimacy.[5] There are other reports of this changing social practice.[6–8]

We began using Google Scholar as the primary literature search tool because of its obvious advantages with relevance to the patient's concern and clinical question. We found it to be very quick and useful. After choosing the most useful article from Google Scholar, it is always possible to find that same reference in PubMed and hit 'related citations.' This will match all of the keywords in the article chosen to the extensive body of literature in the PubMed database with identical keywords. This combines the 'specificity' of Google Scholar with the 'sensitivity' of PubMed. By doing them sequentially, you can find all the relevant literature quickly. You may or may not feel the need to do this based on the confidence you have from the results of the Google search. As we discussed above, digital publication and retrieval is a rapidly changing social phenomenon. The wide variety of medical journals that are included in Google searches reassure us that any reputable/journal will be accessible through Google.

Medical librarians have clearly noted the change in practice and have included Google Scholar as a digital resource.[2] They have concerns about the lack of comprehensive searches. As mentioned above, we typically find the best article possible using Google Scholar and then locate that article in PubMed. By using the 'related citations' feature of PubMed, we engage a database search based on the Medical Subject Headings (MeSH) which is the underlying structure of Medline. These two methods are complementary, and between the two, we have found it to be both time efficient and comprehensive.

Searching, Finding, and Retrieving

In the language of evidence based medicine, this step in the process is called 'foraging.' That is a good descriptor. Foraging conjures up images of wandering around, searching, trying to visually discern things of value, and following leads or information that probabilistically is related to what we are looking for. This section of the process may seem haphazard for that reason. Do not use the case example as a strict formulaic approach; rather, try to get the gist of the general principles and then try it out on your own and self-evaluate how the process works for you. Do not get discouraged, we both do this consistently with success, but before doing it successfully, we had our share of failures. It is an acquired skill. Although we present the information in a somewhat linear manner, we do that as a skill building way of explanation. In actuality, we use the 'copy and paste' function and usually have multiple windows open while toggling between Google Scholar, PubMed, and EBM websites. Metaphorically, however, you need to learn the melody before playing a fugue. Thus, this activity does take on the seemingly haphazard, direction changing qualities communicated by the word 'foraging.' Again, use this chapter to learn how different search strategies work for you. Share with your colleagues and friends the results of your most successful searches.

When we began sharing this process with our colleagues, we got requests to solve the unsolvable. The clinical question was obscure and before we even started to look for information, we had a sinking sense that we were on a wild goose chase. In retrospect, the question probably originated from the clinician and not the patient because it dealt with obscure pathophysiology. Expectations were unrealistic and we looked like fools instead of experienced doctors. In retrospect, before foraging, we should have made a mental estimation of whether the question is answerable. Additionally, we were not grounding the question closely enough into a real patient narrative – patients simply do not ask about rare diseases. With more experience, we have acknowledged that there probably isn't information available and use the foraging process to confirm that. A lot of this comes with experience in the types of questions and the utility of the process. It is very easy to get lost when doing a search because hyperlinks never end. Stay focused and be systematic when foraging. So, in general, the steps we recommend before you go off wandering through Google Scholar are:

1 Choose key words from the clinically relevant question.
2 Try out those key words as search terms in Google Scholar.
3 Do a quick search using different versions of the keywords, looking for acronyms or synonyms that might be substituted for the keyword you started with, but seem to be standard or frequently used keywords in article titles that Google Scholar will capture in the next query.
4 Re-search using the highest relevant keywords.
5 Begin evaluating the Google Scholar summaries as they are displayed on the screen.
6 Choose which link you will follow first by evaluating the Google summary.
7 Repeat the last step until you have a sense of the range of literature available.
8 Explore the Google Scholar summaries that you want to further evaluate by following the hyperlink to the journal article abstract or paper.
9 Using Google Scholar filters, search 'all related' and date ranges of articles.
10 Get a PDF image of the most promising article and review the methodology.
11 Scan the references of that article looking for related articles.
12 Pick the best summary of the literature, usually from one to five articles for complete evaluation.

Finding the most recent information is vital for a complete analysis of the literature. To overcome this limitation, we have also discovered that the search can be further refined by dates of publication. By selecting 'Advanced Search' on the Google Scholar page, the publication dates used in the search can be selected, thereby limiting the search to the years selected. We often use this process to insure that we have a complete search, including the recent literature that has not yet been able to accumulate a large number of 'cited by' [other articles], to help our patient make their decision. We will demonstrate this process in the following application to clinical scenario. Thus, by examining heavily cited literature, we quickly establish the 'standard' to which other research is compared and by looking for recent publications, we can determine if that standard has been updated. Including words such as 'randomized controlled trial' or 'meta-analysis' in the search terms can also screen for higher quality of evidence.

We are able to use Google Scholar quickly and effectively, allowing this process to occur during the patient encounter. It can be difficult at first. When we started, we often left the room during the Google Scholar search in case we got stuck. We did not want to get stuck with the patient staring at us, while we stared at the computer screen. However, through lots of practice, we have refined our foraging process so that we can locate the most relevant information quickly. Again, it is important to engage the patient in this process, so we talk out loud about what we are doing and why we chose to do it that way. This 'self disclosure' allows the patient to understand the doctor's experiences and analytical processes, building confidence and trust in the process. After all, most of our patients already search Google on their own. Our experience shows us that time efficiency is maximized by evaluating the search results carefully before choosing the first article since it is easy to get lost in the interrelated linking internet web structure.

What Keywords to Use

Choosing the right keywords will make the difference between an easy search and a difficult one. We usually try to avoid acronyms as many articles will not use the acronyms; therefore, the most relevant articles might not reach the top of the search results page. If the author of the most relevant article does not use the term CAD, then Google would not recognize the article at a high level of relevance and we might not find it.

For therapeutic searches, we usually start with words directly from the PICO question. For example, searching for the answer to the question, 'Does clopidogrel in addition to aspirin reduce mortality in patients with a recent acute myocardial infarction,' we started with the following keywords: recent, acute, myocardial, infarction, clopidogrel, and aspirin. Notice how we did not use MI for myocardial infarction or ASA for aspirin. In this case, the most relevant article was on the first search results page.

Diagnostic keyword selection is much simpler. We start with the diagnostic test, what the test is being used for, and the terms for the test characteristics. For the question, how accurate is MRI in the detection of osteomyelitis in the foot, we will use the keywords magnetic, resonance, imaging, osteomyelitis, foot, sensitivity, and specificity.

We continue to emphasize the importance following this process in sequence and avoiding mistakes early in the process. If attention was not used during the patient encounter, then the patient's concern might not be understood and the wrong question would be asked. With the wrong question, the wrong keywords would be selected resulting in the return of irrelevant medical literature.

The Google Scholar Search Results Page

After selecting our keywords and pressing the 'Search' button, Google Scholar proceeds to the Google Scholar Results Page. This really is not any different than the Google results page that everybody is familiar with. But, it is important to discuss this page as the article selection process actually begins with this page. For each article link, Google displays a truncated title, a partial listing of the authors, a very brief abstract excerpt. Also included is the URL, which provides information regarding the source of the information. We preferentially select .nih or .edu file extensions, or major medical journals' URLs.

While examining the Google Scholar search results page, it is helpful to look at the link information provided on the screen. The evaluation process begins here. Article links can be deemed as irrelevant or might look useful based on this information. The truncated title and the brief abstract excerpt (the Google summary) give a lot of information to help with this decision. For example, if we are looking for information on clopidogrel and aspirin for secondary prevention of coronary artery disease employing only medical management, and in the Google Scholar summary, it states that the patients had an angioplasty, then the article is not relevant to our search because we were not looking for the benefits of clopidogrel and aspirin in patients that had an angioplasty. That is a different question. Thus, this link can be skipped.

The Role of Regular Google

Patients often bring in newspaper clippings or internet search results about some type of treatment. They are often looking for their doctor's opinion about whether or not it would be a good idea, reflecting a healthy skepticism while being an informed patient. If we recognize it as a legitimate medical treatment we usually proceed directly to Google Scholar. However, patients often bring in alternative treatments with outlandish claims. In this case, it is best to start with regular Google search. The first step in evaluating it is the proper motive for selling these products, an analysis of the ingredients and/or manufacturer, and the therapeutic benefits claimed by the product. If there are no references on the website, we usually make some assessment regarding the relative safety of the product (since these are rarely FDA approved), help the patient evaluate the cost, and caution them regarding the unknown efficacy.

For example, a patient of ours was using 'Stanback' for her headaches. She wanted to know if it would interact with her blood pressure medications. We had no idea what ingredients were in Stanback. It is doubtful that this trade name would be listed in Google Scholar. We used regular Google search to look up the product information and then discussed with the patient that the caffeine might increase her hypertension, however, since her blood pressure was under very good control, likely it was safe for her to take. If the patient's concern was the effectiveness of this product, we would use Google Scholar with the chemical names of the main ingredients to search for relevant information.

Who Uses Google? Everybody

Our patients all use Google to self diagnose. When a patient starts to use medical jargon or asks esoteric questions about a particular disease, we sometimes ask, 'What else did you find on the web?' We know our patients well enough that if we guessed wrong, we can recover easily enough, but usually, we get sheepish grins and a flood of narrative dilemmas based on the patient's inability to evaluate the information. In fact, that is exactly why they made the appointment. As a doctor they are looking for your analysis and ability to relate the information to their particular case in a way someone without medical training cannot do.

Patients use the internet frequently for dietary information, drug information, etc.[9] Doctors use Google frequently. Their use seems to be limited to similar concerns as well as treatment side effects and drug safety information. Eighty six percent of physicians use the internet for medical information and 21% of physicians responded that they use Google searches while in the exam room with the patient.[10] What we are talking about here is converting from casual use to a more sophisticated evidence based quality standard of use for Google to access medical literature.

STORY TIME

We were volunteering at a 'free-clinic,' one that provided services for patients without insurance or access to medication. A resident in training from a program across town was also volunteering that same evening. She made the statement that, 'This patient needs to be changed to full dose aspirin because he's had an angioplasty.' Since we do not change our patients from 81 mg of aspirin to 325 mg of aspirin simply because they have had an angioplasty, we challenged the statement, wondering if there was any evidence for such management. The resident was adamant that she was correct. That type of certainty is always suspect so we used the only computer in the building, which was reserved for the clinic manager, to quickly scan the literature. In less than three and a half minutes, we were convinced that there was no high quality evidence and told that to the resident. We inquired what evidence she was aware of and she replied, 'Every cardiologist in our hospital does it.' We stated that there might be a well-reasoned pathophysiologic reason or some disease oriented evidence, but no patient oriented clinical evidence was available on our quick search. She insisted, provoking our standard clinical wager of 5¢. She promised to email the evidence to us, but nothing was forthcoming. The next month, we asked her precepting attending why she did not email us with the answer and he said, 'She couldn't find any evidence.'

The point of the story is ... once you learn the search protocols, information retrieval can be very quick.

NARRATIVE ASPECTS OF ACCESSING INFORMATION

Remember, this process is a co-constructed narrative. When we do a physical exam we often say things like, 'I'm examining your thyroid, which is a gland in your neck ...' This includes the patient in the process. Similarly, we typically say about the computerized medical record and the computer screen, 'Nothing in here is a secret ...' and tilt the screen so that the patient can see the same things we are looking at when we are looking at it. They have become so much of the process that they often point with their finger and say, 'What's that?' In this way, we look at laboratory data, X-rays, and progress notes together. We look at their electronic medical record together, graphing laboratory data over time and re-checking what the specialist told the patient compared to what the specialist wrote in the medical record. When we begin accessing information, we also talk through the process – saying things like, 'I'm going to check if this research has been updated by looking for articles published this year ...' The advantage is that nothing remains a mystery to the patient. They can carry the narrative thread as long as the doctor shares the journey with them. As we mentioned, you might want to test it out to gain confidence before you totally incorporate it into the clinical encounter.

The important point is that this is a co-constructed narrative. The doctor entered the world of lived experiences while listening to the patient's story and now the patient enters the world of the doctor's source of information. Historically, the definition of a 'profession' included specialized knowledge. By using this process, we have changed the 'specialized knowledge' from purely content to include analytic skills. This is why the patient goes to a doctor; they need the doctor's ability to contextualize the information, interpret the information, and relate the information to the illness story. When you listen carefully, the patient's illness stories often include a description of a previous doctor and what that doctor did or did not do, such as exams, statements, etc. In the same way, the computer 'searching' becomes part of the illness story. It is vital to 'de-mystify' the process enough so the patient can include it when they re-tell their story of the office visit. Because it is a process of discovery for the doctor and the patient, the 'journey together' is a metaphor for the rest of the management plan and indeed for the relationship itself.

What we are actually doing is foraging for information that will be used to write the next episode in the narrative. This is the emergent part of the story. We do not yet know at this point what choice the patient will make about further testing, but we need to contribute to the story by giving the range of dramatic or narrative choices that are also clinically appropriate. Remember when we talked in the first chapter about trying not to direct the patient into what we think is important, but to discover what the patient thinks is important? That same guiding principle is manifest in this process. By avoiding disease oriented evidence and by double checking that the actual research selected to bring back into the story is consistent with the patient's narrative dilemma, we maintain the narrative grounding for the evidence based approach. We demonstrated this same principle when trying to convert the narrative dilemma into a clini-cally relevant question – does it match? So the question for us now is the same – does the research match the narrative-clinical dilemma? We consistently for-age until we are able to make some statement out loud in the presence of the patient relating to the patient's narrative dilemma to the contents of the research articles. Only if we are convinced that we are accurately reflecting the patient's concern do we proceed to the next step. This is the time to check back with the patient to assess for agreement. If not, we keep foraging until we con-vince ourselves that there is no information available.

APPLICATION TO OUR CLINICAL CASE SCENARIO

1. Choose Key Words from the Clinically Relevant Question

Returning to our example, we need to take the clinically relevant question and Google Scholar search terms that will maximize the relevance of evidence to the clinical question. In our example, we are attempting to find the test charac-teristics of a specific test for a specific diagnosis. Remember that test characteris-tics for different diseases using the same test will vary. Again, this demonstrates the utility of following this process in sequence because the search terms are derived from the clinical question.

As you recall, the clinically relevant question to our patient's concern was:

'What is the sensitivity and specificity of CT coronary angiography to detect clinically significant coronary artery disease in patients with moderate risk for coronary artery disease?'

From this question, we typically name the test as the first search term. 'CT' as a search term could use the acronym or spell out the term computed tomography. We had the experience where successful searches depend on finding the exact keywords. It is worthwhile trying it in a couple of different ways and quickly assessing the results of the search. For example, let us try the keywords: computed, tomography, coronary, angiography, sensitivity, specificity, coronary, artery, disease.

2. Try out Those Key Words as Search Terms in Google Scholar

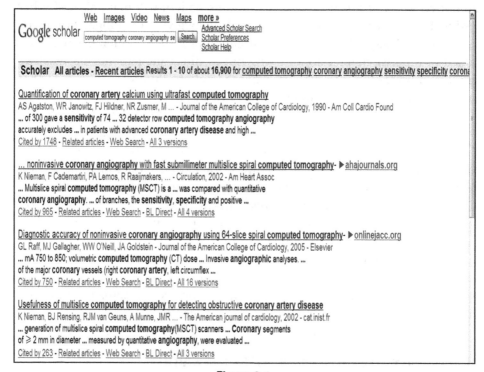

Figure 3.1

Notice that the first article refers to coronary artery calcium screening, which is totally unrelated to our clinical question. Since listing coronary artery disease as separate entities, the search included all varieties and types in that category that is additive. By using the acronym, CAD, we are trying to limit it to a specific medical condition and hopefully avoid some of the articles on screening. Because we are only assessing the utility of our keywords, it is useful to try several versions such as spelling them out versus using the acronym. At this point, we are still trying to find the optimal search terms, so, let us repeat the same search using the keywords: CT, coronary, angiography, sensitivity, specificity, CAD.

3. Do a Quick Search

Using different versions of the keywords, looking for acronyms or synonyms that might be substituted for the keyword you started with, but seem to be standard or frequently used keywords in article titles that Google Scholar will capture in the next query.

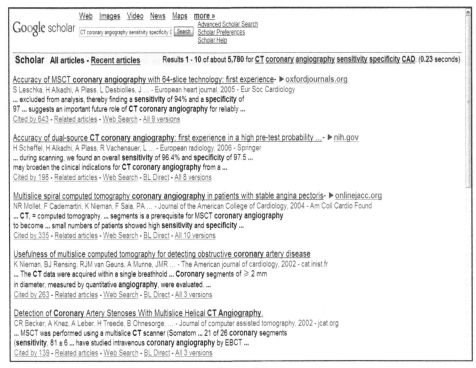

Figure 3.2

Notice that the first article uses the term MSCT. This stands for multi-slice CT, which is a clue to an alternative key word that might be important while foraging to ensure that we find the relevant literature. By using MSCT, we are further refining our search to help ensure a high level of accuracy. Before this process, we did not know that the acronym, 'MSCT' even existed, because we do not use it in our institution. It is worth taking the time early in the process to work with your keywords and sample various Google Scholar search results before committing to the next step of the process. Notice, once again, this is a process that requires starting from the beginning so that the patient's concern is answered accurately and completely. If the steps are done in the wrong sequence you will wind up with a different result and that will affect our patient's care later in the process.

In this example we were able to reach saturation in only three attempts. The number of attempts will vary. Sometimes we get lucky and are confident our search is complete with less attempts. For other searches, we need to spend more time.

4. Re-search Using the Highest Relevant Keywords

So, lets try it a third time using the keywords: MSCT, coronary, angiography, sensitivity, specificity, CAD.

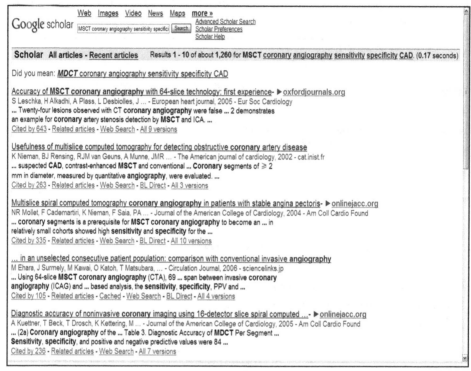

Figure 3.3

What we are demonstrating here is how to refine the foraging methodology to ensure we find the medical literature most related to the clinical question. The cognitive process used during foraging borrows a methodology from qualitative research called 'saturation'. Saturation is defined where any further refinements yields no additional information. Another way of saying this is we have a fair level of confidence that we have sampled the available literature to ensure validity of the search. Notice that the difference between our second and third search is very small. This is where we decided that our search had reached saturation. Sampling in this way is a process that yields higher accuracy than attempting an exhaustive list. Again, this is the difference between algorithmic Google Scholar search and a PubMed database search.

5. Begin Evaluating the Google Scholar Summaries as They are Displayed on the Screen

Now that we have selected a Google Scholar results page, we next need to evaluate the individual search results in the page selected. This is where we look for file extensions, such as .edu, .nih, .cdc, etc. Notice that in our search, we primarily have individual academic journal articles.

The next step in the foraging process is to evaluate the information provided on the Google Scholar results page. This includes the title, publication year, number of times cited, and abstract fragment. We are looking to see if our test was used, multi-slice CT, and if it was used in the detection of the disease we are looking for, coronary artery disease. Again, these criteria reflect our search terms that were derived form the clinical question, which in turn was derived from the patient's concern. Notice the layering of this process which has its foundation in the patient's story. (We have a saying in our teaching program, 'Repetition is the mother of learning.' So you might hear this theme again as we proceed.) Let us evaluate each article in turn.

6. Choose Which Link You Will Follow First by Evaluating the Google Summary

Accuracy of **MSCT coronary angiography** with 64-slice technology: first experience- ▶ oxfordjournals.org
S Leschka, H Alkadhi, A Plass, L Desbiolles, J ... - European heart journal, 2005 - Eur Soc Cardiology
... Twenty-four lesions observed with CT **coronary angiography** were false ... 2 demonstrates
an example for **coronary** artery stenosis detection by **MSCT** and ICA. ...
Cited by 643 - Related articles - Web Search - All 9 versions

Figure 3.4

This looks highly relevant and is worth going to the next step of following the link and evaluating the abstract. At this point, we are simply choosing which hyperlinks are worth investing more time to find the appropriate medical literature. Remember, it is easy to get lost and finding the correct keywords along with choosing articles worth evaluating further by looking at the Google Scholar summary are vitally important in making this process fast enough to do at the point of care. We learned the hard way that if you are not careful in prioritizing what to evaluate next, you wind up wasting a lot of time. At this point, we have 'placed a mental bookmark' on this article and will return to evaluate the abstract by following the hyperlink after we finished reviewing the other Google Scholar summaries on this screen. Let us now check the next Google summary.

7. Repeat the Last Step until You Have a Sense of the Range of Literature Available

Usefulness of multislice computed tomography for detecting obstructive **coronary** artery disease
K Nieman, BJ Rensing, RJM van Geuns, A Munne, JMR ... - The American journal of cardiology, 2002 - cat.inist.fr
... suspected **CAD**, contrast-enhanced **MSCT** and conventional ... **Coronary** segments of ⩾ 2
mm in diameter, measured by quantitative **angiography**, were evaluated. ...
Cited by 263 - Related articles - Web Search - BL Direct - All 3 versions

Figure 3.5

This also looks relevant, but has far less information. At this point, we are unsure if it is a study or just a review article. It is still useful to follow the hyperlink and evaluate the abstract., but lets review more Google Scholar summaries first.

Multislice spiral computed tomography coronary angiography in patients with stable angina pectoris- ▶ onlinejacc.org
NR Mollet, F Cademartiri, K Nieman, F Saia, PA ... - Journal of the American College of Cardiology, 2004 - Am Coll Cardio Found
... coronary segments is a prerequisite for **MSCT coronary angiography** to become an ... in
relatively small cohorts showed high **sensitivity** and **specificity** for the ...
Cited by 335 - Related articles - Web Search - BL Direct - All 10 versions

Figure 3.6

This Google Scholar summary states 'relatively small cohorts ...' This statement confirms our suspicion that the body of literature related to this topic is likely to contain many studies with few cases, limiting the definitive nature of any one particular study. So, a larger definitive study or meta-analysis will be our eventual endpoint of foraging. This is useful information; however, this particular study does not match our clinical question, and our patient's story, the study population (stable angina pectoris). Notice, that although we will not invest more time reviewing this particular study, since it would just be a waste of time, the Google Scholar search has helped formulate the parameters for identifying the most relevant clinical literature. We are very selective about which hyperlinks to investigate further, again for efficiency purposes. This summary does not need to be 'bookmarked.' Let us proceed to the next Google Scholar summary.

... in an unselected consecutive patient population: comparison with conventional invasive **angiography**
M Ehara, J Surmely, M Kawai, O Katoh, T Matsubara, ... - Circulation Journal, 2006 - sciencelinks.jp
... Using 64-slice **MSCT coronary angiography** (CTA), 69 ... span between invasive **coronary**
angiography (ICAG) and ... based analysis, the **sensitivity**, **specificity**, PPV and ...
Cited by 105 - Related articles - Cached - Web Search - BL Direct - All 4 versions

Figure 3.7

This is a more recent study (2006) and has methodological merit in that it is a population based study with an excellent gold standard. Since the medical literature is cumulative, the more recent studies will cite all previous knowledge accumulated to date. This is an efficient way to evaluate articles published prior to 2006. We need to ensure that the population used is similar to our patient and does not include asymptomatic individuals. Otherwise the prevalence of the disease is different, introducing spectrum bias. We will invest the time and review this article abstract below. Meanwhile, we proceed in evaluating the next Google Scholar summary.

Diagnostic accuracy of noninvasive **coronary** imaging using 16-detector slice spiral computed ...- ▶ onlinejacc.org
A Kuettner, T Beck, T Drosch, K Kettering, M ... - Journal of the American College of Cardiology, 2005 - Am Coll Cardio Found
... (2a) **Coronary angiography** of the ... Table 3. Diagnostic Accuracy of **MDCT** Per Segment ...
Sensitivity, **specificity**, and positive and negative predictive values were 84 ...
Cited by 236 - Related articles - Web Search - All 7 versions

Figure 3.8

This article is irrelevant as the test is outdated. (16-slice CT versus 64-slice CT.) We do not need to evaluate this article any further.

We continue this process through the first page, and sometimes the second page of the Google Scholar results, building a general sense of 'the body of literature.'

Let us take a second to review the foraging process up to this point and see how close we are to having a sense of what is available in the literature base. We started with the terms from our clinically relevant question (computed, tomography, coronary, angiography, sensitivity, specificity, coronary, artery, disease). During our Google Scholar search, we needed to modify our search terms in order to find all of the relevant information. We did this until our search reached saturation. Then, we examined the search results by first looking at the journal source, web extensions, and reviewing the Google summaries.

8. Further Explore the Google Scholar Summaries that You Want to Further Evaluate by Following the Hyperlink to the Journal Article Abstract or Paper

Notice that we have not yet followed any hyperlink to the actual journal article abstracts or papers. It is now time to look further at the abstracts that passed our screening described above. We want to further evaluate the first, second, and fourth article from our last Google Scholar search.

We selected the first Google Scholar summary and followed the hyperlink to the following article abstract.

European Heart Journal (2005) 26, 1482–1487
doi:10.1093/eurheartj/ehi261

Clinical research

EUROPEAN
SOCIETY OF
CARDIOLOGY®

Accuracy of MSCT coronary angiography with 64-slice technology: first experience

Sebastian Leschka[1], Hatem Alkadhi[1], André Plass[2], Lotus Desbiolles[1], Jürg Grünenfelder[2], Borut Marincek[1], and Simon Wildermuth[1*]

[1]Department of Medical Radiology, Institute of Diagnostic Radiology, University Hospital Zurich, Rämistrasse 100, 8091 Zurich, Switzerland; and [2]Clinic for Cardiovascular Surgery, University Hospital Zurich, Switzerland

Received 17 December 2004; revised 7 March 2005; accepted 15 March 2005; online publish-ahead-of-print 19 April 2005

See page 1451 for the editorial comment on this article (doi:10.1093/eurheartj/ehi322)

KEYWORDS
Computed tomography;
Conventional coronary
angiography;
Coronary artery disease

Aims The aim of our study was to investigate the accuracy of 64-slice computed tomography (CT) for assessing haemodynamically significant stenoses of coronary arteries.
Methods and results CT angiography was performed in 67 patients (50 male, 17 female; mean age 60.1 ± 10.5 years) with suspected coronary artery disease and compared with invasive coronary angiography. All vessels ≥1.5 mm were considered for the assessment of significant coronary artery stenosis (diameter reduction >50%). Forty-seven patients were identified as having significant coronary stenoses on invasive angiography with 18% (176/1005) affected segments. None of the coronary segments needed to be excluded from analysis. CT correctly identified all 20 patients having no significant stenosis on invasive angiography. Overall sensitivity for classifying stenoses was 94%, specificity was 97%, positive predictive value was 87%, and negative predictive value was 99%.
Conclusion Sixty-four-slice CT provides a high diagnostic accuracy in assessing coronary artery stenoses.

Figure 3.9 Reproduced from *European Heart Journal.* 2005; **26**:1482–7. Leschka, *et al.* Accuracy of MSCT coronary angiography with 64-slice technology: first experience. Reproduced by permission of the European Society of Cardiology.

In the methods section of the abstract, there were only 67 patients in the entire study. This limits its usefulness, so we keep it in mind and continue foraging. What we will be looking for is consistency of the results across multiple small studies like this.

Then, we looked at the second article's abstract, which follows.

Usefulness of Multislice Computed Tomography for Detecting Obstructive Coronary Artery Disease

Koen Nieman, MD, Benno J. Rensing, MD, PhD, Robert-Jan M. van Geuns, MD, PhD, Arie Munne, RT, Jurgen M.R. Ligthart, RT, Peter M.T. Pattynama, MD, PhD, Gabriel P. Krestin, MD, PhD, Patrick W. Serruys, MD, PhD, and Pim J. de Feyter, MD, PhD

The latest generation of multislice spiral computed tomography (MSCT) scanners is capable of noninvasive coronary angiography. We evaluated its diagnostic accuracy to detect stenotic coronary artery disease (CAD). In 53 patients with suspected CAD, contrast-enhanced MSCT and conventional angiography were performed. The CT data were acquired within a single breathhold, and isocardiophasic slices were reconstructed by means of retrospective electrocardiographic gating. Coronary segments of ≥2 mm in diameter, measured by quantitative angiography, were evaluated. In 70% of the 358 available segments, image quality was regarded as adequate for assessment. The overall sensitivity, specificity, and positive and negative predictive values to detect ≥50% stenotic lesions in the assessable segments were 82% (42 of 51 lesions), 93% (285 of 307 nonstenotic segments), and 66% and 97%, respectively, regarding conventional quantitative angiography as the gold standard. Proximal segments were assessable in 92%, and distal segments and side branches in 71% and 50%, respectively. Including the undetected lesions in nonassessable segments, overall sensitivity decreased to 61% but remained 82% for lesions in proximal coronary segments. MSCT correctly predicted absent, single, or multiple lesions in 55% of patients. Thus, despite potentially high image quality, current MSCT protocols offer only reasonable diagnostic accuracy in an unselected patient group with a high prevalence of CAD. ©2002 by Excerpta Medica, Inc.
(Am J Cardiol 2002;89:913–918)

Figure 3.10 Reproduced from *The American Journal of Cardiology*. **89**/8: 6. Nieman K, *et al*, Usefulness of multi-slice computed tomography for detecting obstructive coronary artery disease. Copyright (2002), with permission from Elsevier.

This study only has 53 patients in the entire study. Again, this limits its usefulness and we are building a sense for what type of information is available. In this situation, we generally make scratch notes about the sensitivity and specificity to compare amongst these small studies to get a sense of the range, a proxy for dispersion of more accurate data.

Next, we looked at the fourth article's abstract. Remember, this is the most recently published to date and we are looking for a study that has a larger number of cases (N). Unfortunately, this image was not available for reproduction, but in the methods section of the abstract it states, 'Methods and Results Using 64-slice MSCT coronary angiography (CTA), 69 consecutive patients, 39 (57%) of whom had previously undergone stent implantation, were evaluated'[11] This article shows again a very small number of patients (69) and also many of the patients had previous coronary angioplasty. Putting these two pieces of information together we get a sense that there are multiple small published studies. This is important information as we continue to explore the domain of available literature. Thus, the study is not only small, but the study population does not match our patient.

9. Using Google Scholar Filters, Search 'All Related and Date Ranges of Articles'

The next phase of foraging is to continue to refine the search protocol, attempting to get the next layer of relevant clinical trials. This is when we use the 'Related articles' hyperlink (located at the bottom of the Google summary). We want to use the most relevant article for this function. Of the three abstracts that we evaluated, the first article is the most relevant. This function selected 101 articles out of the previous 1260 articles that matched our keywords.

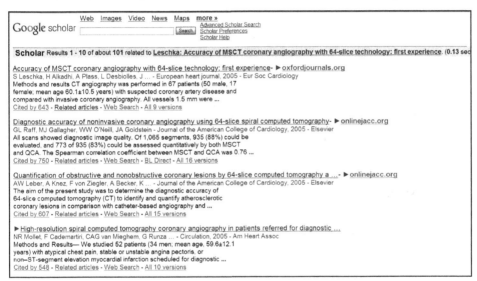

Figure 3.11

This is an iterative process, so we need to review the titles and short Google Scholar summaries for relevance. This time, we will add scanning of the publication dates as an additional screen. Notice, the first article is the same as the article we selected for 'Related article.' This is always the case.

The second article states, 'Of 1,065 segments, 935 (88%) could be evaluated and ...' in the portion of the summary seen on the Google Scholar results page. This is obviously a coronary artery segment based study, which is disease orientated evidence and not patient orientated evidence that matters. Thus, this article is not very relevant to our patient's concern. In a segment based analysis, the researchers count the number of segments evaluated by the CT. Hence, they count multiple segments for each patient, which provides a larger number to use in their statistical analysis. A patient with coronary artery disease could have four diseased segments, which would count multiple times in the segment based analysis.

The third article's Google abstract looked relevant, so further evaluation could be helpful in our search. The abstract is as follows:

Journal of the American College of Cardiology
© 2005 by the American College of Cardiology Foundation
Published by Elsevier Inc.

Vol. 46, No. 1, 2005
ISSN 0735-1097/05/$30.00
doi:10.1016/j.jacc.2005.03.071

EXPEDITED REVIEWS

Quantification of Obstructive and Nonobstructive Coronary Lesions by 64-Slice Computed Tomography

A Comparative Study With Quantitative Coronary Angiography and Intravascular Ultrasound

Alexander W. Leber, MD,* Andreas Knez, MD,* Franz von Ziegler, MD,* Alexander Becker, MD,* Konstantin Nikolaou, MD,† Stephan Paul, MD,* Bernd Wintersperger, MD,† Maximilian Reiser, MD,† Christoph R. Becker, MD,† Gerhard Steinbeck, MD,* Peter Boekstegers, MD*

Munich, Germany

OBJECTIVES	The aim of the present study was to determine the diagnostic accuracy of 64-slice computed tomography (CT) to identify and quantify atherosclerotic coronary lesions in comparison with catheter-based angiography and intravascular ultrasound (IVUS).
BACKGROUND	Currently, the ability of multislice CT to quantify the degree of coronary artery stenosis and dimensions of coronary plaques has not been evaluated.
METHODS	We included 59 patients scheduled for coronary angiography due to stable angina pectoris. A contrast-enhanced 64-slice CT (Senation 64, Siemens Medical Solutions, Forchheim, Germany) was performed before the invasive angiogram. In a subset of 18 patients, IVUS of 32 vessels was part of the catheterization procedure.
RESULTS	In 55 of 59 patients, 64-slice CT enabled the visualization of the entire coronary tree with diagnostic image quality (American Heart Association 15-segment model). The overall correlation between the degree of stenosis detected by quantitative coronary angiography compared with 64-slice CT was r = 0.54. Sensitivity for the detection of stenosis <50%, stenosis >50%, and stenosis >75% was 79%, 73%, and 80%, respectively, and specificity was 97%. In comparison with IVUS, 46 of 55 (84%) lesions were identified correctly. The mean plaque areas and the percentage of vessel obstruction measured by IVUS and 64-slice CT were 8.1 mm² versus 7.3 mm² (p < 0.03, r = 0.73) and 50.4% versus 41.1% (p < 0.001, r = 0.61), respectively.
CONCLUSIONS	Contrast-enhanced 64-slice CT is a clinically robust modality that allows the identification of proximal coronary lesions with excellent accuracy. Measurements of plaque and lumen areas derived by CT correlated well with IVUS. A major limitation is the insufficient ability of CT to exactly quantify the degree of stenosis. (J Am Coll Cardiol 2005;46:147–54) © 2005 by the American College of Cardiology Foundation

Figure 3.12 Reproduced from *Journal of the American College of Cardiology*. **46**/5 155. Leber A, *et al*, Quantification of obstructive and non-obstructive coronary lesions by 64-slice computed tomography: a comparative study with quantitative coronary angiography and intravascular ultrasound. Copyright (2005), with permission from the American College of Cardiology Foundation.

This study is very small, only 59 patients. We are looking for a larger study. At that point, we hit the 'back' button and continue to evaluate the original search. We continued to evaluate the articles and they were all consistently small. Google uses an algorithmic prioritization that heavily weighs the number of times an article has been cited. The result of this method is that more recent articles, which have not had a chance to accumulate citations, will have a lower priority. Thus, not easily found.

At this point, we are not confident that we have found the most relevant information (at the time we did this search). There seems to be two barriers. First, CT coronary angiography is a new technology. Thus, the most relevant study could have been published so recently that it has not been cited enough to make the top of the Google Scholar search. Therefore, it would be helpful to search only the recently published articles. This can be accomplished by going to 'Advanced Scholar Search' found at the top of the Google results page and typing in a more recent date range. In our case, we used 2008–2009. Even if the search seems adequate, we actually recommend searching for more recent publications if all of the major references are more than two years old. We have spent nearly 20 minutes searching for our article. This is a difficult search. Most searches does not require this much time and effort.

The second barrier to our first several Google searches seems to be many small studies. We did not come across a meta-analysis, but we have to convince ourselves that a larger randomized controlled trial is not available before we proceed. Therefore, the next search strategy will be focused on locating more recent, larger prospective trials. Keywords associated with larger trials include 'prospective, multi-centered, Meta-Analysis.' Lets try the following keywords: MSCT, coronary, angiography, sensitivity, specificity, CAD, multicenter prospective meta analysis, and also include a more recent time frame. We are going set the search dates, located in the advanced scholar search tab to 2008–2009.

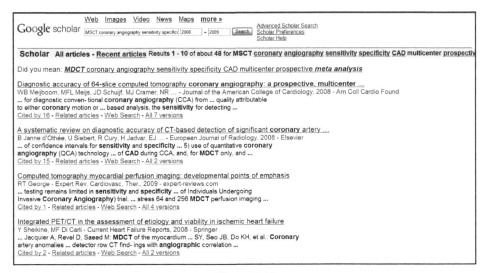

Figure 3.13

The first article looks very promising. It uses the gold standard, coronary angiography, as the comparison in addition to being recent and using a 64-slice computed tomography coronary angiography. The abstract is as follows:

Diagnostic Accuracy of 64-Slice Computed Tomography Coronary Angiography

A Prospective, Multicenter, Multivendor Study

W. Bob Meijboom, MD,*† Matthijs F. L. Meijs, MD,§‖ Joanne D. Schuijf, MD, PhD,¶#
Maarten J. Cramer, MD, PhD,§ Nico R. Mollet, MD, PhD,*† Carlos A. G. van Mieghem, MD,*†
Koen Nieman, MD, PhD,*† Jacob M. van Werkhoven, MD,‖# Gabija Pundziute, MD,‖#
Annick C. Weustink, MD,*† Alexander M. de Vos, MD,§‖ Francesca Pugliese, MD,*†
Benno Rensing, MD, PhD,** J. Wouter Jukema, MD, PhD,¶ Jeroen J. Bax, MD, PhD,¶
Mathias Prokop, MD, PhD,‖ Pieter A. Doevendans, MD, PhD,§ Myriam G. M. Hunink, MD, PhD,†‡
Gabriel P. Krestin, MD, PhD,† Pim J. de Feyter, MD, PhD*†

Rotterdam, Utrecht, Leiden, and Nieuwegein, the Netherlands

Objectives	This study sought to determine the diagnostic accuracy of 64-slice computed tomographic coronary angiography (CTCA) to detect or rule out significant coronary artery disease (CAD).
Background	CTCA is emerging as a noninvasive technique to detect coronary atherosclerosis.
Methods	We conducted a prospective, multicenter, multivendor study involving 360 symptomatic patients with acute and stable anginal syndromes who were between 50 and 70 years of age and were referred for diagnostic conventional coronary angiography (CCA) from September 2004 through June 2006. All patients underwent a nonenhanced calcium scan and a CTCA, which was compared with CCA. No patients or segments were excluded because of impaired image quality attributable to either coronary motion or calcifications. Patient-, vessel-, and segment-based sensitivities and specificities were calculated to detect or rule out significant CAD, defined as ≥50% lumen diameter reduction.
Results	The prevalence among patients of having at least 1 significant stenosis was 68%. In a patient-based analysis, the sensitivity for detecting patients with significant CAD was 99% (95% confidence interval [CI]: 98% to 100%), specificity was 64% (95% CI: 55% to 73%), positive predictive value was 86% (95% CI: 82% to 90%), and negative predictive value was 97% (95% CI: 94% to 100%). In a segment-based analysis, the sensitivity was 88% (95% CI: 85% to 91%), specificity was 90% (95% CI: 89% to 92%), positive predictive value was 47% (95% CI: 44% to 51%), and negative predictive value was 99% (95% CI: 98% to 99%).
Conclusions	Among patients in whom a decision had already been made to obtain CCA, 64-slice CTCA was reliable for ruling out significant CAD in patients with stable and unstable anginal syndromes. A positive 64-slice CTCA scan often overestimates the severity of atherosclerotic obstructions and requires further testing to guide patient management. (J Am Coll Cardiol 2008;52:2135–44) © 2008 by the American College of Cardiology Foundation

Figure 3.14 Reproduced from *Journal of the American College of Cardiology.* **52**/25: 2135–44. Meijboom W, *et al.* Diagnostic accuracy of 64-slice computed tomography coronary angiography: a prospective, multi-center, multi-vendor study. Copyright (2008), with permission from the American College of Cardiology Foundation.

This abstract highlights many good points. First, it has 360 patients in the study. This is a lot larger than the other studies that we found. Second, the article does a 'patient-based analysis.' The other abstracts reviewed were 'segment based analysis.' Remember, in a segment based analysis, the researchers count the number of segments evaluated by the CT. Hence, they count multiple segments for each patient, which provides a larger number to use in their statistical analysis. This puts the emphasis on the Disease Oriented Evidence compared to the Patient Oriented Evidence.

10. Get a .PDF Image of the Most Promising Article and Review the Methodology

11. Scan the References of that Article Looking for Related Articles

12. Pick the Best Summary of the Literature, Usually From One to Five Articles for Complete Evaluation

These last three steps are included for completeness. We only use them if we are unsatisfied with the information we found up until this point. Remember, saturation is the criteria for determining whether to keep foraging or deciding with a reasonable probability that you have a sense of what the research literature can tell us.

Another vitally important guide to making this decision is to make an assessment of whether the information we found while foraging can answer the clinical question and whether it is relevant to the narrative dilemma. In this case, we passed through both those thresholds and decision points and concluded our search. (Remember, if you were to repeat the same process today the information available will have changed.)

Our patient wants to know if she has any disease, not the number of segments that could be diseased. In the 'patient-based analysis,' the test is either positive, if there is any coronary artery disease, or negative if there is not any disease. This is what our patient wants to know about herself and therefore directly answers the patient's narrative dilemma. This was the only article we looked at that had this type of analysis. The researchers were able to do this type of analysis because there were enough patients in the study to make this analysis statistically significant. At this point, we are confident that this is the best evidence available to help our patient make her decision. Thus, we will use this article for further assessment.

USING PUBMED TO CONFIRM THE COMPREHENSIVENESS OF THE SEARCH

As mentioned earlier, once we have found the most relevant article in Google Scholar, re-locate that same article in PubMed and use the 'related citations' option.

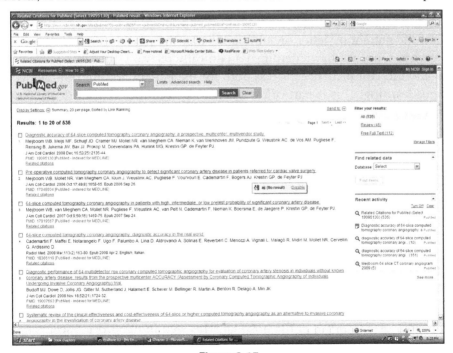

Figure 3.15

Reviewing the first three pages of PubMed results, we found eight other research studies comparable to the one we found in Google Scholar.[11-18] All used coronary angiography as the gold standard and performed a per-patient analysis. One was a systematic review from 2002–2006, pre-dating our study and confirmed the sensitivity and specificity of the article we selected. Four studies had smaller patient populations and also confirmed the sensitivity and specificity of the article we selected. One smaller study had questionable methods and results differed slightly, but wouldn't have changed the answer to the patient's narrative dilemma. There was one report of a 320-row CT coronary angiogram that also confirmed the sensitivity and improved the specificity; this test was not available to us at the time, demonstrating how rapidly technology changes. One study used a study population that did not match our patient population. In summary, we have compelling evidence that we have conducted a thorough literature review and have the best quality information available at the time. We are going to proceed on that basis.

A NOTE ABOUT TIME MANAGEMENT

We have emphasized repeatedly the efficiency of this process. We also said that it takes practice to achieve that efficiency. We use the process routinely on teaching rounds in an inpatient setting. We use it often in the outpatient clinic. We can almost always 'guestimate' the quality of the evidence enough to make a clinical decision during the process of care. Sometimes, we tell the patient that we will do a more thorough search later and get back to them. After patient care is completed, we spend the few extra minutes to complete the search and either inform the patient by letter or summarize it at the next routine or scheduled office visit. Once we have identified a clinically relevant question, we feel an obligation to complete the process both for the patient and for our own continuous learning. This is part of the process of becoming and evidence based practitioner. Often when dictating the progress note, we identify the specific research article and state how it affected decision making for that patient visit. Helping state clearly the basis for decision making enhances the collaborative interaction with our consultant network.

Others have pointed out the difficulties of practicing narrative medicine;[12] we find that the initial investment in time usually pays off with greater efficiency in future appointments with that patient.

A CONTINGENT, EMERGENT, SITUATED, AND CONTEXTUAL MEDICAL KNOWLEDGE

We have been describing a process of care that occurs with the patient in the exam room or on rounds at the hospital. This step in the process seems more 'scientific' because we are searching for research articles. Despite the aura of 'science' we include in this section of each chapter a new perspective of what medical knowledge is – not something that exists as truth, but something that is used together with the patient 'in the moment.'

Accessing for information is *contingent* because we are comparing multiple different sources of information and sorting them mentally. Our judgments, guided by our patient's narrative dilemma are just that – judgments. After choosing which article to investigate further, the potential journal articles lose their *contingency* as 'possibly related' and are put into the category of 'not related.' It is the ability to hold three or four choices in mind simultaneously (such as when we were evaluating Google Scholar summaries) that creates the *contingent* nature of the medical knowledge.

Foraging (accessing information) is *emergent* because of the processual nature of the activity. You go forward in time, making choices, evaluating choices, and winding up with information that up until this point we did not know existed – it *emerged* in the process of foraging. The relevant medical knowledge emerges in this process of care and is separated from the irrelevant medical knowledge by its relationship to the narrative dilemma and clinical question. This is different than starting with all there is to know about measuring coronary heart disease and working backwards to apply it to patient care. That would be the older version of practice when specialists were capable of knowing all the information. Of course, we are describing a different epistemology where 'facts' are only facts if they *emerge* as relevant to the patient care described here.

Accessing information is *situated in time*. The scientific literature is unstable as more is created continuously. We very rarely use textbooks anymore – they are outdated. Most important, accessing information is also *situated within the patient's narrative dilemma* and the clinical question. That type of situated knowledge shifts with each new patient or for that matter, each new concern of the same patient. Although we have emphasized the patient's perspective, remember this is a co-constructed narrative, so the doctor's concerns and worries also create the locus in which this medical knowledge is *situated*.

We have often told our medical students that all health care is delivered within the *context of a relationship*. This relationship is the context of care. Different doctors with differing approaches and beliefs change the *context* of care. Again, we struggle to understand who this patient is, what is it like to be the doctor for this patient, and what type of doctor does this patient need. We describe a cognitive process. Some patients are not at all interested in numbers and research, assuming the doctor is responsible for all of that. We still believe the process is valid, but the format and delivery needs to change. The context of the medical knowledge, however, is still defined by the greater *social context* and the doctor–patient relationship.

REFERENCES

1 http://scholar.google.com/intl/en/scholar/about.html (accessed December 10, 2010).
2 Vine R. Google Scholar. *J Med Libr Assoc.* 2006; **94**(1): 97–9.
3 Ebell M. Information mastery. *FP Essentials, AAFP Home Study Edition No 318.* Leawood, KS: American Academy of Family Physicians; 2005.
4 Brownlee S. *Overtreated: why too much medicine is making us sicker and poorer.* New York, NY: Bloomsbury; 2007.
5 Ebell M. How to find answers to clinical questions. *American Family Physician.* 2009; **79**(4): 293–6.
6 Tang H, Ng JHK. Googling for a diagnosis – use of Google as a diagnostic aid: internet based study. *BMJ.* 2006; **333**: 1143–5.
7 Prendiville TW, Saunders J, Fitzsimons J. The information-seeking behaviour of paediatricians accessing web-based resources. *Archives of Disease in Childhood.* 2009; **94**: 633–5.
8 Steinbrook R. Searching for the right search – reaching the medical literature. *New England Journal of Medicine.* J2006; **354**(1): 4–7.
9 Schwartz K, Roe T, Northrup J, *et al.* Family medicine patients' use of the internet for health information: A MetroNet study. *Journal of American Board of Family Medicine.* 2006; **19**(1) 39–45.
10 Dolan PL. 86% of physicians use Internet to access health information. *American Medical News.* January 11, 2010.
11 Ehara M, Surmely J-F, Kawai M, *et al.* Diagnostic accuracy of 64-slice computed tomography for detecting angiographically significant coronary artery stenosis in an unselected consecutive patient population comparison with invasive angiography. *Circ J.* 2006; **70**: 564–71.
12 Kalitzkus V, Matthiessen PF. Narrative based medicine: potential, pitfalls, and practice. *IJNP.* 2009; **1**(1): 56–64.

CHAPTER 4

Assess the Quality of the Information

KEY CONCEPTS TO REMEMBER

➤ After acquiring a basic knowledge of research study design, continuous learning and practice is required to sharpen these skills.

➤ Different types of research designs are susceptible to different types of bias and varying ability to determine cause and effect relationships.

➤ There are standardized questions to evaluate the quality of research articles about diagnostic tests.

➤ We use the SORT criteria, which is a grading system for the quality of research.

➤ Being able to assess the quality of the medical literature helps the co-constructed narrative because you can avoid creating a story that is simply not believable, for the patient or the doctor.

LEARNING ABOUT ASSESSING THE QUALITY OF RESEARCH

Introduction

At its core, the medical literature is similar to other types of literature; there is a 'narrator' (the authors), a target audience, and the story of how the research was conducted. That story is either believable or not. That's what this chapter is about. Although we mention the standardized ways that 'evidence' is graded, it is equally reasonable to view a research study as a story. One of the problems with the medical literature is the 'narrator' is often a pharmaceutical company with a profit motive, which changes the way the story is told. This is often called 'spin.' The story is often simply, but subtly made up by changing the initial primary outcome measure to other outcome measures[1] – storytelling with a social purpose, just like we mentioned in chapter one on 'narrative.' By understanding medical literature from this perspective, it levels the playing field and facilitates the task of integrating narrative medicine and evidence based medicine – the two stories have to be understood within their respective frameworks and then a larger story created by including the two perspectives. That is what we mean by 'integrating.' Keep this concept in mind as you read this chapter, but for learning purposes, we will present the 'standard EBM concepts' before tackling the more difficult task of creating a co-constructed narrative.

Narrative in Science

In order to interpret clinical literature, the reader needs some basic understanding of classic research designs: epidemiologic exploration, retrospective cross sectional study, cohort design, natural experiments, non-randomized controlled trials or open label trials, case controlled studies, randomized controlled trials, and ultimately meta-analysis of randomized controlled trials. (Notice the linguistic use of the word 'interpret' which takes us right back to Chapter 1, when we discussed multiple possible 'interpretations.' The same is true of the medical literature.) This explains how different doctors can come to vastly different conclusions from the same research article. The classic case for this is the NINDS trial.[2] During Journal Club, we examined one of the outcome variables, the NIH Stroke Symptom Scale and found its variability/reproducibility was as large as the definition of 'improvement,' leading to the conclusion that the study results could have been explained by chance alone. We further looked at the scale itself for 'face validity' and most of the residents recognized that the range of inter-rater reliability in an Emergency Department was high enough to determine that 'statistically significant' would not translate to 'clinically significant,' based on their own experience. It was also concerning that in Table 1, the placebo group received far less aspirin, making the study group not comparable to the placebo group. Yet, the study is widely accepted as 'positive' or 'evidence of benefit.' We even have billboards advertising that our Emergency Room has STROKE accreditation. Our colleagues staunchly defend the conclusions of this study in which the authors support the use of thrombolytic therapy in the setting of early non-hemorrhagic stroke. The point is we are each allowed to form our own opinions of the relative strength of the benefit versus the harm based on the actual methods and results of the clinical trial.

The Research Endeavor

This step in the process requires practice and continuous learning. Our goal in this book is to outline the basics as described by the standard texts of evidence based medicine.[3-9] It is very easy to critique or find fault with any individual research article. The reason for that is that researchers work with limited resources and must make real life choices, often between two suboptimal practical methods. There are many different research methods to answer any particular question, so the actual research article is more a reflection of what resources the authors had available and the choices they made about measurement and variables which results in the particular study design eventually chosen. Our experiences have been that we often find partial evidence or information that is suggestive but not definitive. These are the realities of clinical decision making. The purpose of this chapter is to demonstrate how to make a decision about the quality, validity, or 'truth value' of a research article.

Primary Care Medical Abstracts

After learning basic 'book knowledge' about assessing the quality of research studies our continuous learning and practice came in the format of a medical reading service called 'Primary Care Medical Abstracts,' featuring Jerome Hoffman, MD and Richard Bukata, MD. This subscription reviews 40 articles a month. The articles are selected from all the major high impact journals, but also from hundreds of journals published world-wide. They are chosen based on the utility to primary care doctors in practice. They also include topics that we should be knowledgeable about from various specialties so that we can explain them to our patients. Not only do they go over the content of current controversies in medicine, their special emphasis is on critiquing the research methodology and identifying the biases of the study. After years of listening, we have a good sense of what is in the literature, which helps in foraging, but most importantly for this topic – how to assess the validity of the literature. Again, we'd like to point out that we have fore-grounded research articles on diagnosis and therapy, but there are many other types of research published. These other studies provide good background information, but we have embarked on a very specific purpose in this book.

The alternative standard format for most physicians has been 'Journal Club.' This is also a good way to continually practice 'assessing the literature'; we just want to emphasize that it takes continual practice.

Reasonable Physicians Disagree

For this reason, reasonable clinicians can arrive at different recommendations or beliefs. The utility of this skill set, however, is that it facilitates conversations between physicians about how and why they recommend a specific course of action. The ability to have this discussion at the level of an evidence based format enhances clinician to clinician communication. As primary care physicians, we are often faced with patients who have conflicting recommendations from two separate specialists. This system flaw is disconcerting for patients and part of primary care is to assist the patient in integrating their illness experience, recommendations from specialists, and help them progress through the process of care. The ability to understand the basis of the specialist recommendations is a tremendous help in the co-creation of the narrative illness experience.

Research Design

We will try to describe the distinguishing features of each of the following study designs. The reader will ultimately understand that the inferential strength or validity of the findings of the study results in a grading system that reflects how close we believe the research reflects 'reality.' Each of these study designs is more or less susceptible to bias or confounding which detracts from 'truth value' of the study. In the description of the different types of the methodology, we can highlight strengths and weaknesses that will show the reader the utility of each of these study types.

Also in this chapter, we list a series of specific questions that can be applied to individual research articles. These will identify the strength and/or weaknesses of the study. After reviewing the literature available, the clinician must generate some sense of what we know and what we do not know. This assessment is what we need to bring back to the patient to continue the co-constructed narrative. The critical point is that some clinical decision has to be made regardless of our knowledge or ignorance. We still have a patient in front us requiring a decision about what to do next.

If you are already an evidence based medicine guru, you can probably just skim the following two sections. We include them here for the beginner who needs a basic grounding in research study methodology. Remember, this basic knowledge is required, since every sequential step builds on the previous one and affects the ones to follow.

If you are a novice and this material seems 'too much like research' to be relevant, do not give up. You wouldn't be reading this book and have gotten this far if you were not interested. For you, we suggest picking only one topic and practicing that same topic repeatedly until you feel confident that you can incorporate it into an office visit. Pick a topic most of your patients are interested in. Go to Journal Club. Find a buddy; find a mentor; practice and explore. It is fun, really. Residents finally realize that it is fun *after* they have done it. Besides, we believe strongly that the doctors of the future MUST have these skills, so it becomes a sooner or later decision. Do not procrastinate.

Study Design

There is a typical sequence in which new knowledge is created. The exploratory and least expensive designs are usually done first as they provide preliminary data that justifies the cost of more expensive randomized controlled trials with greater degree of ability to infer cause and effect. Let us go through the different common study designs in the medical literature.

Case Reports

When rare conditions occur, it is helpful for other physicians to know about them. This type of publication is to alert the medical community to a particular condition and to have other clinicians increase their awareness of possible new or rare conditions. The body of literature related to HIV disease originally started as a case report. Case reports can be considered 'letters' to your colleagues, trying to inform them about something potentially important. This works well with identifying rare complications of treatments that do not surface during randomized controlled trials (RCTs) of therapy. By design, RCTs are not powered (do not have enough participants) to find rare complications. An example of this is case reports of mandibular joint necrosis with bisphosphonates. When we first had to deal with this clinical question, there were only scattered case reports. Case reports serve to heighten awareness and encourage other practitioners to also report similar experiences. Eventually one of the other study designs may augment this knowledge, but the question has to originate somewhere, such as a case report.

Epidemiologic Exploration

Epidemiologic exploration studies look for associations between factors that affect the outcomes. In this type of study the data collection plan specifying variables is determined earlier in the study planning. Types of data collection can vary. A good example is when AIDS first became recognized but public health officials had no idea the cause of the illness. They hypothesized multiple associations, going through multiple iterations before correctly identifying the etiologic agent. These types of studies are most appropriate when there is no clear understanding about what the important clinical variables might be. They are exploratory studies. Typically, many different variables are measured and the resulting data are reviewed for statistically significant associations. These associations guide hypothesis development for subsequent studies with other types of research designs. The ability to infer cause and effect is probably the least for epidemiologic explorations of the study designs mentioned. These types of studies serve as a springboard for further research.

With the advent of large databases, there are many published reports of associations of variables that were measured for some reason other than the research being reported. This is a variation on a classical epidemiologic study because the range of measured variables is constrained by the structure of the database. These studies are sometimes derogatorily referred to as data dredging or data snooping. They have a purpose; assigning their relative value is what this chapter is about.

Retrospective Cross Sectional Study

A retrospective cross sectional study is a study in which the preexisting data are reviewed looking for associations. The advantages of this type of study are that they are very inexpensive and methodologically relatively easy to perform. Typically there is only one group and the researcher chooses multiple variables with hypothesized associations. They then look for associations between the variables (outcomes). For example, in a group of male obese patients, some take aspirin daily while others do not and a researcher will look to see if the mortality rate is associated with aspirin. The fact that the variables are limited to what has already been collected decreases the flexibility of the types of questions that can be asked. Similar to epidemiologic studies this only demonstrates an association between variables and cannot infer cause and effect, so these studies are used for hypothesis generation to guide further research.

Often, these types of studies are done by chart review. Chart review is highly susceptible to bias and the results are almost meaningless unless proper methods are used. The proper way to conduct a chart review is described by Gilbert, et al.[10]

Cohort Design

A cohort is a group of individuals (cases) measured across an interval of time (as opposed to a single slice of time in a cross sectional study). This type of study is done prospectively. With the advent of large databases, sometimes data from the past is examined, but the concept that the exposure precedes the outcome of interest is preserved. The study identifies two groups (or cohorts), one with a predisposing factor and the other without that factor within the larger population. After a certain interval of time, the outcome is measured for both groups searching for a difference between the groups. The underlying logic is to relate the exposure to the outcome. The weakness of this study design is the large potential for biases. Specifically, what other factors are associated with the predisposing factor (exposure), but not accounted for in the control group? This bias limits the ability to infer cause and effect.

Non-randomized Controlled Trials

These are typically pharmaceutical industry sponsored studies. Many times they are exploring the use of 'off-label' indications. These are often post marketing explorations of expanded uses of different pharmaceuticals. In general, the design itself results in poor quality evidence with limited clinical usefulness.

Case Controlled Studies

These studies are used for extremely rare conditions where it would otherwise be impossible to enroll a sufficient number of cases into another type of study design. A collection a cases with the target disorder are collected first and a matched group without the disorder is designed around them which controls for age, gender, co-morbidities, etc. The problem is that controlling for bias is extremely difficult. The utility of these studies is that they allow us to explore rare diseases or side effects. If questionnaires are used to collect data, expect 'recall bias' which means that people with vastly different experiences remember those experiences differently, confounding the 'data.'

Randomized Controlled Trials

These are typically more expensive, often requiring major funding sources and multi-center studies. Justification for institutional review board approval requires demonstration of pilot data to balance the risk of benefit versus harm of the clinical trial, which is often in the form of research using the study designs described above. Often safety monitoring committees are part of the study design. The most important feature of these types of studies is the randomization, which is a process to distribute the confounding variables equally between the two (or more) groups. This feature is the most important component of maximizing the ability to infer cause and effect.

Meta-analysis of Randomized Controlled Trials

A meta-analysis begins by doing a literature search in the topic area. It then specifies strict criteria for sorting which studies will be included and excluded. It is important to realize that the meta-analysis is only as good as the studies included in the analysis. When multiple meta-analyses on the same topic are compared, it is easy to see how the investigators themselves can influence the conclusion. This is especially true for pharmaceutical industry sponsored studies. If you are combining data from poor quality studies, then there is no added benefit. Selecting only the best quality studies, the meta-analysis combines the data and repeats the analysis on the combined data set. This is a methodology to greatly enhance the power of the study (because it results in a large number of cases in the trial.) A well done meta-analysis of high quality randomized controlled trials is considered some of the best evidence available. The constituent studies are represented in graphical form with mean, number of cases and a measure of variability such as the 95% confidence interval all displayed against a line that defines benefit verses harm for the outcome variable. We should caution the reader that many publications describe the studies included as 'poor quality' and then proceed to analyze the combined data set anyway. This type of information is of limited value. Other problems arise when large studies are combined with smaller trials; the larger trial has undue influence on the conclusion.

An editor for an evidence based medicine publication once took us to task for making the comment that a large well done RCT was sometimes better than a meta-analysis believing that a meta-analysis is always better. In addition to the problems listed in the above paragraph, there is another critical flaw in the medical literature that is amplified by doing meta analysis: publication bias. Ramsey, *et al* demonstrated that on average, only 17.6% of trials registered in the ClinicalTrials.gov database were eventually published.[11] There was a very high bias for 'positive' trials (65%). One can imagine that most of the negative trials were in the 83% of trials that were unpublished. Others have commented on the limitations of meta-analyses.[12]

Systematic Review

In many ways this is similar to a meta-analysis. However, the conclusion comes not from combining the data sets but by evaluating the relative contribution from each data set to the composite answer to the research question. This must be done by someone that is very knowledgeable in research methodology. A gold standard would be the Cochrane Review Group.

Being familiar with these different types of study designs is important for efficient information foraging. Often, multiple small cross sectional studies will be found and subsequently a larger randomized controlled trial or meta-analysis will be available. At that point, the clinician can focus simply on the latter types of studies and safely ignore the smaller exploratory studies.

Others

Our readers should know that there are other research study designs that get more complex, but are not covered here. Again, our goal is simply to get started with a working knowledge to start using the process of care we describe.

Clinical Example Illustrating Study Designs

We recently had a patient come into the office who said that she discontinued her alendronate because of she heard on the television that long term use caused stress fractures of the femoral shaft. We had heard about the same topic, but were not really familiar with the evidence. The medical student working with us said that the professor who gave the lecture on that topic presented an elegant pathophysiologic explanation based on over suppression of bone turnover from prolonged bisphosphonate therapy and concluded with the statement, 'I tell my patients to stop taking the medicine after five years.' That same afternoon in clinic, we had another patient that stopped her alendronate 'because my previous doctor told me not to take it after five years.' Using the information scavenging methods described in Chapter 3, we quickly found many case reports or case series describing the problem.[13] We found two case controlled trials[14, 15] which referenced a randomized controlled trial with 2027 participants.[16] The fascinating part was that there was a clear distinction between 'morphometric' (radiographically identified fractures) and 'clinically apparent fractures.' This is an example of DOE and POEMs. The fractures the patient was concerned about seemed to be described as DOE case reports. Part of the purpose of knowing about different types of study designs is to evaluate the strength and weakness of the evidence. The authors of one of the case controlled trials concluded, 'Still, a treatment-associated incidence density of 1/1000 is acceptable, considering that bisphosphonate treatment is likely to reduce the incidence density of any fracture by 15/1000 according to a large randomized trial.' Although we believe these authors are correct, they compare apples and oranges and the real incidence of sub-trochanteric fractures (a rare condition) could be better estimated using a cohort design. At our institution, there are corporate databases that can identify patients who have consistently filled a bisphosphonate prescription for more than five years and generate a comparator group naive to bisphosphonates. All relevant fractures could then be identified in the electronic medical record and a more accurate assessment of risk of harm versus risk of benefit could be generated. Thus, a cohort trial is higher quality evidence than a case series or a case controlled trial and able to generate relevant information that is impossible to obtain using a randomized controlled trial because the N (number of cases) required to identify this rare complication is impractical using a RCT. This type of information is vital to correctly writing the co-constructed narrative as our process continues. This is an example where we made the best decision at the time, but fully expect the medical literature to continue to evolve, highlighting the need to remain curious and attentive. The question was important and we will be on the look-out for further information as it becomes available.

Questions for Evaluating a Research Study

In the next section, we will review relatively standard, well acknowledged questions that assist the clinician in determining the quality of the research articles generated by the search. The familiarity with these questions is an essential part of Journal Club and finding the answers in the text of the article requires practice. Our experience shows that beginners often get bogged down in details and extraneous material giving the impression that the medical literature is difficult to read. In actuality, in a well written, well structured article the answers should be easy to locate. The most important overview is an explicit statement regarding the purpose or research question that was studied. By identifying this first, it helps eliminate extraneous information and makes extracting the answers to the following questions much easier. The following questions should be asked directly of the research question. Sometimes publications are 'bulked up' with sub group analysis or secondary outcomes, all of which should be ignored. This type of text and scientific writing can be referred to as 'data dredging.' The research question should be found in the abstract. If it is not explicitly stated, then perhaps you should not read the article.

Diagnostic Article Research Questions

1. Was There an Independent 'Blind Comparison' with a 'Gold Standard'?

There are really two questions embedded in this question. The first question refers to the 'gold standard.' Every diagnostic test has to be compared to 'truth.' How truth is determined in these types of articles is based on what is called the 'gold standard,' which is a different diagnostic test that is generally considered the most accurate available. In clinical practice, the gold standard cannot always be used as it is usually expensive, difficult to perform, or dangerous. For example, a heart catheterization is the typical gold standard for the diagnosis of coronary artery disease. It carries a risk of arterial perforation, arrhythmiagenesis, infection, and death. In studies that determine how accurate the stress test is, they compare the stress test results to the results of a cardiac catheterization. By definition in a study, the gold standard is always correct. There are not any false positives or false negatives in the gold standard. The astute reader will recognize that this assumption is not always true, but it is a compromise we make so that we can evaluate these alternative tests.

Unfortunately, using a high quality gold standard is not only expensive, but also must be justified ethically. As a result, sometimes you will see combination endpoints used instead of the gold standard. For example, in PIOPED II,[17] which studied the accuracy of spiral CT scan for the diagnosis of pulmonary embolism, the researchers used a composite reference which was a series of tests including ventilation-perfusion scan, Doppler ultrasound, and the probability of disease based on clinical presentation. The researchers only used a pulmonary angiogram, which is the gold standard in the diagnosis of pulmonary embolism (PE), when the other tests could not sufficiently diagnose the disease. Upon evaluating the quality of the PIOPED II study, we would have to evaluate the quality of this composite reference standard. Is it good enough to replace the gold standard of pulmonary angiogram? *It is crucial that upon evaluation of the literature the 'truth' value of the gold standard is also assessed.*

The second part of the question refers to blinding. Diagnostic tests being evaluated should be assessed without knowing the results of the gold standard test. This is known as a blind comparison. Obvious bias is introduced if the result of the comparison is known in advance. Specific statements by the authors of the research study should convince you that the interpretation of the diagnostic should be blinded to each other, usually requiring two different people, one to assess each test at the time we need to decide whether to begin therapy.

2.   Was the Setting for the Study as Well as the Filter Through which Study Patients Passed, Adequately Described? (Inclusion/Exclusion Criteria)
The first part of this question refers to the study setting. The description of the setting is important because the research may have taken place in such a highly controlled environment, as such the replication of that ideal environment is not practical. An example of this is the NINDS, in which the effectiveness of thrombolytic agents for acute ischemic strokes were studied.[2] The radiologists (not ER physician) were able to provide a reading of the head CT scan quickly (less than three hours). Similar services might not be available at your hospital.

The second part of this question refers to the inclusion/exclusion criteria. It is usually described in the method section. It is important to make sure that the patients similar to your own are not systematically excluded during this process. One should also identify or consider the specific reasons why study participants were included or excluded. The fairness of these judgments can be questioned. Once again, this is often done for practical purposes, but might limit the research findings. Sometimes, an unfair selection is introduced For example, in *The effect of Carvedilol on morbidity and mortality in patients with chronic heart failure* study,[18] patients were given carvedilol for two weeks prior to the study to see if they could tolerate the medication. The researchers excluded patients who did not follow the medication regimen during this two week period. This methodology selects patients that could tolerate the medication. But what about the patients that could not tolerate it? What if the patient stopped taking the carvedilol because they were experiencing a side effect? Those patients were excluded because they did not complete the run-in period. However, in practice, we do not have a similar advantage of only treating the patients that can tolerate the drug (or test).

3. Did the Patient Sample Include an Appropriate Spectrum of Patients to Whom the Diagnostic Test will be Applied in Clinical Practice?

In other words, has the diagnostic test been evaluated in a patient sample that included an appropriate spectrum of mild and severe, treated and untreated disease, plus individuals with different but commonly confused disorders?

This is often a significant problem in the medical literature since most publications come from large tertiary hospitals. It has been demonstrated multiple times that these patients do not reflect patients seen in general practice. In fact only one in a thousand patients with complaints is evaluated in such an academic setting. This introduces something called 'spectrum bias,' which means the diagnostic test may perform differently in different subgroups of the population. Therefore, readers should carefully assess the description of the study population and determine the similarity of the patients cared for in their own practice. Because of this discrepancy we have selectively chosen how to proceed with analysis (described in the next chapter), using likelihood ratios instead of positive or negative predictive values because likelihood ratios are not dependant on the prevalence of the disease in the population whereas positive and negative predictive values incorporate this bias into the analysis. It is more valid to assign a probability of disease using all the clinical information available at the time than to assume the prevalence of the disease in your patients is the same as where the original study was performed. We will discuss this in more detail later. For now, be aware that the study population is an important part in evaluating medical literature about diagnostic tests.

4. Have the Reproducibility of the Test Result and its Interpretation been Determined?

This question refers to an 'operator dependent bias,' which means that if a radiologist can consistently produce similar readings with similar films. This is often difficult to control and research studies often describe the diagnostic test being interpreted by two independent blinded readers. The degree that these two interpretations of the same test agree over and above random chance (50/50) is called a Kappa statistic. Generally, a Kappa value greater than 0.8 is acceptable. When there is a disagreement, the author should describe a recon-ciliation process to determine if the test was positive or negative. This some-times involves a third reader or conferencing for a consensus reading between the two readers. This seems most obvious in imaging tests, but is also an ele-ment in other types of diagnostic test such as rapid antigen detection, blood values, etc. The amount of routine variability in these routine tests should be described. Additionally, an adequate description of what is considered a posi-tive test should be provided by the authors.

5. Have the Tactics for Carrying out the Test Been Described in Sufficient Detail to Permit their Exact Replication?

The test should be standardized and recognizable, usually described elsewhere in the medical literature. If this is not the case, then closer scrutiny of how the test was performed should be made to determine if the test can be performed at your home institution. This will affect how you describe the evidence to the patient.

SORT Criteria

There are many grading systems to label the quality of the evidence. We pre-fer the SORT (an acronym standing for Strength of Recommendation Tax-onomy) because it includes the concepts of DOEs versus POEMs discussed above.[19] We also like it for its simplicity. *A-level recommendation* is based on consistent and good quality patient-oriented evidence; *B-level recommenda-tion* is based on inconsistent or limited quality patient oriented evidence; and *C-level recommendation* is based on consensus, usual practice, opinion, disease-oriented evidence, or case series. This pretty easily sorts out what we know from what we do not know. It is used consistently in the family medicine literature and quickly summarizes the most relevant parameters of how we judge the literature. When evaluating individual studies, the SORT criteria uses a similar system, but with the numbers 1, 2, 3 to grade the level of evidence presented in the individual paper. Level 1 is good quality patient-oriented evidence, Level 2 is limited-quality patient oriented evidence, and Level 3 is other evidence.

Strength of Recommendation Taxonomy (SORT)

In general, only key recommendations for readers require a grade of the "Strength of Recommendation." Recommendations should be based on the highest quality evidence available. For example, vitamin E was found in some cohort studies (level 2 study quality) to have a benefit for cardiovascular protection, but good-quality randomized trials (level 1) have not confirmed this effect. Therefore, it is preferable to base clinical recommendations in a manuscript on the level 1 studies.

Strength of recommendation	Definition
A	Recommendation based on consistent and good-quality patient-oriented evidence.*
B	Recommendation based on inconsistent or limited-quality patient-oriented evidence.*
C	Recommendation based on consensus, usual practice, opinion, disease-oriented evidence,* or case series for studies of diagnosis, treatment, prevention, or screening.

Use the following table to determine whether a study measuring patient-oriented outcomes is of good or limited quality, and whether the results are consistent or inconsistent between studies.

Study quality	Diagnosis	Treatment/prevention/screening	Prognosis
Level 1—good-quality patient-oriented evidence	Validated clinical decision rule SR/meta-analysis of high-quality studies High-quality diagnostic cohort study†	SR/meta-analysis of RCTs with consistent findings High-quality individual RCT‡ All-or-none study§	SR/meta-analysis of good-quality cohort studies Prospective cohort study with good follow-up
Level 2—limited-quality patient-oriented evidence	Unvalidated clinical decision rule SR/meta-analysis of lower-quality studies or studies with inconsistent findings Lower-quality diagnostic cohort study or diagnostic case-control study§	SR/meta-analysis of lower-quality clinical trials or of studies with inconsistent findings Lower-quality clinical trial‡ Cohort study Case-control study	SR/meta-analysis of lower-quality cohort studies or with inconsistent results Retrospective cohort study or prospective cohort study with poor follow-up Case-control study Case series
Level 3—other evidence	Consensus guidelines, extrapolations from bench research, usual practice, opinion, disease-oriented evidence (intermediate or physiologic outcomes only), or case series for studies of diagnosis, treatment, prevention, or screening		

Consistency across studies	
Consistent	Most studies found similar or at least coherent conclusions (coherence means that differences are explainable) or If high-quality and up-to-date systematic reviews or meta-analyses exist, they support the recommendation
Inconsistent	Considerable variation among study findings and lack of coherence or If high-quality and up-to-date systematic reviews or meta-analyses exist, they do not find consistent evidence in favor of the recommendation

*—Patient-oriented evidence measures outcomes that matter to patients: morbidity, mortality, symptom improvement, cost reduction, and quality of life. Disease-oriented evidence measures intermediate, physiologic, or surrogate end points that may or may not reflect improvements in patient outcomes (e.g., blood pressure, blood chemistry, physiologic function, pathologic findings).
†—High-quality diagnostic cohort study: cohort design, adequate size, adequate spectrum of patients, blinding, and a consistent, well-defined reference standard.
‡—High-quality RCT: allocation concealed, blinding if possible, intention-to-treat analysis, adequate statistical power, adequate follow-up (greater than 80 percent).
§—In an all-or-none study, the treatment causes a dramatic change in outcomes, such as antibiotics for meningitis or surgery for appendicitis, which precludes study in a controlled trial.

Figure 4.1 Reprinted with permission from American Family Physician. February 1, 2004. Strength of recommendation taxonomy (SORT): a patient-centered approach to grading evidence in the medical literature. Copyright (2004), American Academy of Family Physicians. All Rights Reserved.

STORY TIME

After a long day at the office, I was walking out the door and one of the medical assistants ran after me and handed me a glossy reprint from the New England Journal of Medicine of a study of Namenda® that she had gotten from a pharmacy representative that provided lunch. (I had not had lunch because I do not ever talk to pharmacy representatives.) I took the article and quickly scanned the 'METHODS' section of the paper. I found a 200 question, non-validated scale on quality of life for patients with Alzheimer's disease used as the outcome variable. Additionally, the comparator group was placebo – not standard therapy or combination therapy or other environmental or cognitive training, reminder aid-type of interventions. The most impressive part was that the authors reported a four-point difference in the mean score that was 'statistically significant.' Although the authors claimed this as a major breakthrough in the treatment of Alzheimer's, I handed the article back to the medical assistant, totally unimpressed, thinking that I considered it a negative study. There must have been a large advertising budget at that time because the next day, a family brought their loved one in asking if they should put him on Namenda. When I asked a bit more of the story, I discovered that resources were scant, medications were not covered benefit, and it would be a sacrifice to even buy the medicine. I said, 'I just saw a research trial on that topic and I can tell you that I think your loved one would be better off if you used the money for some other aspect of his care.'

The point of the story is ... being able to assess the quality of the research literature changes the way the doctor assists the dramatic choices patients and families have to make.

THE NARRATIVE ASPECTS OF ASSESSING THE QUALITY OF THE INFORMATION

A good story ought to be convincing. This is especially true if you have to live the story you helped create. The importance of knowing how to evaluate study design and quality is to judge whether or not to believe the information the study purports to suggest. In the office, we have often said, 'There is only one small study with only a few patients. The methods are not that good, so I wouldn't use this to decide how you want to handle your situation. I think we should look at other things to help us make this decision.' Alternatively, if there is a solid literature base with consistent results and high quality studies, then it deserves to become part of the narrative of the office visit. If the evidence is a sub-plot in the co-constructed narrative, we have to know how much emphasis to give it and how extensively the sub-plot needs to be developed. This will vary with what you find in this step of the process. Remember, the whole purpose of this process is to help the patient write the story of his/her life. We are supplying the narrative tools and raw material for that story. Too often, we present medical information in terms of black and white, yes or no, or simply, 'Do this.' Stories often have more ambiguity and uncertainty that the characters must resolve. In order to portray the next episode – the clinical decision – accurately, we need to know the quality of the evidence. We have heard doctors portray 'medical knowledge' as if they are far more certain of 'the correct treatment' than the research literature supports. When this happens, the patient often accepts what the doctor says. Alternatively, patients often return to our office after seeing a specialist, asking permission to disagree with the specialist's advice. Rather than contradict our consultants, we say, 'Let's explore what evidence is available that led them to that recommendation.' This allows the specialist to remain authoritative and also for the patient to decide whether or not the specialist's advice applies to their life situation.

APPLICATION TO OUR CLINICAL CASE SCENARIO

The descriptions of how to evaluate an article are generalized to evaluate a variety of study designs. To give our readers a sense of how to apply this to a specific journal article, we are going to use the same questions but apply to the article we chose to answer our patient's question.

1. Was There an Independent 'Blind Comparison' with a 'Gold Standard'?

There are two questions embedded in this first criterion. The easiest refers to the 'gold standard,' which in this case is coronary angiography. This study directly compared CT coronary angiography with conventional angiography, by catheterization. Thus, the gold standard was used. This means we are comparing an anatomic test to another anatomic test which seems appropriate. Furthermore, one of the reasons why we chose this article was because it was considered either positive or negative by patient, not by coronary artery segment. We think that this patient based analysis is the most appropriate gold standard (compared to segment based analysis.) Although researchers can compare any test to any other test, the real question is did they use an appropriate gold standard. In our opinion, the researchers chose a good, appropriate gold standard.

The second question refers to a blind comparison; did the interpreter of the CT coronary angiogram know anything about the clinical history (i.e. risk factors such as age, sex, tobacco use, previous coronary disease, etc.) or the actual result of the coronary catheterization angiogram. On page 2137 the authors state, '... experienced observers ... unaware of the results of the CCA [Conventional Coronary Angiography] evaluated the CTCA [Computed Tomographic Coronary Angiography] datasets.' This indicates appropriate blinding for the study.

2. Was the Setting for the Study as Well as the Filter Through Which Study Patients Passed, Adequately Described? (Inclusion/exclusion)

Study group. From October 2004 until June 2006, 433 symptomatic patients with stable or unstable anginal syndromes who were between the ages of 50 and 70 years were enrolled in 3 university hospitals. To avoid radiation exposure in young patients, who have a higher lifetime attributable risk than older individuals receiving the same dose, patients enrolled in the study were age 50 years or older (17). A maximum age limit was set to minimize the presence of severe coronary calcifications, which especially occur in the elderly and are known to hamper precise coronary stenosis evaluation. Sixty-two patients denied (written) informed consent, and 11 patients were excluded because of CT-related criteria (5 scanner malfunction, 3 poor intravenous access, 2 contrast extravasation, and 1 second-degree atrioventricular block because of beta-blockers). Thus, the remaining study population comprised 360 patients (Fig. 1).

Patients with stable chest pain were categorized as having typical or atypical angina pectoris. Typical angina was defined when the following 3 characteristics were present: 1) substernal discomfort; 2) precipitated by physical exertion or emotion; and 3) relieved with rest or nitroglycerine within 10 min. Atypical angina pectoris was defined when only 1 or 2 of these 3 symptom characteristics were met. Patients presenting with an acute coronary syndrome were categorized as having unstable angina pectoris (in the absence of a troponin increase as measured at 2 separate time intervals) or as non–ST-segment elevation myocardial infarction whenever troponin levels were elevated. Only patients with an acute coronary syndrome that did not require an urgent invasive strategy were included.

Patients with a previous history of percutaneous coronary stent placement, coronary artery bypass surgery, impaired renal function (serum creatinine >120 μmol/l), persistent arrhythmias, inability to perform a breath hold of 15 s, or known allergy to iodinated contrast material, were excluded.

Figure 4.2 Reprinted from *Journal of the American College of Cardiology*, 52/25, Meijboon W, *et al.* Diagnostic accuracy of 64-slice computed tomography coronary angiography: a prospective, multi-center, multi-vendor study, pages 2135–44, Copyright (2008), with permission from the American College of Cardiology Foundation.

In reference to Figure 4.2, the authors have a separate subsection specifically describing the study group, one of the strengths of the article. They used patients with stable or unstable angina, patients aged 50–70 years old, and who were candidates for coronary angiogram. They give explicit descriptions and criteria for atypical angina pectoris and acute coronary syndrome. In addition, the authors also described the exclusion criteria and gave specific parameters such as describing renal failure as a creatinine greater than 120 umol/l. Some studies will only state that patients with renal failure were excluded, but that can be difficult to interpret as they could be referring to end stage renal disease or anyone with at least stage III chronic kidney disease. This study was very specific.

3. Did the Patient Sample Include an Appropriate Spectrum of Patients to Whom the Diagnostic Test will be Applied in Clinical Practice?

In other words, has the diagnostic test been evaluated in a patient sample that included an appropriate spectrum of mild and severe, treated and untreated disease, plus individuals with different but commonly confused disorders?

There is a wide range of patients with differing clinical presentations, risk factors, gender, physical exam findings and previous evidence of disease. Unfortunately, the age range studied is rather restricted. The study did not include younger or older individuals. They justify this by preventing radiation exposure in young patients and to avoid more coronary calcium deposits in older patients, which would adversely affect the test characteristics (sensitivity/specificity). Remember, this is the first large trial attempted, so one must be understanding of the study design. *The real question is do we believe the patients in this study are similar enough to our patient to apply the results to her situation.* We believe the answer is yes.

Although we were aware of radiation exposure from diagnostic tests from other papers, this specifically discusses the issue. We would typically point this out right in the exam room while reviewing the literature with the patient present (helping the patient to enter into the doctor's 'way of knowing,' but keep this in mind as we proceed with our case example.

4. Have the Reproducibility of the Test Result and its Interpretation Been Determined?

In this particular study, they had multiple trained interpreters and they specifically report a kappa statistic in the result section of the study. Recall that kappa is the inter-observer variability above chance. In this study it ranged from 0.66–0.69. What this means is that different people looking at the scans did not always agree. That is why they used a consensus reading amongst three experienced individuals for the actual measurement. Although we would hope for a higher kappa, this is very similar to our own institution where a radiologist and cardiologist review the films simultaneously sitting side by side. The fact that the kappa is relatively low means that there is an operator dependent bias in reporting the results and is a weakness of the test and limits the 'truth' of the test results.

5. Have the Tactics for Carrying Out the Test been Described in Sufficient Detail to Permit Their Exact Replication?

> **Scan protocol.** Each center used a 64-slice CT scanner from a different vendor (Sensation 64, Siemens, Forchheim, Germany; Brilliance 64, Philips Medical Systems, Best, the Netherlands; Toshiba Multi-Slice Aquilion 64 system, Toshiba Medical Systems, Tokyo, Japan). Patients with a heart rate exceeding 65 beats/min received either additional oral or intravenous beta-blockers.
>
> A nonenhanced scan to calculate the total calcium score was performed before the CTCA. The scan parameters of the scanners are shown in Table 1. A bolus-tracking technique was used to synchronize the start of image acquisition with the arrival of contrast agent in the coronary arteries.
>
> The effective dose of the nonenhanced scan and the CTCA was estimated from the product of the dose-length product and a conversion coefficient (k = 0.017 mSv/[mGy × cm]) for the chest as the investigated anatomical region (18).

Figure 4.3 Reprinted from *Journal of the American College of Cardiology*, 52/25, Meijboon, W *et al.* Diagnostic accuracy of 64-slice computed tomography coronary angiography: a prospective, multi-center, multi-vendor study, pages 2135–44, Copyright (2008), with permission from the American College of Cardiology Foundation.

Even during our search for information it became apparent that there were many specific machines, techniques, and protocols. Remember this technology was evolving rapidly when we were preparing this manuscript. In this article the authors give exquisite detail in the follow categories: scan protocols, image reconstruction, quantitative coronary angiography, CT image evaluation. The standard is whether this study could be repeated. From the information provided, the answer is a resounding yes because all of the details have been provided.

Application of the SORT Criteria

Using the SORT criteria, this article has many of the features to achieve a level 1 rating, including, it is a well designed cross-sectional study with adequate size (power), and blinding. However, the spectrum of patients is not very broad secondary to the age restrictions, and the kappa was low. Although we would rank this a SORT level 2 strength of evidence, we are convinced by our thorough foraging technique that this is the best information available for this patient at this time. Perhaps by the time you read this book there will be another large multi-center study or a well done meta-analysis. Again, this is the way the medical literature evolves.

A CONTINGENT, EMERGENT, SITUATED, AND CONTEXTUAL MEDICAL KNOWLEDGE

In this chapter we discussed the concept that the medical literature is a text that can be understood by reader response theory – every time someone reads the text, it means something to that individual reader at that time. Perhaps it would mean something else at a different time and with a different reader. We phrased it as 'is the story told by the research article believable?' The doctor's (and patient's) response to the article is *contingent* upon whether they believe the study was well performed and the interpretation of the data matches the actual results. We also discussed the contingent nature of how the medical literature is produced – we are not being told the whole story due to publication bias. The unknown trials and whether they are reported or not creates a contingency of knowledge. In our case example, we have dealt with the contingency of the patient's perspective compared to the doctor's belief in 'vulnerable plaque'. Both perspectives are part of the co-constructed narrative. This particular article was chosen because it answered the patient's narrative dilemma about the shape and integrity of the coronary arteries. The doctor's concern is also real (you might hear more about it later ...)

The *situated* characteristic of this knowledge is that it is situated in time. This technology was a fad in medicine. We have moved on to 128-slice CT coronary angiograms and the medical literature (at the point of writing) has yet to emerge.

The *emergent* nature of the knowledge is a recognition that the radiation side effects of the technology are still being assessed and will not be known for certain, if at all, until sometime in the future. From the patient's perspective, what is emerging is a concept of how to understand whether or not she has 'clogs' in her arteries. Emerging from her fear is a way of understanding the medical environment in which she participates.

The knowledge is *contextual* because the definition of 'significant' coronary artery disease is defined by the researchers at greater than 50% when all the previous angiography data was reported as greater than 70%. We will discuss how researchers create categories in the second half of the book, but the definition creates a context for describing the world. We need to recognize that 'clinically significant' is in the eyes of the beholder and the context of this knowledge is defined by the categories others have used. They could recalculate the data and present it differently, but that information is not available to us – the way the story of 64-slice CT coronary arteriography was told has a context unto itself.

REFERENCES

1 Ewart R, Lausen H, Millian N. Undisclosed changes in outcomes in randomized controlled trials: an observational study. *Annals of Family Medicine.* 2009; 7(6): 542–6.

2 NINDS. Tissue plasminogen activator for acute ischemic stroke. *New England Journal of Medicine.* 1995; 333: 1581–7.

3 Sackett DL, Haynes RB, Guyatt GH, Tugwell P. *Clinical Epidemiology: a basic science for clinical medicine.* 2nd ed. Boston: Little Brown and Company; 1991.

4 www.cebm.net/ (accessed December 10, 2010).

5 Greenhalgh T. *How to Read a Paper.* London: BMJ Publishing Group; 1997.

6 Riegelman R, Hirsch R. *Studying a Study and Testing a Test.* Boston: Little, Brown and Company; 1989.

7 Fletcher R, Fletcher S, Wagner E. *Clinical Epidemiology: the essentials.* Baltimore: Williams and Wilkins; 1988.

8 Hulley SB, Cummings SR, editors. *Designing Clinical Research.* Baltimore: Williams and Wilkins; 1988.

9 Hennekens C, Buring J. *Epidemiology in Medicine.* Boston: Little, Brown and Company; 1987.

10 Gilbert EH, Lowenstein SR, Koziol-McLain J, *et al.* Chart reviews in emergency medicine research: where are the methods? *Annals of Emergency Medicine.* 1996; 27(3): 305–8.

11 Ramsey S, Scoggins J. Commentary: Practicing on the tip of an information iceberg? Evidence of underpublication of registered clinical trials in oncology. *Oncologist.* 2008; **13**: 925–9.

12 McNutt RA. Evidence-based medicine requires appropriate clinical context *JAMA.* 2010; **303**(5): 454–5.

13 Kwek EBK, Goh SK, Hoh JSB, *et al.* An emerging pattern of subtrochanteric stress fractures: A long-term complication of alendronate therapy? *Injury.* February 2008; 39(2): 224–31.

14 Schilcher J, Aspenberg P. Incidence of stress fractures of the femoral shaft in women treated with bisphosphonate *Acta Orthop.* August 2009; 80(4): 413–15.

15 Lenart B, Neviaser A, Lyman S, *et al.* Association of low-energy femoral fractures with prolonged bisphosphonate use: a case control study. *Osteoprosis Int.* 2009; **20**(8): 1353–62.

16 Black D, Cummings S, Karpf D, *et al.* Randomized trial of effect of alendronate on risk of fracture in women with existing vertebral fractures. Fracture Intervention Trial Research Group. *The Lancet.* 1996; **348**(9041): 1535–41.

17 Stein P, Fowler S, Goodman L, *et al.* Multidetector computed tomography for acute pulmonary embolism. *New England Journal of Medicine.* 2006; 354: 2317–2327.

18 Packer M, Bristow MR, Cohn JN, *et al.* The effect of Carvedilol on morbidity and mortality in patients with chronic heart failure. *New England Journal of Medicine.* 1996; 334: 1349–55.

19 Ebell M, Siwik J, Weiss B, *et al.* Strength of recommendation taxonomy (SORT): a patient-centered approach to grading evidence in the medical literature. *Journal of American Board of Family Practice.* 2004; 17: 59–67.

CHAPTER 5

Apply the Information to the Clinical Question

KEY CONCEPTS TO REMEMBER

➤ The sensitivity and specificity of a particular test for a particular condition are called the test characteristics. They are calculated when the presence or absence of the condition is measured twice simultaneously for each case: once with the particular test and again measured with the 'gold standard.'

➤ Never equate a positive test with the presence of disease or a negative test with the absence of disease. You have to train yourself to think in probabilities.

➤ Likelihood ratios are simple algebraic equations using sensitivity and specificity as the variables.

➤ Using clinical judgment to assign a pre-test probability has less risk than using 'positive predictive value' of a test which assumes your patient population has the same prevalence of disease as the research population.

➤ Diagnostic tests can cause harm not only by technical complications, but also by lack of cognitive skills to interpret the test correctly.

➤ Doctors determine the diagnosis – not tests.

LEARNING ABOUT APPLYING INFORMATION TO CLINICAL QUESTIONS

Introduction

We want to once again emphasize that this is a process of care, which means that the sequence or ordering each of these steps must be kept intact or the final outcome will be suboptimal. (Remember, repetition is the mother of learning.) So far we have invested a lot of time and effort into understanding the missing information or the 'potential next chapter' of the narrative. This section specifically addresses how to use the cumulative information up until this point.

In general, patients bring issues of diagnosis or therapy into the doctor visit. It is important to clearly understand which of these two domains the clinical question involves. In this chapter, we will introduce the concepts of 'test characteristics' for articles on diagnostic tests. Then, in Chapter 11, we will introduce the concept number needed to treat for therapeutic articles. We have selected these specific interpretations of the medical literature because they are best suited for building the co-constructive narrative.

The medical literature is diverse. Much of it is related to disease oriented evidence. This type of research should be thought of as 'theory building,' and not confused with patient oriented evidence. There are also cost-benefit analyses, exploratory studies, editorials, non-systematic reviews, research articles with a very narrow focus that might not be important to your practice, and, increasingly, process of care studies (e.g. benefit or lack of benefit of 'stroke units'). While all these papers make for a well-rounded, well-informed clinician, they are not directly related to the clinical decision making in the exam room with the patient present. Most patients want to know 'What is wrong with me? What can be done about it?' Clinical decision making is closely tied to diagnosis and treatment. It is these two types of papers that we pay particular attention to – they are most relevant to the patient.

The clinician needs to have discernment when approaching the medical literature. You must be able to ignore all of the irrelevant literature. This narrows the focus of what needs to be read and applied, making the lifelong learning task simpler.

Sensitivity/Specificity

The basic research methodology for medical literature about a particular test is to measure a disease outcome twice on each patient – once with a new test that is being investigated and once with a reference standard, ideally, the gold standard. The research is to determine how well the new test works when compared to the gold standard. This structure sets up a classic 2 x 2 table in which the columns are disease present and disease absent (see Table 5.1). The presence or absence of disease is determined by the gold standard being positive or negative as the gold standard is considered to be always correct. The rows of the table are how many times the investigational is test is either positive or negative.

Table 5.1

	Disease Positive	Disease Negative
Test Positive	a	b
Test Negative	c	d

This classic 2 x 2 table is used for many different functions in statistics. It also sets up a numerical definition for sensitivity and specificity. The sensitivity and specificity together are referred to as the test characteristics of the investigational test.

Sensitivity is the percentage of patients with disease who have a positive test for the disease in question.[1]

Meanwhile, specificity is percentage of patients without disease who have a negative test for the disease in question.[1]

These are technical definitions and even we get confused and need to look them up. Do not worry. The common sense definition of sensitivity is how well the test finds the disease in the population. Typical EBM texts say you can remember this with the mnemonic *SnOut*, which means if the test has a high sensitivity a negative test result rules out the diagnosis. This is almost like a mind teaser, but those two phrases are consistent – if the test is good at finding disease and the result is negative, the patient must not have the disease – it is ruled out.

The common sense definition of specificity is that a positive test means that your patient probably has the disease. *SpPin* means that with a high specificity you can rule in the diagnosis. Again these two viewpoints are consistent – specificity is a measure of how many times a negative test represents no disease. If the specificity is high, all the negative tests accurately reflect no disease, so a positive test is really disease; there are few false positives.

Even writing the last couple of paragraphs was confusing for us. Do not worry, at some point, you will have an intuitive understanding of how these numbers work on an interactive basis when applying them to actual practical cases. Do not sweat it; we are using sensitivity and specificity as variables to calculate Likelihood ratios to predict probabilities, which is easier to intuitively understand and more useful for the patients. We do not use the words 'sensitivity' and 'specificity' with patients.

Sensitivity and Specificity can be calculated as shown in Table 5.2:

Table 5.2

	Disease Positive	Disease Negative
Test Positive	a	b
Test Negative	c	d

$$\text{specificity} = a/(a+c) \qquad \text{sensitivity} = d/(b+d)$$

We have good news for you, the authors typically report the sensitivity/specificity for multiple different scenarios in the abstract. We looked at an article about sensitivity/specificity for color flow Doppler ultrasound for diagnosing deep vein thrombosis. The authors reported a series of sensitivities/specificities for a distal DVT, proximal DVT, and all DVT in combination.[2] Likewise the PIOPED II study, you can use the original data to calculate the sensitivity/specificity in patients with low probability/medium probability/high probability of disease.[3] The point is to read the article carefully and make sure the numbers most relevant to your patient are the ones you use. If you really need to, you can take the results section and calculate the sensitivity/specificity yourself. Because we are busy clinicians, we usually accept that the authors and editors use algebra correctly. Only if we are skeptical about how the study is written, or suspicious of conflicts of interest, or a poorly reviewed journal do we re-check the author's algebra. If the actual numbers to do these calculations are not included in the article, then we become suspicious.

We Live in a World of Probabilities

Remember, we are trying to figure out how to use the test (or if the test should be used). We need to do a bit more work to apply the information to our specific patient.

Unfortunately, many clinicians think that if the test is positive, the patient has the disease and if the test is negative, the patient does not have the disease. This type of thinking is dangerous. The whole purpose of exploring the sensitivity and specificity is to help us interpret the results of a test based on probabilities. The reality is we must have been suspicious enough that the patient has the disease to order the test in the first place. After getting the results we can only have our original suspicion confirmed or denied to the extent that the test characteristics are good. The reality is that a positive test only tells us how much increase in the probability the patient actually has the disease after getting the test result. Similarly a negative test does not mean the patient does not have the disease. Depending on the test characteristics, the result of the test only tells us how likely the patient indeed does not have the disease. Understanding this in a general sense is vital to becoming an evidence based medicine physician. We live in a world of probabilities. In order to apply the research to our patient, we need a structured way to take the research data and help us order and interpret tests for our patients. The methodology for doing this is to use likelihood ratios.

Doctors Need to Understand Clinical Epidemiology – No Excuses

Unfortunately, an assessment of how often clinicians use likelihood ratios showed that only 3% of 300 surveyed physicians do use them. The main reason given for not using them was 'non-familiarity'. The other reason was impracticality.[4] Instead, it seems that clinicians make a gestalt judgment about the accuracy of a test using simple sensitivity and specificity – concepts that they are familiar with. This simply isn't good enough. Far too often we have had the entire management discussion totally changed when we converted from vague 'sensitivity and specificity' arguments to actual calculated probabilities. We encourage all physicians to step up to the plate and learn skills that have huge impact for their patients. Our patients deserve the best. Besides, we need to make these calculations to communicate with our patients well enough to create the co-constructed narrative. With the use of computers and interactive nomograms, the issue of 'impracticality' is not justified. We hope the 'nonfamiliarity' problem is changing – that is part of the reason we wrote this book.

Likelihood Ratios

So the next step is to calculate likelihood ratios. There are two different likelihood ratios. One ratio if the test turns out positive; one ratio if the test turns out negative. We always ask our residents to look at the literature, find the sensitivity/specificity, and calculate both likelihood ratios before ordering the test. (This is a great demonstration of contingent.) In this way, we can quickly ascertain whether ordering the test will be beneficial in clinical decision making. If it is not going to be helpful, PLEASE do not order the test. Unnecessary testing can harm patients both through the technical consequences, such as bleeding, infection, etc, and also through providing misleading information that leads to more unnecessary tests and unnecessary complications. It also really negatively impacts the patient's story.

The good news is that calculating the likelihood ratios is very simple. They are simple algebraic transformations using the sensitivity and specificity. A helpful hint – even though the research article will say 'the sensitivity is 97% ...' we always use decimals, which means converting the percent to 0.97. If you have trouble remember the equations, they can be found easily using the center for evidence based medicine (cebm.net), Google, or your favorite website. A word of caution – highly trained doctors frequently make mistakes while doing algebra. Although we review these equations almost weekly, about half the time, resident physicians make algebraic mistakes. They all have calculators on their cell phones and try to combine the steps without writing anything down. Our advice is to write out the equations as you solve them, just the way you were taught in fourth grade. The equations are:

$$LR\ (+test) = \frac{Sensitivity}{1 - Specificity}$$

$$LR\ (-test) = \frac{1 - Sensitivity}{Specificity}$$

$$LR\ (+) = \frac{Sensitivity}{1 - Specificity} = \frac{.9}{1 - .76} = 3.75$$

$$LR\ (-) = \frac{1 - Sensitivity}{Specificity} = \frac{1 - .9}{0.76} = .13$$

For example if a you look in the literature to a find a test for disease 'zebra-itis' with a sensitivity of 90% and a specificity of 76%, then you can calculate the likelihood ratios using the above equations.

Pre-test Probability

In order to use likelihood ratios, the clinician has to estimate the 'pre-test probability' which is simply the probability that the patient has the disease before you order the test. Clinicians do this all the time without even realizing it. The difficulty with selecting the pre-test probability is that you have to assign a number for the probability the patient has the disease. Clinicians are far more comfortable using words like unlikely, rare, remote possibility, probable, likely, almost certainly, etc. The problem is, one person's 'unlikely' could be 0.2% and another person's 'unlikely', for the same patient, could be 10%. In fact, we do not allow the residents to use linguistic descriptors of probabilities. We make them assign a number to it. When we do this on rounds as a group, the results are usually in tightly bunched estimates of pre-test probability. If there are widely disparate estimations it is simply a signal for us to have a discussion about what underlying evidence each participant is using to assign a number. These clinical discussions rapidly aggregate the group's list of pre-test probabilities within a narrow range.

When we started using this methodology with our colleagues, many of them balked at the thought of having to assign a number for pre-test probability. They were used to the typical 'true, false, yes, no' thinking and felt dishonest and, worse yet, were inaccurately guessing. It took many months to change the culture of the department to accept probabilistic thinking. We believe this has to start in medical school and be role modeled in practice.

When we look things up (such as in *Up to Date*), there are often tables showing the frequencies of particular symptoms with certain diseases. Sometimes there are decision rules, such as the Wells Criteria. Most often there are risk factors for certain diseases. All of these sources of information are from epidemiologic studies. There is more out there than you think. The single biggest source of information is the clinical history and the next most important source of information is the physical exam. When we use our clinical skills, we are constantly assessing the probabilities of a particular disease using all of the above types of information. We usually describe this as a 'differential diagnosis'. We all know that not everything on that list is equally probable; just articulate it with numbers, that is called the pre-test probability. Most of us are unaware that we are doing it, but we do it anyway. Trust your clinical skills.

In summary, estimating the pre-test probability is simply using all of your clinical skills and everything you know about the patient, given the clinical circumstances up until the time you're contemplating ordering the test. You are making a prediction about the likelihood of a disease or condition in YOUR specific patient. Believe it or not, this is far more valid than assuming a uniform prevalence of disease across all populations. Give yourselves credit; *clinical judgment is required to make decisions*.

Post-test Probability

So now that we have the pre-test probability and have calculated the likelihood ratios, we have enough information to calculate the 'post-test probability' that the patient has the disease keeping in mind the result of the test. This allows us to interpret the test.

Remember, a positive test does not mean that patient has the disease and a negative test does not mean that the patient does not have the disease. The test results only increases or decreases the probability that the patient has the disease.

Calculating the post-test probability requires complicated mathematics. Fortunately, there is a nomogram which will do the mathematics for you.

Referring back to our suspected 'zebra-itis', our group agreed on a pre-test probability of 30%. The 'zebra-itis' scanner (the test) is either going to be positive or negative. If the test is positive, we would use the positive likelihood ratio and apply using the nomogram[5] below in the following way:

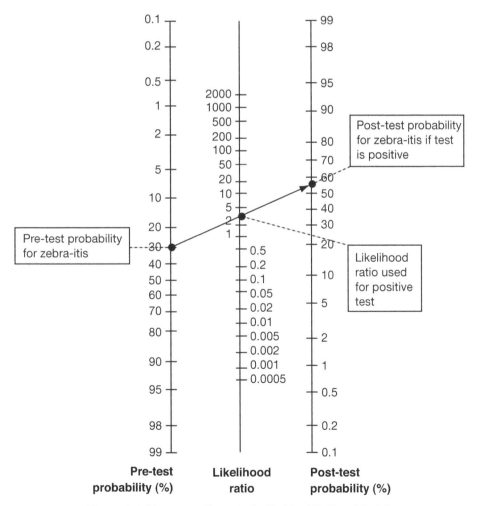

Figure 5.1 (Nomogram Example for Positive Likelihood Ratio). (Figure adapted from Fagan, TJ.[5]).

If the test is negative, then we would use the negative likelihood ratio and apply it using the nomogram below in the following way:

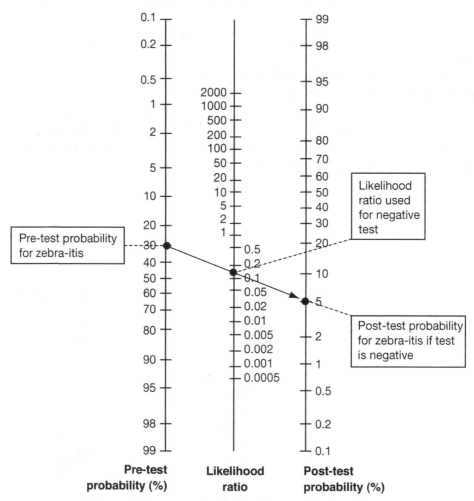

Figure 5.2 Nomogram Example for Negative Likelihood Ratio.

Notice that once you have looked in the literature and calculated the likelihood ratios you have all the information you need to forecast the potential clinical situations after the test has already been performed. It is important to antici-pate the results and interpret them to decide whether or not the test would be helpful. These two potential scenarios are examples of the 'contingencies' of clinical care that exist before the next episode of the 'narrative' emerges. There is a third implied 'next step' – decide NOT to do the test at all. Again, we want to emphasize the importance of, 'Do no harm.' Using these basic precepts of clinical epidemiology you can insure that your patients get all of the tests that would be helpful and can avoid tests that can be useless and harmful.

Assessing the Evidence Continues as You Apply the Evidence

When trying to apply poor quality evidence to patient care it might be reasonable to explore calculating likelihood ratios (LRs) in more depth. For example, if you see a sensitivity with a very wide 95% confidence interval, try calculating the LRs first using the mean and then again using the lower end of the 95% confidence interval. How much difference will this make in clinical decision making? This is a gauge of how emphatic to be when explaining the post-test probabilities to the patient. This is, of course, a judgment, but we want clinicians to make judgments based on evidence and experience. Remember, the resulting medical story should be believable for both the doctor and the patient.

Many times we hear clinicians at our institution talk about the 'positive predictive value' and 'negative predictive value' of a test. We do not use those numbers as they are very highly affected by the prevalence of the disease in the population tested. Most medical literature about diagnostic tests is produced in academic tertiary care centers, the prevalence of disease in these populations is very different than patients you see in the primary care office. Thus the predictive values have limitations and might be misleading.

A Diagnosis is a Clinical Decision

Naively, we think that a test will make a diagnosis. That is absolutely wrong – doctors make diagnoses. They only say them out loud when they are convinced they are true. Unfortunately, what they are really doing is stating that the probability of a certain diagnosis is so high that we believe it to be true. It is never 100% because no test is perfect. Allow us to repeat that – no test is perfect. We do need to make diagnoses despite the fact that we will never be 100% certain. Without a diagnosis (one that the patient can believe in) we can't function as physicians.

Unfortunately, most of us are uncomfortable with uncertainty. We hate to burst your bubble, but it will never go away. Simply be a doctor and make a clinical judgment.

A Cautionary Tale Illustrated by a Clinical Example

In one of our clinics, a young woman presented with mild right lower quadrant pain. After a history and physical, the doctor decided to order a pelvic ultrasound. In retrospect, it is unclear why the test was ordered, but logically, the differential diagnosis includes ovarian cyst, possible torsion of an ovarian cyst, appendicitis, endometriosis, etc. Since this was a resident clinic there is a lot of cross-covering. Someone other than the ordering physician got the radiologist's report that stated, 'Possible abnormality, suggest trans-vaginal ultrasound.' The report of the trans-vaginal ultrasound stated, 'Poorly defined abnormality in the hepatic fossa; suggest ultrasound of the right upper quadrant.' Dutifully following up on the test report, another ultrasound was ordered, which also showed a possible abnormality near the biliary tree; a CT scan was recommended. At this point, the work-up took on a life of its own and the patient subsequently got a CT cholangiopancreatography followed by an Endoscopic Retrograde Cholangiopancreatography. This test has a notoriously high complication rate and indeed our patient suffered necrosis of the pancreas requiring a three week hospitalization complicated by excruciating pain and ultimately initiation of insulin therapy. When the case was reviewed, the patient's initial right lower quadrant pain was completely resolved by the morning after the original pelvic ultrasound. The probably diagnosis was Mittleschmerz, a benign, physiologic condition. We were treating the test reports and not the patient. Fear of uncertainty by the doctors was driving much of the management. No one had ever considered the pre-test probabilities when ordering any of these tests. Although it required a doctor's order for each of these tests, the entire clinical condition was not assessed. The correct next 'test' was to talk to the patient on the telephone. This case highlights the dangers of testing: (1) identification of 'incidentalomas' that require ever more invasive procedures; and (2) just because the test was 'positive' does not mean that the patient has the disease; someone should have recognized the incredibly low pre-test probability of an asymptomatic patient before looking for rare diseases. This unguided ordering of tests is described by Bernard Lown in his book, *The Lost Art of Healing*.[6]

STORY TIME

As we mentioned earlier, the longer you practice in this style, the repetitive clinical situations result in the same relevant questions and the process can become predictable. If there is a mid-range pre-test probability of a valvular vegetation, or endocarditis, then the test characteristics of a trans-thoracic echocardiogram make it a fairly useless test because the post-test probability will not change enough to help you make a decision. This becomes apparent by doing the calculations and plotting it out on the nomogram. If you seriously are considering a valvular lesion, then you need to do a trans-esophageal echocardiogram. We once arrived in the hospital when the residents had ordered BOTH tests because the cardiology fellow requested a TTE and the residents wanted a TEE. As attending physicians, we went berserk! The patient had been through this clinical scenario several times before and understood what was involved in each of the two tests. We made the residents do the calculations and draw lines on the nomograms for both tests to prove to themselves that the trans- thoracic echocardiogram was not going to be helpful. They decided to cancel the TTE, but the cardiology fellow had already written the order and the patient already had the trans-thoracic echocardiogram. It was negative. So what explanation do we give the patient? Your test is negative? That clearly is not the same as 'you don't have valvular vegetation ...' We have been trying to eliminate that type of black and white thinking. Facing up to the cardiology fellow, they re-ordered the trans-esophageal echo and it was positive, resulting in a very high post-test probability of endocarditis, requiring treatment. The residents were gleeful! They couldn't believe this stuff actually works; it made a difference in medical management. The residents had more carefully analyzed the information than someone higher in the hierarchy of medical education.

The point of the story is ... although the residents were gleeful at their diagnostic prowess, the patient was disappointed he had to undergo six weeks of IV antibiotic therapy. Please remember whose story we are in.

NARRATIVE ASPECTS OF APPLYING THE INFORMATION TO THE CLINICAL QUESTION

Although there are formulas, numbers, and calculations in this step of the process, it is important to point out that we are applying the information to the patient's problem. If we have stayed on track, the patient and the doctor should begin to recognize the upcoming clinical decision that has to be made. This will be a very high stakes decision because it will have direct impact on what the patient does next. Because likelihood ratios are 'positive' and 'negative' the best metaphor is 'a fork in the road.' In narrative terminology, this is the dramatic moment where the plot of the story is being decided. Choices are presented. The story must be written with those choices in mind. This part of the process precedes the discussion of how the choices will be made, but the build-up is coming into focus. Applying the information to the clinical question as described in this chapter is a type of 'foreshadowing.' The co-constructed narrative is emerging.

APPLICATION TO OUR CLINICAL CASE SCENARIO

Applying the concepts we discussed above to our patient requires finding the sensitivity and specificity within the article. In some cases authors will not specifically state these numbers with regard to the specific outcome we are interested in. Therefore, sometimes you need to use the 2x2 to calculate these number. In this case, they are explicitly stated in Table 4, on page 2139.

Table 4 Diagnostic Performance of 64-Slice CTCA for the Detection of ≥50% Stenosis on QCA in the Per-Patient Analysis (95% CI)

	Prevalence of Disease, %	n	TP	TN	FP	FN	Sensitivity, %	Specificity, %	PPV, %	NPV, %
Patient-based analysis	68	360	244	73	41	2	99 (98–100)	64 (55–73)	86 (82–90)	97 (94–100)
Stable angina pectoris	63	233	145	56	31	1	99 (98–100)	64 (53–74)	82 (76–88)	98 (95–100)
Non-ST-segment elevation acute coronary syndrome	79	127	99	17	10	1	99 (97–100)	63 (45–81)	91 (85–96)	94 (84–100)
Men	76	245	185	38	20	2	99 (97–100)	66 (53–78)	90 (86–94)	95 (88–100)
Women	51	115	59	35	21	0	100 (100–100)	63 (50–75)	74 (64–83)	100 (100–100)
Typical angina pectoris	70	151	104	31	15	1	99 (97–100)	67 (54–81)	87 (81–93)	97 (91–100)
Atypical angina pectoris	50	82	41	25	16	0	100 (100–100)	61 (46–76)	72 (60–84)	100 (100–100)
Unstable angina pectoris	75	77	57	13	6	1	98 (95–100)	68 (48–89)	90 (83–98)	93 (79–100)
Non-ST-segment elevated myocardial infarction	84	50	42	4	4	0	100 (100–100)	50 (15–85)	91 (83–99)	100 (100–100)

CI = confidence interval; CTCA = computed tomography coronary angiography; FN = false-negative; FP = false-positive; NPV = negative predictive value; PPV = positive predictive value; TN = true-negative; TP = true-positive; QCA = quantitative coronary angiography.

Figure 5.3 Reprinted from *Journal of the American College of Cardiology.* **52**/25: 2135–44. Meijboon W, *et al.* Diagnostic accuracy of 64-slice computed tomography coronary angiography: a prospective, multi-center, multi-vendor study. Copyright (2008), with permission from the American College of Cardiology Foundation.

Table 5 Diagnostic Performance of 64-Slice CTCA for the Detection of ≥50% Stenosis on QCA in the Per-Vessel Analysis (95% CI)

	Prevalence of Disease, %	N	TP	TN	FP	FN	Sensitivity, %	Specificity, %	PPV, %	NPV, %
Vessel-based analysis	26	1,440	354	821	245	20	95 (92–97)	77 (74–80)	59 (55–63)	98 (96–99)
Right coronary artery	39	360	132	170	50	8	94 (90–98)	77 (71–82)	73 (66–79)	96 (92–98)
Left main coronary artery	2	360	5	338	16	1	83 (50–100)	95 (93–97)	24 (8–44)	100 (99–100)
Left anterior descending coronary artery	37	360	133	126	100	1	99 (97–100)	56 (49–63)	57 (51–63)	99 (97–100)
Circumflex coronary artery	26	360	84	187	79	10	89 (83–95)	70 (65–76)	52 (45–60)	95 (92–98)

Bias-corrected 95% CIs from a bootstrap analysis are reported for the vessel analyses and the individual vessel analyses.
Abbreviations as in Table 4.

Figure 5.4 Reprinted from *Journal of the American College of Cardiology.* **52**/25: 2135–44. Meijboon W, *et al.* Diagnostic accuracy of 64-slice computed tomography coronary angiography: a prospective, multi-center, multi-vendor study. Copyright (2008), with permission from the American College of Cardiology Foundation.

We specifically chose Table 4 instead of Table 5, reproduced in Figures 5.3 and 5.4, because Table 4 is a patient based analysis and Table 5 is a segment based analysis. Our patient is really interested in determining if she has any vessel that is diseased and less concerned about specific vessels or multiple vessels. She wants to know if she has disease or not. Notice that when we compare Table 4 and Table 5 there is a difference between the reported sensitivities and specificities.

Because these authors have written a thorough and well designed research trial and publication, the information is easy to find. The sensitivity for 64-slice CTCA for 50% stenosis is 99% [98–100] and the specificity is 64% [55–73]. The numbers in brackets are the 95% confidence interval. If the confidence interval is very narrow, we have a high confidence that it is exactly that number or very close to it. If the confidence intervals are very broad, it means that we have less confidence that it is exactly that number. So, confidence intervals are a reflection of the variability in the data set. For practical purposes, in an office setting, we simply use the mean which is the number stated first.

After identifying the sensitivity and specificity, we can calculate the likelihood ratios for this test for a specific outcome. Although data quality, variability in the data set, different analysis and interpretations are all part of clinical research, we are really only interested in enough valid information to help structure a conversation with our patient. In this case, we have a fairly high confidence that we can portray the risks and benefits accurately enough to give the patient enough information to choose whether or not she wants to proceed with this test. The alternative would be to say 'We don't know' but we would only do that if the study was extremely flawed or we were totally unconvinced of the validity of research literature we reviewed.

$$LR\ (+) = \frac{Sensitivity}{1 - Specificity} = \frac{.99}{1 - 0.64} = 2.75$$

$$LR\ (-) = \frac{1 - Sensitivity}{Specificity} = \frac{1 - .99}{0.64} = .016$$

A rule of thumb for likelihood ratios to be extremely helpful is for a positive test (LR (+)), it should be greater than 10; for a negative test (LR(-)), it should be less than 0.1. Since the positive likelihood ratio is only 2.75, a positive 64-slice CTCA will only marginally increase the probability that our patient has coronary disease. However, with the low negative likelihood ratio, if the CTCA is negative, it will drastically reduce the probability that our patient has disease. Our patient has had a previous negative stress test, but is still worried and what she really wants is confidence that she does not have disease. Hence, this particular test will be able to address our patients concern. The high sensitivity means we will find disease if it is there. This also means that if the test is negative, we can be confident that we can reassure our patient she doesn't have any 'clogs'. (SnOut) The risk is that the test might be positive and we might be stuck figuring out if it is a false positive.

In order to use the nomogram, we have to establish a pre-test probability for coronary artery disease in our patient. Remember, a pre-test probability is a clinical judgment about the probability of the target disease in this particular patient given all previous clinical information at the time. This information is summarized in the table below. Without the prior stress test, her risk is moderate/high, which translated into a probability (which is a number) is approximately 50%. This probability is based on our assessment of the patient's risks and history of her illness. It is our clinical opinion, recognizing that others may differ. However, our patient had a previous negative stress echocardiogram, which has a significant impact in our assessment. Therefore, we have adjusted the pre-test probability to 20%.

Establishing Pre-test Probability for our Case Scenario

Table 5.3 Our patient's cardiac risks to help us determine a pre-test probability

Risk Factor	Data	Relative Risk Assessment
AGE (>55)	58 y/o	↑
Gender	female	↓
Family history	Yes	↑↑↑
Tobacco use	Yes	↑↑↑
Hypertension	Yes	↑↑
Dyslipidemia	Yes	↑
Diabetes	No	↓↓
Nature of pain	Sharp in breast	↔
Radiation of pain	Goes to shoulder	↑
Associated symptoms	Exertional dyspnea	↑↑
Known coronary artery disease	No	↓
Previous tests	Stress echo was negative	↓↓↓↓

Using the Likelihood Nomogram

The usefulness of this process is that the clinician can anticipate the implication and possible meaning of the test result both if it is positive and if it is negative. In Figure 5.5, below, you will notice that the pre-test probability is 20% and if the 64-slice CTCA is positive, then our patient has a post-test probability of coronary disease of 40%. Likewise, if the test is negative, then the post-test probability of coronary disease is approximately 0.4% as seen on Figure 5.6. The next step would be to include this information into a conversation with the patient to help her decide whether or not to proceed with testing.

The Complete Clinician

In our institution, the CT coronary arteriograms are interpreted jointly by a cardiologist and a radiologist. Since our patient is really concerned about having ANY clogs at all, this is a case where we would saunter off to the radiology reading room and ask to review the images together with the radiologist. A 'negative' test is in the eye of the beholder. It is a much more powerful story to tell the patient, 'I looked at the images of your test together with the radiologist and I saw how round and clean the arteries were,' compared to, 'Your test is negative.' In fact, during one of these sessions, the radiologist and cardiologist were discussing whether to characterize a coronary plaque as 'mild' or 'moderate.' I provided the historical information about the patient's anxiety and why the test was ordered, at which point I heard the radiologist dictate, 'Minimal mild plaque seen in the distal left anterior descending artery.' In this case, the co-constructed narrative extended to other consultants, which is the way it should be.

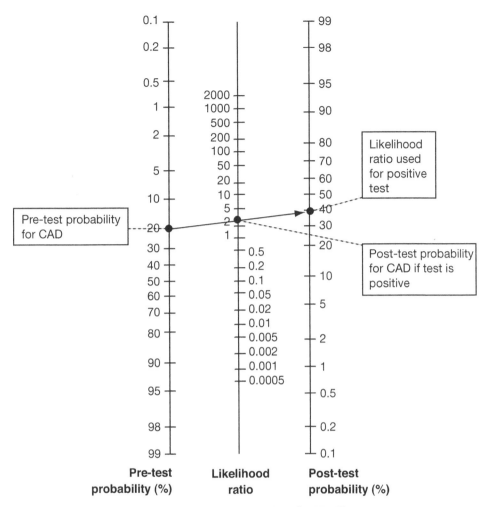

Figure 5.5 CAD Nomogram for a Positive Test.

A CONTINGENT, EMERGENT, SITUATED, AND CONTEXTUAL MEDICAL KNOWLEDGE

The *contingent* nature of looking into the possibilities before ordering the test was highlighted when we said that we should look at both the post-test probability with a negative test and a positive test before deciding whether or not to order the test.

The *situated* component of applying the information is best exemplified by assigning a pre-test probability. This means that a probability has to be assigned in this process of care with exactly the patient, the information we already have about the patient for each test at the time the test is ordered. The exact situation at the time the test is ordered must be assessed, knowing that any other information will change the situation and the pre-test probability.

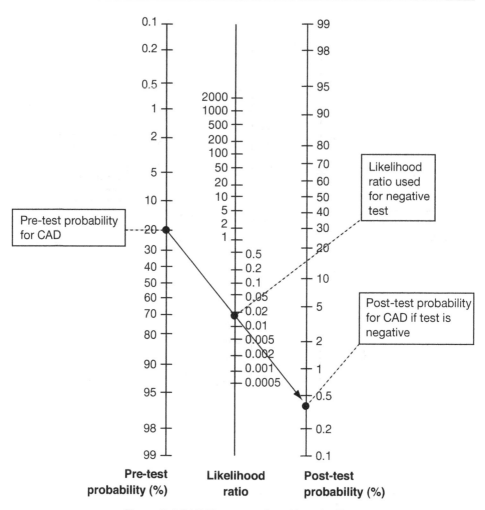

Figure 5.6 CAD Nomogram for a Negative Test.

The *emergent* nature of the process again refers to the chronology of care. During the example recorded in story time, the diagnosis emerged by using this process compared to using the process of 'expert opinion.' By recognizing that a trans-thoracic echocardiogram is insufficient to apply evidence to the clinical question resulted in a different, additional test being used. Notice that what would have emerged in the two different scenarios called for two very different courses of action with all the attendant complications of each.

The *contextual* nature of applying the information is one again highlighted by assigning a pre-test probability. Not only does the patient specific information have to be considered, the pre-test probability has to be assigned within the context of what we know about the target disorder as well. This is where the typical signs and symptoms learned in medical school for specific conditions helps to form the context of this process.

REFERENCES

1 Ebell M. Information mastery. In: *FP Essentials, AAFP Home Study Edition No 318.* Leawood, KS: American Academy of Family Physicians; 2005

2 Lensing AWA, Doris CI, McGrath FP, *et al.* A comparison of compression ultrasound with color Doppler ultrasound for the diagnosis of symptomless postoperative deep vein thrombosis. *Archives of Internal Medicine.* 1997; **157**(7): 765–8.

3 Stein P, Fowler S, Goodman L, *et al.* Multidetector computed tomography for acute pulmonary embolism. *New England Journal of Medicine.* 2006; **354**: 2317–27.

4 Reid MC, Lane DA, Feinstein AR. Academic calculations versus clinical judgements: practicing physicians' use of quantitative measures of test accuracy. *American Journal of Medicine.* 1998; **104**(4): 374–80.

5 Fagan T. Nomogram for Bayes's Theorem. *New England Journal of Medicine.* 1975; **293**(5): 297.

6 Lown B. *The Lost Art of Healing.* New York, NY: Ballantine Books; 1996.

CHAPTER 6

Assist the Patient in Making a Decision

KEY CONCEPTS TO REMEMBER

➤ Doctors demonstrate and share their expertise – not in knowing every-thing – but by being able to quickly locate relevant information and manipulate it analytically so that it is useful for the patient in the exam room.

➤ The narrative and the evidence are blended (integrated) by going back to where the patient left off – the narrative dilemma – and showing how the evidence fits within that context; the evidence thus becomes situated and contextualized within the narrative framework.

➤ The concept of a 'decision threshold' is important when migrating from narrative and evidence to a clinical decision – 'a fork in the road' as the story continues.

LEARNING ABOUT MAKING DECISIONS

Introduction

We have spent a lot of time finding data and information that will be used to assist the patient in making a decision. In the outpatient setting, there are computers in the exam room with the patient and we simply explain to the patient what we are doing throughout the process so that they can feel included as we access the information. Patients do expect doctors to be 'experts.' What we demonstrate to the patient is our expertise in using the most up to date information available and our ability to evaluate research trials. It also gives a good opportunity if we wind up on a commercial website to use it as a teaching method with patients to instruct the patients what information on the web should not be used.

The next step is one of the most difficult transitions in the process of care. Studies have consistently shown that patients want to be given information and doctors underestimate the amount of information patients want to receive.[1] The patient communication literature has reached no consensus about how that should be done. In fact, we believe there is no 'one best way' because every patient is different. In this chapter, we will be sharing methods that we used successfully, but they are only our recommendations as the literature is inconsistent.

We will defer reviewing the literature on conveying uncertainty and risk to patients until the final chapter in Section II, but for now, we will continue to emphasize how to integrate narrative medicine and evidence based medicine into the co-constructed narrative.

Relationship Centered Care

It is amazing that one of the frequent responses in allowing the patient to tell the story in their own words is to thank the doctor. We believe they are actually thanking the doctor for facilitating the process of self discovery in a safe environment; everybody has a need to be known. This process often helps them clarify their own expectations, fears, and emotions related to the clinical problem.

The current best standard of care is described by Beach and Inui in their article 'Relationship centered care,'[2] which is a refinement on patient centered care. Relationship centered care is as unique as each of our patients and that is why we believe there is no best standard of communicating uncertainty or risk inherent in medical research. We are quite comfortable with relationship centered care based on our description of the process of care as we have described it so far. This last step in the process highlights this because we enter into a discussion of risks and uncertainties within the context of the patient's stories and through exploration of the story, the patient's values, and the narrative elements; we help the patient create the 'co-constructive narrative.' Right there in the exam room, we help them write the next chapter of their life. This requires a continuity of the story and a blending of the clinical information and expertise of the doctor as well as the patient's expertise and resources. This is the essence of relationship centered care where we openly acknowledge the vulnerabilities of the patients and the doctors as well as the moral dimensions in creating that next chapter in the patient's life.

Introducing Evidence into Relationship Centered Care

With the increased literature base, increased evidence, and increased availability of evidence in medicine, the problem becomes how both to find relevant information and then share that information with our patients. In years gone by, patients simply trusted the doctor's decisions. Those social expectations have changed, even if a residual of the sentiment remains. Although we present our method of accomplishing this task within the framework of the process presented, we must note that there is little evidence on which we base our recommendations. In the literature, the term, 'shared decision making' is used. Although we agree that shared decision making is better care, it falls somewhat short of a co-constructed narrative as implied by relationship centered care. One of the most helpful distinctions we have seen to make this distinction is the difference between the *logic of choice* and the *logic of care*.[3] Although we present communication strategies in Chapter 11 to help patients make a choice, the entire premise of this book exemplifies the logic of care, which implies a mutually shared responsibility for decision making. We hope that our readers can see that the ordinary tools of narrative medicine and evidence based medicine which are already available can be used to create relationship centered care which is a form of the logic of care. These practices are integrally related to what we later describe as the social practice of healing.

The Narrative Turn (A Twist in the Plot)

We have tried to highlight the sharing and explaining that occurs in the exam room during earlier steps in the process. This was to keep the patient's attention to the 'storyline' for things that one might assume are the business of the doctor. We have now reached the point where the evidence needs to be re-contextualized into the patient's illness narrative. Building on a firm shared knowledge base, it is time to convey the meaning of the evidence to the patient's specific concern.

Other clinicians have frequently voiced their perplexity in how to introduce evidence into the office visit. For us it has always been easiest to use the narrative component and go back to the patient story where the patient left off, saying something such as, 'As you were telling me about the pains in your chest I understood that your most important concern was ... we now have some new information, so lets see how it fits into your thoughts about how you would like to proceed.' By grounding the evidence based medicine deeply into the patient's story we consistently are able to establish the appropriate context for data, which is one of the recognized problems in how to explain uncertainty and risk to patients. By embedding the data in the narrative context, it makes it easier to understand, because patients have an intuitive knowledge of their own story. By allowing them to participate as the evidence was generated, patients can understand how the evidence relates to their story that they shared with the doctor. This will generate questions from their perspective as well as help the doctor understand how to present the information in a way that will make sense to the patient. Depending on the story, a one in 50 chance may sound great to one patient and dangerous to another.[4]

De-contextualized evidence lacks meaning.

Explaining the Meaning of the Test Before Ordering the Test

In the last chapter, we mentioned that as we calculated the probability of disease for both a positive test and the probability of disease for a negative test before the test was ordered was a good idea. Remember we talked about the 'fork in the road?' This is the time to allow the patient to reflect with the advantage of 'anticipatory retrospection.' How would you feel if it turned out that this is the probability of the disease? Could you live with that? If the test showed a probability of disease of this, would you be willing to accept the risks and benefits of treatment with only that level of being able to be sure? Would more tests be needed? These questions have different answers for different people. This is where the concept of 'the decision threshold' comes up. How sure does the patient need to be before they can proceed to a decision about where their story is going next. All of this can be done with imaginative conversations, probing and exploring different possible directions or outcomes.

STORY TIME

When I was in college, I noticed a bump on one of my fingers that I had never noticed before. I went to the student health service and had the doctor look at it. He told me it was just a normal bone. I was perfectly willing to accept that. Then he said that there was a 1 in 10 000 chance it could be some abnormal growth of the bone and asked if I wanted it X-rayed. I thought he was a lunatic because he seemed to be talking about someone other than me – I got out of there as fast as possible. In retrospect, I realize he was harboring a fear that the bump was a sarcoma. In later years, I re-examined that bump and realized it was simply a boney prominence on my metacarpal bone.

The point of the story is ... be careful whose anxiety and tolerance for uncertainty you include in the co-constructed narrative.

NARRATIVE ASPECTS OF ASSISTING THE PATIENT TO MAKE A DECISION

This whole part of the process is narrative. It is the co-constructed narrative in its purest form. Neither participant has totally dominated the process, both have participated in all aspects of the process and now is when the narrative thread of the patient's life and the contribution of evidence based medicine is fully developed. It is time to make a decision. The decision needs to be made together, it needs to emerge out of the relationship.

APPLICATION TO OUR CLINICAL CASE SCENARIO

1 *Doctor:* So when we were talking earlier, *you wanted to know if you*
2   *had any clogged arteries.* You were telling me that you were
3   afraid that you were going to get a blood clog and something
4   unexpected was going to happen in the future. The newspaper
5   article you showed me describes one of the machines in
6   the hospital called a 64-slice CT angiogram. This is an X-ray

7		machine that takes a picture of the shape of your arteries. So
8		for now on we are going to refer to it as the X-ray that takes
9		a picture of the shape of your arteries. All of those computer
10		screens that I was showing you gave me enough information
11		so that we can have a very careful discussion of the advantages
12		and disadvantages of you having one of those tests. The
13		first thing I have to tell you is that there are no absolutes or
14		certainties in life or medicine and the best we can do is make
15		a good decision at this point. I feel so strongly about that that
16		I think it was worth taking the 10 extra minutes to find out
17		what medical research tells us about that scanner described in
18		the newspaper article.
19		You are afraid of dying suddenly by a clog, but this scanner
20		can only tell us of the shape of your arteries and whether or
21		not there is build up on the side walls of those pipes. We call
22		that atherosclerosis, but people typically call that 'hardening
23		of the arteries.' Let me show you a picture (Doctor is pointing
24		to a picture found on Google Image of the pathophysiology
25		of coronary artery disease). If you look at this picture, the
26		wide open pipe has a larger diameter than the one with the
27		hardening of the arteries.
28	*Patient:*	There is the clog I was telling you about.
29	*Doctor:*	You're right, that is a build up of cholesterol and fats with other
30		cells on the side of the artery. I am actually worried about a
31		different type of clog ... If this thin wall breaks and the fatty
32		goop is exposed to the blood, it will form a clot, a different
33		type of clog, which suddenly blocks the entire pipe, usually
34		causing a heart attack. I want to make sure you understand the
35		difference between build up on the side of the artery wall and a
36		clot that causes heart attacks and sudden death.
37	*Patient:*	Yeah. But if there is no build up on the side of the wall, it
38		won't break and cause that clot, right?
39	*Doctor:*	You have a good point there. But one of the important things
40		about this X-ray that takes a picture of the shape of your
41		arteries is that it doesn't tell us anything about the buildup
42		breaking and clogging the artery. It will only tell us if the
43		artery is open or not.
44	*Patient:*	That is exactly what I want to know. I can't relax until I know
45		that my arteries are super clean. If they are not super clean I
46		want a roto rooter.
47	*Doctor:*	I remember you making that statement earlier in this
48		discussion. What you really want to know if you have any

49		blocked arteries. I really want us to think this through
50		together, but first I want to make sure you understand what
51		this test can and cannot show us. This is only a picture of the
52		shape of the arteries. It can't really predict the future. But, like
53		you said, if your arteries are perfectly normal I am going to
54		recommend that you try to relax. But that brings up the point
55		about how to deal with the possibility that there might be
56		some blockage. What do you think about that?
57	*Patient:*	I don't want to think about that now doctor. To be quite
58		frank, just hearing you talk about it makes me uncomfortable
59		and scared.
60	*Doctor:*	That's fine as long you promise me you will be courageous if
61		we need to have that conversation later.
62	*Patient:*	I trust you doctor; right now I am hoping this test will show
63		no clogs.
64	*Doctor:*	I have to be honest with you, the fact that this is so important
65		to you and so scary makes me want to be more careful
66		about making sure there are no problems with your arteries.
67		When you told me about the pains you were having in your
68		shoulder I knew that the chances that there might actually
69		be something in your arteries was a bit higher. So even
70		though we ran that heart test two years ago, now might be
71		a good time to check again. Before we do that, you need to
72		understand the risks of getting the X-ray that takes a picture of
73		the shape of your arteries. It's my job to tell you these things.
74		In general the test is quite safe. But some people get an
75		allergic reaction to the fluid they put in the IV. If that happens
76		they will have to give you Benadryl® and other medicine
77		and watch you carefully. To prepare for the test, I want you
78		to drink lots of fluids both before and after the test to flush
79		fluid through the kidneys which is a way of protecting them.
80		Occasionally, we see a short drop in kidney function but this
81		almost always returns to normal. Have you understood what
82		we have talked about so far?
83	*Patient:*	Yeah, I can get an allergic reaction or my kidneys can be
84		stressed out. How bad is that kidney problem?
85	*Doctor:*	In someone like you there's a small chance that you could
86		have problems with your kidneys and even a smaller chance
87		that you will have to be watched in the hospital. But I have
88		never known someone like you to have a severe, permanent
89		problem with this test. None of my partners have ever told me
90		that any of their patients have had this type of severe reaction,

91		so it must be pretty rare as we have all been in practice for a
92		long time.
93	*Patient:*	I am more afraid of not knowing than having those
94		complications that you were telling me about.
95	*Doctor:*	I know that you want to know if you have any blocked
96		arteries, but before I feel comfortable ordering one of these
97		tests, there is one more potential complication that I also
98		want to make you aware of. This X-ray that takes a picture of
99		the shape of your arteries has a lot of radiation and when we
100		check your heart, the X-rays have to go through your breast to
101		get pictures of your arteries. Radiation exposure is one of the
102		risks for breast cancer. We are all exposed to radiation on a
103		daily basis, except a test like this is a more concentrated form.
104	*Patient:*	Do you really think that I'll get cancer?
105	*Doctor:*	Like I said at the beginning, I can't predict the future and
106		making a decision is always about choosing between one
107		risk versus a different one. Unfortunately, there is no way to
108		completely eliminate the risk of something bad happening to
109		your health in the future.
110	*Patient:*	Nobody in my family has ever had cancer. Unless you think it
111		is really dangerous, I still need to know about the arteries in
112		my heart.
113	*Doctor:*	Thanks for letting me share the potential risks with you.
114		The purpose of doing that is to share information so you
115		understand what my concerns are and I understand what your
116		concerns are. What I am hoping for is that together we can
117		decide what is best for you.
118		I just want to make sure that you fully understand what your
119		choice really is. What I'd like to do now is talk about how we
120		are going to use the information this test will give us. I am
121		assuming you want to proceed and get the test, is that right?
122	*Patient:*	That's right.
123	*Doctor:*	If the test shows some buildup or clogs we still won't be
124		certain that your arteries are blocked. In fact, it will be about
125		a 50/50 chance. That means that if the test is positive, we
126		are going to have to do more testing and might have to do a
127		cardiac catheterization to figure out your condition properly.
128		Have you ever heard of a cardiac catheterization?
129	*Patient:*	Yeah, George at work had one and he wouldn't shut up about
130		it. He told everybody step by step what happened. He said
131		that they poked a hole in his groin and pushed this wire up
132		into his heart. He actually saw pictures while his heart was

133		beating. He said that he had a really hot flush sensation and
134		there were a lot of bright lights, doctors, and nurses running
135		all over the place. It was busy but it only took about 20
136		minutes.
137	*Doctor:*	So if the test was positive, you might have one of those
138		experiences and that test also has potential risks. It's a little
139		like opening Pandora's box. You have to willing to accept the
140		risk of this test and the ones that might come after it to make
141		sure that you really want to get this X-ray that takes a picture
142		of the shape of your arteries
143	*Patient:*	This sure is complicated. Are you just trying to scare me?
144	*Doctor:*	You were scared when you came into this office. What I heard
145		you say you needed to know whether there were any clogs.
146		Another way of asking this question is how much risk you
147		are willing to take to answer that question. I just don't want
148		you to think that this is a magical test that will answer your
149		question without any potential problems. Do you think
150		getting this test will be worth it for you?
151	*Patient:*	You reminded me about my daddy when we were talking
152		earlier. That's when I realized how important this was for me.
153		I need to know if there is a chance that the same thing might
154		happen to me because if there is I need to sit Jason down and
155		go over some things with him. I hear what you say, but I have
156		done lots of scary things in my life. I really do want to know
157		so I am just going to have to be brave; it's worth it for me.
158	*Doctor:*	Thanks for being so honest with me. And thanks for
159		being patient with me when I listed all those potential
160		complications. I know you didn't want to go through that but
161		I appreciate your willingness to hear me out. I just want to be
162		honest with you too. Whatever happens, we'll get through this
163		together.
164	*Patient:*	You're welcome. You know I don't put up with any of that
165		crap from anyone but you. I trust you.
166	*Doctor:*	Now I would like to share with you the good news. If this test
167		is negative, like your stress test was, the chance that you have
168		any clogged arteries is only 0.2%. That is about as sure as we
169		can get when dealing with this type of problem. If I hear you
170		right, a negative test is exactly what you're hoping for; it will
171		help you get on with your life.
172	*Patient:*	That's exactly what I wanted to hear, doctor, please say a
173		prayer for me that my test is negative. I just need to know.
174	*Doctor:*	I'll not only say a prayer but light a candle too.

NARRATIVE INTERPRETATION OF CLINICAL CASE

The narrative picks up after a brief interlude when the doctor was using the computer to access information. Although the patient was watching, this is participating by watching – it is the mental tracking that we think is important.

Lines 1–4: In order to reintroduce the patient as a 'character' in the unfolding story, the doctor connects the beginning of this dialogue tightly to the ending of the last one by using the patient's statement word for word, 'You want to know if you have any clogged or blocked arteries.' Narratively speaking this keeps the story flowing and allows the reader/patient to follow the story line. It also foreshadows the context of the subsequent conversation.

Lines 4–18: At the end of the last 'episode' the patient handed the doctor a newspaper article. The doctor applies a medical label to something described in the lay press (namely 64-slice CT angiogram). This medicalizes the technology described in the newspaper and connects it to the medical literature the patient and doctor were viewing on the computer. The doctor then explains why the medical information is important to continue the conversation, and introduces the concept of harm and benefit. Trying to avoid medical jargon, the doctor calls it the advantages and disadvantages of the patient having the X-ray that takes a picture of the shape of your arteries. Notice how the narrative floats back and forth across the border between the patient's experiences and the domain of medical knowledge. It is the merging of these two worlds that are often kept distinctly apart that creates the interdependent nature of narrative medicine and clinical epidemiology. The doctor goes on to point out that uncertainty is part of life.

Lines 19–36: The next segment again straddles the patient's need to know if there are any blocked arteries with medical terminology and colloquial cultural knowledge of atherosclerosis and hardening of the arteries. In order to bridge this gap, the doctor uses an image and the conversation shifts to describing the picture. Unspoken, but assumed, is that this might be a picture of the patient's artery. The patient is able to make the connection and states 'there's the clog I was telling you about.' The doctor responds by introducing a concept the patient has not yet experienced and, in laymen's terms, describes plaque rupture. Highly attentive to the patient's 'thought categories,' the doctor differentiates blockage from rupture with subsequent clot.

Lines 37–46: The patient uses this new information but concludes that plaque rupture cannot occur if there is no plaque. The patient has taken this story back to her own idiosyncratic thought categories regarding atherosclerosis and coronary artery disease and dichotomizes into blockage or no blockage. At this point, it would be inappropriate for the doctor to try to change the patient's story and impose a different way to think about the patient's perception of illness. The offer to understand it in a new way was made and declined and from a narrative point of view, this is simply a clue in a mystery novel that turns out to be a dead end.

The doctor does not contest the patient's blockage/no blockage point of view, but rather confirms the patient's interpretation at which point the patient says, 'that is exactly what I want to know,' allowing the narrative to progress into the next chapter.

Lines 47–63: The doctor then foreshadows the conversation into the future of about how to deal with the test results and the patient decides not to pursue that storyline. The doctor follows the lead of the patient, recognizing that although this is a collaborative endeavor, it is still the patient's story.

Lines 65–70: The next segment demonstrates the doctor doing self disclosure and stating that the patient's concern has affected his/her own decision making. This is what is meant by mutual influence according to Beach and Inui. Because the patient is so scared, it has an impact on how the doctor thinks about the pre-test probability of coronary disease demonstrating that the patient's story has influenced the doctor's thinking. The pre-test probability of coronary artery disease was shifted slightly upward. Again, this shows the interdependent nature of narrative and clinical epidemiology and is a demonstration of the co-constructed narrative.

Lines 71–112: The next segment relates to informed consent and the patient allows the doctor to share information but reinterprets the risks of the test into her primary concern about needing to know if she has any blocked arteries. When the discussion drifts towards radiation exposure and cancer, the patient repeats the same process from her perspective. Note that her life experiences draw from her family members and she interprets cancer risk not numerically, but in terms of her family life experiences. (Contextual medical knowledge.) She steadfastly brings the doctor back to her primary concern.

Most of this informed consent addresses the needs of the doctor more than the needs of the patient. It is important that both members of this 'co-constructive narrative' gets their needs met. Having fulfilled his professional obligation, the doctor overtly thanks the patient for letting him get his needs met by sharing the other half of the harm and benefit potential. The question comes up whether the patient has appropriately considered the risks. It is important to note that the patient uses narrative logic and not numbers to judge the relative importance between risk of harm and risk of benefit.

Lines 113–163: The doctor then explains the limitations of the test, but checks back with the patient to verify that she understands the meaning of a cardiac catheterization. The doctor appropriately asks 'Have you every heard of a cardiac catheterization?' Without prompting, the patient verifies that she has a good understanding of the procedure from her co-worker's experiences. Again, the doctor challenges the strength of the patient's decision by asking for a commitment. This provokes the patient to resume control of the narrative and discursively takes control of the conversation and ends the discussion of harm and benefit by reminding the doctor of how the story began. The patient acknowledges the doctor's worries by making a commitment to 'be brave' and the doctor, once again, thanks the patient for her honesty.

Lines 164–174: Throughout this discussion, control and power within the conversation switched, starting by the doctor ceding control to the patient by active listening followed by the discussion being dominated by the doctor's obligation to get informed consent from the patient. The doctor acknowledges the patient's discomfort and his/her own needs to provide informed consent. Thanking the patient is a way of acknowledging 'the logic of choice' while honoring the 'logic of care' in the trusting relationship. There is a shift in the narrative structure when the patient takes control back and finalizes the decision to get the test. At this point, the doctor simply provides a happy ending by telling the patent if the test is negative they would be able to directly answer the patient's primary concern: are there any blocked arteries? By acknowledging the inherent uncertainties, the doctor and patient proceed with a prayer and a candle.

A CONTINGENT, EMERGENT, SITUATED, AND CONTEXTUAL MEDICAL KNOWLEDGE

The doctor was describing *contingencies* when he talked about the possibility of the test being positive, provoking the need to do further tests. Helping the patient understand this contingent outcome is part of clinical decision making.

The decision to pursue ordering the test *emerged* from both the patient and the doctor getting their respective needs met during this interaction. Consider an alternative outcome: the doctor could have simply said, 'That test won't tell you anything important.' Such a response uses the authority of the white coat to re-write the story of the process of care. In order to keep the balance of power in the relationship appropriate, we abide by the concepts of the *logic of care* and *relationship centered care. These two attributes define where the process of care emerges from.* Alternative decisions that do not share these qualities run the risk of abuse of power. It is always reasonable for clinicians to ask themselves what drives the process of care; for this, self reflection is required.

The *situated* nature is illustrated by the informed consent and the needs of the doctor being met as well as the needs of the patient. The doctor provided some self disclosure. (To an appropriate degree, he shared his concerns which were based on the patient's need to know.) Since no two doctors or patients are identical, the needs of the participants are not identical. The medical knowledge that is shared, discussed, and processed is situated within this relationship at this time.

The *contextual* nature of the medical knowledge is demonstrated by the patient using the family history to prioritize what she is more or less afraid of – she wants to know about clogs, but discounts the risk of cancer. The perception of risk of benefit versus the risk of harm is thus altered by the family context.

REFERENCES

1   Lipkus IM. Numeric, verbal, and visual formats of conveying health risks: suggested best practices and future recommendations. *Medical Decision Making.* 2007; **27**: 696–713.

2   Beach MC, Inui T. Relationship-centered care – a constructive reframing. *Journal of General Internal Medicine.* 2006; **21**: S3–8.

3   Mol A. *The Logic of Care: Health and the Problem of Patient Choice.* London: Routledge; 2006.

4   Mangset M. 'Two percent isn't a lot, but when it comes to death it seems quite a lot anyway': Patients' perception of risk and willingness to accept risks associated with thrombolytic drug treatment for acute stroke. *J Med Ethics.* 2009; **35**(42).

PART II

The Process of Care for a Therapeutic Narrative Dilemma

CHAPTER 7

Acquire Enough Information to Understand the Patient's Concern

KEY CONCEPTS TO REMEMBER

➤ There is a natural narrative connection between 'What is the explanation of the symptoms or sensations I'm experiencing,' and 'What do I do about it?'

➤ We view labeling a patient as 'non-compliant' as a narrative failure.

➤ Empathy is a complex cognitive, socio-cultural phenomenon essential to narrative. Understanding the patient's emotions, our own emotions, and how they interact is necessary for storytelling and story listening.

➤ We recommend using the same process for answering questions about therapy as we use for answering question about diagnosis – the process outlined by the six As. There will be different emphasis and methods for each step of the process, but the fundamental sequence that builds upon the patient's story and is tightly structured around this guiding principle is the same. We will highlight some of the differences in methods as we go along in the second half of the book.

➤ It is sometimes useful to survey the range of possible therapies and 'pre-sort' them into something the patient would consider. Remember this process can only be used for one question, one therapy at a time. The entire process has to be repeated for each different therapy, which is why we said some 'pre-sorting' enhances efficiency.

➤ In order for the therapy to work, there has to be a belief that it will work; consider the placebo effect as a useful therapy. The way the doctor interacts with the patient is as important as any other 'drug' according to Michael Balint.

LEARNING ABOUT UNDERSTANDING THE PATIENT'S CONCERN
Introduction

When doctors want to test the abstract reasoning capabilities of patients, they ask them to interpret a proverb, such as, 'What does it mean when we say,

"People who live in glass houses shouldn't throw stones?"' If the patient says that rocks are harder than glass and the glass will break, we assume the patient cannot grasp the abstract meaning of the phrase about blaming others while being blind to our own faults. As a simple thought experiment, suppose a patient tells a complex, multi-layered story and asks the doctor what it means. If the doctor says, 'That's because you have Lupus,' do you suppose the patient might think that the doctor cannot understand the abstract, social meaning of the story and give the doctor a poor grade for mental status?

In this section, we are going to take a more in depth look at how people understand one another to better understand what it means for the doctor to 'understand the patient's concern.'

Non-compliance, Non-adherence

When patient management is difficult or there seems to be difficulties with follow through on management plans, some doctors get frustrated and say the patient is 'non-compliant.' This immediately categorizes the patient as 'at fault,' probably on the basis of breaking one of Talcott Parsons rules when he defined the 'sick role;' the patient is supposed to seek professional advice and comply with that advice in an attempt to recover and re-enter society without restricted social obligations that accompany the sick role.[1] This concept lives on in medical practice by creating social expectations between doctors and their patients. It also re-establishes the hierarchy of power, where the doctor tells the patient what he or she 'must do.' In the language we have been using, the co-constructed narrative embraces the differential experiences of the doctor and of the patient, allowing a safe framework within which it all becomes part of the story. Different perspectives do not create conflict or suffering for the patient because it can be absorbed into the story. In our experience, the 'non-compliance' story always ends badly. We would consider it a *narrative failure*. The doctor that really wants to understand the patient's concern needs to understand the patient's story. Thus, the question becomes, 'When we last talked, we agreed that you would start the new medication. Can you tell me what happened and what you were thinking so that I can understand why that never occurred?' The narrative approach to patient interviewing always assumes there is a reason for something that happened or did not happen. If the doctor is not judgmental, but trying to understand, the patient is usually willing to explain the reasons. Non-adherence refers to the patient's response to the treatment plan – not the patient's response to the doctor. Too often doctor's take non-adherence personally and feel offended (even though we pretend not to be offended). When threatened in this way, doctors pull rank and assume the 'power up' position and label the patient as non-compliant. We are suggesting that any time the agreed treatment did not materialize, there is *always* a narrative task for the doctor and patient to complete.

Empathy

In a succinct, well written article, Platt and Platt demonstrate the cognitive, social shift from non-compliance to non-adherence using 'empathy.' The article is titled, 'Empathy: a miracle or nothing at all?'[2] In a written dialogue, the nurse reports that the patient refuses his evening insulin, causing frustration for the nurse. The next day the doctor has a three minute conversation with the patient where the story of low blood sugar reactions is offered by the patient and his wife. The doctor interviews them in a narrative way, using what we call 'empathetic stepping stones.' These statements are simply reiterations of what the patient said, ala Carl Rogers, or quiet waiting while acknowledging listening ('I see.') This type of 'listening for the story' gives the patient the time and space within the interview to explain the story further. (Recall that doctors interrupt and direct patients away from the story.) The patient realizes the doctor is listening and feels safe enough to share an emotion: 'It's awful. You wake up sweaty and confused ... Maybe not wake up at all.' The doctor has to recognize the dramatic climax of the story signaled by the emotion conveyed, and replies, 'Pretty scary.' By naming the emotion (empathy), the patient immediately knows that the doctor understood the illness experience story and only then can they agree on a management plan for insulin. When the doctor leaves the room he asks what just happened. The intern who observed the morning's encounter said, 'Nothing, he changed his mind.' The intern's statement is like telling your patient, 'Rocks are harder than glass and glass breaks,' a statement void of abstract thinking on the part of the doctor; this is a demonstration of narrative incompetence. The nurse says, 'It was a miracle.' Actually, it was a demonstration of a storyteller and a doctor who understands how to listen to a story. It was less of a miracle than simply medicine practiced well.

Platt and Platt quote Coulehan and Block,[2] 'The empathetic physician is also the scientific physician because understanding is at the core of objectivity.' *It is important to note the science in narrative demonstrated by this sentence.* Empathy is a social act that demonstrates effective communication in the affective world. Emotions are a type of cognition that impacts social behaviors. This is why we emphasized self reflection so heavily – it is easy to confuse your own emotions with the emotions of the patient. The process of transference and counter-transference is ubiquitous, whether or not we allow ourselves to acknowledge it. Understanding emotions is a necessary skill to be able to use narrative in medicine; emotions create the dramatic moment of the story. Without understanding emotions, you can't understand a story…you can't practice narrative medicine.

Part of the culture of medicine is to protect the doctor from experiencing too much of the patient's emotional pain as a survival technique when dealing with suffering, death and disease. This is probably counter-productive part of the culture of practicing medicine.[3] Empathy is often confused with 'feeling the patient's pain.' It is not that at all – empathy is *understanding* the patient's pain. If we allow ourselves to approach these inner experiences of our patients, we more quickly arrive at the narrative dilemma and this is formalized in an empathetic statement. The true protection from burn-out in the field of medicine is self reflection and allowing the doctor to *experience* his or her *own* emotions.

The Science in Narrative

Throughout this book, we have tried to break down the barriers and stereotypes of narrative not being scientific and science as the path to 'truth.' The explanation for why empathy is so important to narrative is based on the *Theory of the Mind*, which is recognized by a large variety of disciplines. Michael Tomasello gives a succinct description.[4] He claims that humans recognize other humans as intentional, purposeful beings that share a mental life similar to one's own. Humans understand the world in these terms, allowing for one person to understand how the other feels in certain circumstances, and to predict how they might act (or think) in these causal terms. Embedded in these simple assumptions is the narrative framework. Stories are an artifact of our shared cognitive abilities and cultural creations. Tomasello's second premise is that humans can engage in 'joint attention.' In our particular case, both the patient and the doctor can focus on the story and mutually engage in that experience. These two fundamental abilities allow for cultural storytelling and shared understandings.

Once again, to highlight the science in narrative, neuroscientists have rediscovered what cognitive scientists already demonstrated. Humans have something called 'mirror neurons,' which allow for people to understand the feelings of others and to anticipate how another human might respond in a given situation. 'Thus, pre-motor mirror neuron areas ... previously thought to be involved in action recognition are actually also involved in understanding the intentions of others.'[5] This convergence of bio-science and social science is the fundamental premise of this book. Each way of knowing is necessary, but insufficient alone; the seemingly disparate ways of knowing can be integrated using the underlying meta-language represented by these two epistemologies. Although that last sentence was a mouthful, put simply it means we're asking doctors to bring their full humanity and all its dimensions into the process of care. Being willing and able to do this safely makes a doctor into a healer.

Reviewing the Overall Process for Integrating Narrative Medicine and Evidence Based Medicine

As discussed in the preface, the process of care outlined by the six As – (1) **Acquire** enough information to understand the patient's concern; (2) **Ask** a clinically relevant question; (3) **Access** information to answer the clinically relevant question; (4) **Assess** the quality of the information; (5) **Apply** the information to the clinical question; and (6) **Assist** the patient to make a decision. –can be used for either diagnostic tests or treatment decisions. The above conversation with the patient included sharing information about the diagnostic test which is an important part of the 'co-constructive narrative,' but also serves as the first step in understanding the patient's concern about how to respond to the information, especially, whether or not therapy is indicated. This will require discussion of the risks of harm and risks of benefits. Once again we use the same process to find, evaluate, and apply the medical literature to our patient's specific concerns. Just to make this perfectly clear, we will be repeating the same process of care; however, this time the focus will be on therapy whereas the previous section was on a diagnostic test. The fact that the two sections of the book are connected by a continuing conversation with the patient emphasizes our main thesis: The beginning and end of every patient encounter involves a meaningful conversation with the patient that evolves over time. The story is in the relationship.

Keeping Track of the Narrative Thread

Once again, it is important to allow the patient to define which therapies they are willing to consider. The process does not work well if you are trying to compare one therapy to another. If you wanted to do that, you would have to start at the beginning and run through all six steps for both of the therapies under consideration. It gets far too confusing to do more than one at a time. Anticipate foraging for information when you are trying to consider multiple questions. Rarely are these decisions so urgent that you can't take one at a time or one at each office visit. Remember, narrative has structure. No matter how complex the story becomes, you should be able to analyze the structure of the story.

The Narrative Basis for Understanding the Patient's Concern

Sometimes patients simply want to know what is going on in their body. Just knowing that the diagnosis is not dangerous may be enough to satisfy the patient and resolve the narrative dilemma. Sometimes, a trivial cosmetic problem may be causing much distress. Sometimes the diagnosis and therapy are related (as in our case scenario) and sometimes they are not. Remember, you must let the patient take the lead and direct the story wherever it is meant to go. Listening on several levels may be necessary. As we proceed, we find that our patient's concern spans the spectrum from diagnosis through therapeutic concerns. If the patient brings the concern into the clinical interview, there is usually enough motivation to be adherent to the therapy. By engaging the patient into helping create the co-constructed narrative, you build a natural 'buy in' that increases adherence. Patients have a sense that they are enacting their own story that they helped to write. This intention and belief in improvement gives any therapy the added benefit of the placebo effect over and above the therapeutic effect of the particular therapy – they can be additive.[6] We will gladly accept anything that helps the patient.

STORY TIME

We saw a patient who brought in a 'laundry list' of topics, none of which seemed terribly important. The patient wanted to share recent accucheck readings and blood pressures and report back from things specialists had told him. The last thing on his list was a minor arm pain in the triceps area. The history and physical were completely benign. Experience told us that he was not reassured by a simple musculo-skeletal explanation the way most patients are. We identified an unspoken feeling – and said, 'Since you seem really concerned about your arm, we should talk about whether or not you think an X-ray today would be helpful.' The patient replied, 'I'm so glad you said that. I know it seems silly, but I was worried that I might have a sarcoma in my arm.'

The point of the story is ... the emotion quickly uncovered the narrative dilemma and changed the management.

APPLICATION TO OUR CLINICAL CASE SCENARIO

1	*Doctor:*	Hi Mrs Smith. How are you doing?
2	*Patient:*	I have been absolutely wonderful since you called me and
3		told me that my test was normal.
4	*Doctor:*	I still think that it's important that we spend a few minutes
5		understanding what the results of the test mean for you. Can
6		you tell me about that?
7	*Patient:*	I am glad that I had the test done. When you were going
8		over all of the risks, it made me realize how badly I needed
9		to know. I am overjoyed that my test was negative and that I
10		didn't have any problems. I'm blessed. I feel like that I can get
11		on with my life.
12	*Doctor:*	If you remember way back at the beginning I mentioned that
13		there were actually two separate issues. The most pressing
14		concern was whether or not you had any clogs, but the other
15		one was the difficulty you were having with Jason. How's that
16		going?
17	*Patient:*	I spent a lot of time thinking about what happened to my
18		daddy and I told you that I was worried about what might
19		happen to me. I guess that stirred up a lot of memories. I

20		always told you about how much I depended on him to help
21		baby-sit while I was at work. I couldn't even imagine getting
22		through that part of my life without his help. But now that
23		I think about it, he wasn't perfect. There were times that I
24		needed him and he was out at the bar. I always made excuses
25		for him because I thought that helped him deal with the loss
26		of his wife. You know I never knew my mom, so for me, I
27		thought that it wasn't that big of a deal, but it wasn't the same
28		for him. I always knew that it was really hard on him, which
29		is why I made excuses. I guess that day he died was the one
30		thing I couldn't excuse him for, leaving me all alone like that.
31		This might sound a little funny, doctor, but I never missed my
32		mom until the day he died. It was just a sensation of being all
33		by myself and not knowing how I was going to survive.
34	*Doctor:*	That sounds overwhelming.
35	*Patient:*	I don't know how I made through those first few years. In fact,
36		I don't remember much from then. But, I kept my job and
37		raised my son. He was on the football team and I had to miss
38		the games, but I would sit him down at night and explain to
39		him that all we had was each other and that I wish I could
40		have been there. But, he needed to understand that I was
41		working two jobs for him.
42	*Doctor:*	It sounds like you gave him the freedom to be a kid, which is
43		surely a wonderful gift.
44	*Patient:*	That's the gift I never got. With mom dying early and dad
45		missing her while raising me, I guess I realize now how much
46		responsibility I had to take when I was a kid. When daddy died
47		I think it was so hard on me because I finally realized that I not
48		only lost him, but I lost the chance to ever have a mother and
49		in some ways, I lost my chance to ever be a kid. Don't take this
50		the wrong way, but when you told me my test was normal and
51		my arteries were clean, I actually felt angry at my daddy.
52	*Doctor:*	You talked a little bit about sacrifice and the gifts parents give
53		to children. I think you just gave yourself a wonderful gift.
54	*Patient:*	What do you mean by that?
55	*Doctor:*	You've never allowed yourself to be angry at your dad, but,
56		by facing up to your fears of heart problems you're finally
57		able to express part of the grief of losing your parents. By
58		acknowledging those feelings I think you get to claim part of
59		yourself back. I'm looking forward to having more of these
60		kinds of discussions in the future so I can better understand
61		your experience.

62	*Patient:*	Thanks for understanding doctor. So I can go now?
63	*Doctor:*	Not yet. So far we've found out that you don't have any heart
64		clogs, but you are still young. Remember our conversation
65		about cholesterol pills?
66	*Patient:*	Not that again. I told you that I don't want any chemicals in
67		my body.
68	*Doctor:*	What else do you want?
69	*Patient:*	You're trying to trick me again?
70	*Doctor:*	What do you mean by that?
71	*Patient:*	After my last heart test, we talked about chemicals in my
72		body and before I knew it I promised you that I would stop
73		smoking.
74	*Doctor:*	So how did that work out?
75	*Patient:*	I know you were right. I was thinking that my test might not
76		be normal if I had smoked these last four years. I sure did
77		save a lot of money, which helped with buying things for my
78		grandchild. I guess it's like the high blood pressure pills, I
79		know I should do it and I have been procrastinating.
80	*Doctor:*	Having just gone through a major heart test is a good time to
81		think about it again. Remember our conversation about cracks
82		in the wall of the arteries causing sudden blood clots?
83	*Patient:*	Yes.
84	*Doctor:*	That's the reason you are taking the aspirin. In case that
85		would happen, the aspirin can help you by protecting you
86		from forming a complete clot in the artery. We also think that
87		cholesterol pills 'toughen up' the lining of the arteries and
88		make them less likely to crack. I'm still talking about our major
89		theme of preventing something unexpected and catastrophic.
90	*Patient:*	Do you really think that cholesterol pills can do that?
91	*Doctor:*	Let's take a look at the medical literature and see what we find.

NARRATIVE INTERPRETATION OF CLINICAL CASE

This interview starts with a greeting which reestablishes the ongoing relationship. In terms of narrativity, we also think about a *beginning*, a *middle*, and an *ending*. Although each chapter or episode has a beginning, middle, and end, the patient's life at this point only has a beginning and a middle. The co-constructive narrative talks about multiple competing possible endings and so narrative medicine deals with contingent endings.

Lines 2–11: After the greeting, the patient states that she is 'absolutely wonderful' because the test was normal. The physician perceives a potentially cause and effect relationship because of the feeling of 'being wonderful' and the fact that the test being normal. His response is to 'unpack' the embedded meanings for the patient and states that he feels that it is important to understand the results of the test, inviting the patient to elaborate. The patient responds reflectively, giving affirmation to the patient's concern about 'needing to know,' and moves the narrative forward in time by saying she can get on with her life.

Lines 12–34: The doctor also reflects that the original interview contained more than one issue and facilitates the *subplot* of difficulties with her son, Jason. This provokes further reflection which in a narrative sense becomes *flashbacks*, widening the 'frame' of the story. The patient reminisces about her father; her sense of being overwhelmed, but also recalls a fuller picture of her relationship with her father. In a medical sense, we will call this working through denial, but in a narrative sense we will call it development of the *plot*. The twist in the plot comes when the patient states, '... but I never missed my mom until the day he died.' The plot deepens when the patient brings up the existential fear of survival and the doctor responds with an empathetic statement, allowing the patient to continue the story about raising her son. The doctor then takes on the role of narrator and interprets the patient's revelations and adds a value judgment, namely 'a wonderful gift.' This highlights the ethical and moral context of narrative.

Lines 35–51: By simply following the storyline the patient moves the plot forward developing the issues of grief and loss of the relationship of her mother and *metaphorically* connects her own lost childhood with the subplot of raising her son Jason. She also brings the two threads of the narrative together by stating, '... when you told me my test was normal and my arteries were clean, I actually felt angry at my daddy.' The power of narrative medicine is demonstrated by the patient's ability to create *coherence* in her life story, connecting her coronary arteries to her relationship with her father (mother).

Lines 52–61: The doctor responds with an interpretive moment and the patient asks him to explain the *tension*. Allowing the patient to tell the story and making up the story for the patient is a tension that is always part of the co-constructive narrative. Because of the unequal power positions of the social relationship, doctors need to use extreme caution whenever making an interpretation, especially if it leaks into the clinical encounter instead of being used only as a way of thinking. In this instance, the doctor simply uses the story elements provided by the patient and reflects them back to the patient in the context of the relationship. He verbally acknowledges the healing power of narrative by stating, '... by acknowledging those feelings I think you get to claim part of yourself back.' The doctor then invites the patient to continue the process.

Lines 62–91: The patient feels a sense of closure and wants to end the interview, but the doctor also is part storyteller, reminding the patient about previous conversations having to deal with cholesterol pills. There is a conversational interaction triggering a parallel process to a previous episode in the patient's life regarding lipid lowering medicines, smoking, and managing high blood pressure. The doctor responds by using this moment to create a 'narrative twist.' With the heightened sense of *drama* reflected in the test for coronary artery plaque the doctor pushes the narrative both forward by a discussion of cholesterol lowering pills by using the narrative form of 'desire,' stating 'I'm still talking about our major theme of preventing something unexpected and catastrophic.' Notice that this is our original narrative dilemma discovered during the initial interview assisting the patient to develop the theme when she asks, 'Do you really think that cholesterol pills can do that?' So the story continues by venturing back into the medical literature.

A CONTINGENT, EMERGENT, SITUATED, AND CONTEXTUAL MEDICAL KNOWLEDGE

Examining the larger frame for this patient story, the possibility of using drug therapy for treating the patient's hypercholesterolemia has been talked about in the past, but remained *contingent* upon the right time and situational motivation that was brought out in this clinical interview. Although it was never acted upon in the past, the contingent nature of the discussion created the potential for action as illustrated in this patient encounter.

The *emergent nature* of the medical knowledge is demonstrated by the doctor saying, 'Let's take a look at the medical literature and see what we find.' By applying the research information to the new situation of having been tested for coronary disease and the concomitant emotional discoveries that occurred during that discussion, re-opens the possibility for medication to emerge as a viable management plan.

Again, the therapy is *situated* in the narrative – a narrative that the patient and the physician co-constructed. The meaning of the research data is only relevant to this situation at this time; this recognizes that in a different situation, the same research data assumes a different meaning.

The *context* of the medical knowledge recognizes why the research was done initially, what popular culture informs the patient about 'high cholesterol' and heart disease, the alternative therapies, the patient's belief about how much control she has over her diet and how that affects the cholesterol and risk of heart disease. The patient's values about 'chemicals' and natural products are part of the context within which the knowledge will be interpreted by the patient and the doctor together.

REFERENCES

1 Parsons T. *The Social System*. London: Routledge; 1991 [1951].
2 Platt FW, Platt CM. Empathy: a miracle or nothing at all? *Journal of Clinical Outcomes Management*. 1998; 5(2): 30–3.
3 Engel JD, Zarconi J, Pethtel LL, *et al. Narrative in Healthcare: Healing Patients, Practitioners, Profession, and Community*. Oxford: Radcliffe Publishing, Ltd; 2008.
4 Tomaello M. *The Cultural Origins of Human Cognition*. Cambridge: Harvard University Press; 1999.
5 Iacoboni M, Moinar-Szakacs I, Gallese V, *et al.* Grasping the intentions of others with one's own mirror neuron system. *PLoS Biology*. 2005; 3(3): 379.
6 Moerman D. *Meaning, Medicine and the 'Placebo effect'*. Cambridge: Cambridge University Press; 2002.

CHAPTER 8

Ask a Clinically Appropriate Question Based on the Patients Concern

KEY CONCEPTS TO REMEMBER

➤ Active listening identifies 'emotionally loaded' content, which often is closely related to the narrative dilemma.

➤ Patients sometimes share their idiosyncratic health beliefs; we usually try to honor these rather than contest them – it just seems like the narrative thing to do.

➤ Only one question can be answered at a time. The whole process needs to be repeated if you try to evaluate two different therapies.

➤ To structure the clinically relevant question, we use PICO format. By matching the patient population to our patient, it maintains relevance to our patient's story.

LEARNING ABOUT ASKING CLINICAL QUESTIONS

Review of Transitioning from a Patient's Concern to a Relevant Clinical Question

Remember that this requires very active listening. The narrative dilemma is often embedded in a very emotional context. For instance, if a patient ever uses the words 'worried,' 'anxious,' or 'stressed,' we always look for the under-lying plot or dramatic moment, such as worried about what? What is being threatened? How does the patient think it will happen? What consequences (next episodes) does the patient think will happen? *Remember, these questions are important because the medical literature has to be reviewed not only for the test or treatment, but also for the target disorder.* A single treatment may be used for seizures and for peripheral neuropathy, but the evidence and how we use it is vastly different. That is why the narrative information is so important – we need to capture it in the clinically relevant question.

It astonishes us when we hear the surprises about patients' worries. Often these worries have been created by things that other doctors said, but did not explain. Other times, they seem as non-sequiturs – and we wonder how patients put two unrelated concepts together. An example would be when we had a patient present with a skin lesion (or perceived skin lesion), but his real narrative dilemma was his concern about growing hair on his palms of his hands if he masturbated. In these cases, we acknowledge that the patient had a reason to associate a symptom with a certain condition and all we have to do is explain that medically, there is not and cannot be medical causation. At times, that is all the patient needs to answer the narrative dilemma. We would, however, expect him to return with the next logical narrative dilemma fairly soon. Usually, these types of questions can be embarrassing for the patient to voice. By reviewing the narrative of how the patient got to such a point in the story (making the concern part of the patient's real experiences) and adjusting the narrative in the office visit is a very non-threatening way to handle concerns such as these.

Sometimes we uncover 'idiosyncratic health beliefs.' These are beliefs that are so outlandish and not shared by anyone else that they are simply bizarre. From a narrative standpoint, we always honor these beliefs and do not try to take them away from the patient. After all, this is the way they understand the world and their place in it. We will try to weave an alternate narrative thread into this belief system and continue working with the patient on their terms. That is why it is so important not to assume anything, but practice listening to the whole story. Remember that narratives have an internal cohesion as a series of causal events that lead from episode A to episode B. The story has to make sense to the patient; otherwise, all the medical knowledge in the world will not relieve the patient's suffering.

Formulating a Clinically Relevant Question Using PICO Structure

As mentioned in Chapter 2, a clinically relevant question regarding therapy is formatted using PICO, which is an acronym that stands for patient population, intervention, comparison, and outcome. The key component of constructing this question is making the question relate to the patient's dilemma that we discussed above. It has to be relevant to the patient's concern based on the conversation listed when we were acquiring enough information to understand the patient's concern. Once again, before we embark on a long process, it is important to make sure that we are answering the patient's clinically relevant question. At times, physicians also have questions that they need to answer to provide good care, but we want to make absolutely certain that we do not answer the physician's question while avoiding the patient's question. This is a process that must stay narrow and focused. Asking too many clinical questions simultaneously will become frustrating and unproductive. Strict criteria to keep the focus on the patient's concern will not only simplify the process, but also be an invaluable guidepost to keep the process on track.

STORY TIME

We once had a patient who complained about a scratching feeling 'under her heart.' It only lasted a second, so it was quite atypical and something a doctor would dismiss as inconsequential. By following the narrative thread, we were able to ask, 'What is it that you are afraid of?' To which the patient replied, 'I think I'm about to have a heart attack when that happens.' This answer was a surprise to us, since that wasn't even being considered in the differential diagnosis. By providing an alternative explanation, the patient replied, 'I am so relieved.' The cardiologist who had been previously consulted had reviewed the chart only – not spoken to the patient – and called to say that he thought the patient's condition was completely explained by a chronic pulmonary condition. We explained that the patient's real concern was these transient bodily symptoms that seemed to us to be associated with PVCs, an issue that the patient wanted addressed by a cardiologist. We had to tell the cardiologist that he actually had to talk (listen) to the patient and answer the question we raised in the consult.

The point of the story is ... you need to listen to the patient to discover the narrative dilemma; it can't be done with a medical chart or results of tests only.

NARRATIVE ASPECTS OF ASKING A CLINICAL QUESTION ABOUT THERAPY

There is a qualitative difference between experiencing and understanding symptoms and actively doing something to change the body, such as take medications or consider surgery. Changing the body seems to have a higher threshold – or greater narrative task – than simply understanding what is going on. After all, if we change the body then we change ourselves. We have noted that it often takes time for patients to 'warm up' to potential therapies. We always allow the patient time to accept the new narrative thread of changing their body by taking a pill. Although we prescribe medications on a routine basis, consider the narrative task of the patient – they have to understand their body and themselves in a different way, going from 'being healthy' to 'needing a pill to maintain health.' That is not an easy transition to make. By giving the patient time to consider this transition, it seems that adherence is improved in the long run. After all, if the story does not make sense to the patient, why would they act on it?

APPLICATION TO OUR CLINICAL CASE SCENARIO

Our patient is very concerned because of her family history. She is afraid that what happened to her loved ones is going to happen to her. Although we discussed risk factors and we evaluated her clinical status as low probability of coronary disease present at this time. She is concerned about preventing disease in the future and replicating the abandonment she felt in the past for her son Jason, whom she thinks needs her help raising his child. The doctor has tried to discuss cholesterol lowering pills in the past, but the patient was never interested in those 'chemicals.' Now, that she has dealt with her concern about coronary artery disease, she is more open to the discussion about what she can do to prevent having a heart attack. In this case, our conversation led us to the fact that our patient needs to decide whether to treat with lipid lowering medicines, specifically statins, as a primary prevention in a moderate risk patient. As clinicians, we know that lack of stenotic coronary arteries is not the same as protection against future heart attacks.[1] Notice how the doctor's concern and the patient's concern have converged from clogs versus vulnerable plaque to both the doctor and the patient are concerned about preventing future events. It is clear that the patient was not ready to address this issue until her fear of 'clogs' was addressed. Now she is 'on the same page' with the doctor about vulnerable plaque and the chances of her being adherent to this type of therapy skyrocketed because the story has evolved; this is the co-constructed narrative.

The structure of question using the PICO format using the following:

P = Patient Population: Patients at risk for coronary artery disease.
I = Intervention: Statins.
C = Comparison: Placebo.
O = Outcome: Mortality reduction.

Using these terms we can formulate our patient's concern in the following PICO question: *in patients at risk for coronary artery disease, do statins reduce mortality?*

A CONTINGENT, EMERGENT, SITUATED, AND CONTEXTUAL MEDICAL KNOWLEDGE

The *contingent* nature of asking the question about statins is that the patient may or may not decide to proceed and initiate treatment; both possibilities are possible at this point in the process. The question does help to frame the actual choices that are part of the contingent issues the doctor and the patient are exploring.

The clinically relevant question is *situated* within the narrative after the emotionally difficult decision to have a test for coronary artery disease and before a contingent future of illness or disease and early death. Although the doctor initiated the discussion of statins (remember that the patient asked if she could go now ...), the doctor raised the question within the narrative framework that the patient and doctor are co-constructing. This question is relevant to the patient's ongoing narrative concerns.

The clinical question *emerged* out of the background of the patient's concerns. It *emerged* because of the ongoing story. This discussion is based on what happened before. Had the CT coronary angiogram been positive for disease, the issue of taking statins would have emerged in a completely different way – and the clinical question would have changed. The medical literature associated with treating established CAD is a completely different body of literature. This story would be quite different.

We live in a society where 'knowing your cholesterol' is common practice. Consider a different *context*, such as sub-Saharan Africa – who cares what your cholesterol is if you face the difficulties of life as lived there?

REFERENCE

1   Nissen SE. Limitation of computed tomography coronary angiography. *Journal of the American College of Cardiology.* 2008; **52**: 252145–7.

Access Information Relevant to the Question

KEY CONCEPTS TO REMEMBER

➤ Google Scholar performs the best amongst the current technology to find relevant medical literature. PubMed performs best to locate the comprehensive bibliography.

➤ Continuous learning is required to stay current with technological advances. The skills necessary to evaluating the scholarship of the medical literature remains timeless.

➤ Foraging has evaluative elements embedded in it. It is important to know how to evaluate medical literature to forage for information efficiently.

➤ You can stay current in your medical knowledge when you use this process to investigate tips and leads from patients and consultants. Stay curious.

➤ It is important to understand the strengths and weaknesses of EBM databases and websites.

LEARNING ABOUT ACCESSING INFORMATION

Using Google Scholar while Foraging for Therapy Information

As demonstrated previously, we will rely on Google Scholar, using all of the specific search techniques discussed in Chapter 3. As we mentioned, technology changes and at this point we are using Google Scholar. During the writing of this book, a new search engine, BING, was launched. We tested using the search terms both in the diagnosis section and in the therapy section. In the first instance we got only consumer related sites and none related to original research. For the therapy section, we did get some scholarly journals, but the relevance of the articles was very low. Remember that we liked Google Scholar because the specificity of the search results was so high. For the foreseeable future, Google Scholar seems to be in the lead. Remember, this is where keeping up to date with new technologies is vitally important – who knows what technological development will replace Google Scholar. It should be pointed out that the actual scholarship parts of the process will maintain their relevance, so learning this method is still based on the doctor–patient relationship and the ability to access and manipulate, analyze and apply information at the site of care for the benefit of our patients.

A Closer Look at Foraging for Information

Since this is the second time we are addressing the issue of foraging, it is fair to point out that we really are evaluating the information as we are searching for the information. This is to make the foraging more efficient. Pharmaceutical industry sponsored papers are easy to spot because the intervention is often not matched with an appropriate comparison group of patients. If it is matched with placebo and not the prevailing standard of care, we call these papers 'straw man analysis,' since the comparison group is so easy to knock down. We also are eliminating papers with poor methods and inadequately powered studies. So, that means that having a good knowledge base of how to evaluate medical literature is necessary to forage for information efficiently. Remember, it takes practice. If it does not work the first couple of times, ask yourself where you got off track. It is always a good idea to think carefully before following any hyperlink. Remember it is easy to get lost.

Another useful situation for foraging is when a specialist recommends an unrecognized or bizarre therapy. It is always good to check it out and see for yourself the basis of the recommendation. As mentioned before, the truth value of the information needs to be part of the honest story we tell the patient. Never pretend our recommendations are worth more than they actually are. We will talk more about this when we discuss the SORT Criteria for ranking the quality of the evidence. (You narrativists out there will recognize this as 'fore-shadowing,' or hinting at things that might lie in our near future.)

EBM Websites and Databases

Over the past five years, we have consistently used the Centre for Evidence Based Medicine.[1] To date, there has been nothing to make us change our fundamental preference. This site offers a wealth of information. We do not have to memorize the URL – simply type in the name in a Google search and you'll find it. We do not memorize EBM equations; they are always available within a couple clicks of the mouse. For beginners there is an excellent glossary and review of research methodologies (similar to Chapter 3). There is also a chart used to grade evidence that is tied more closely to study type and quality; we propose the alternative, simpler method to grade the quality of the evidence (the SORT method),[2] but you should be aware of both systems. The website is updated frequently and has great depth of information as well as information on continuing education.

For us, the most useful tool is the interactive Nomogram for using Likelihood Ratios. This is an interactive version of the Fagan nomogram[3] that allows you to quickly compare a range of pre-test probabilities and on a contingent basis decide if it will change medical decision making. This is useful if you or your group of colleagues come up with different estimates of the pre-test probability.

As we mentioned earlier, if the studies for a given test are small (small N or number of cases studied), the 95% confidence intervals will be large. We can easily check what would happen to the clinical decision if the original research was skewed and the real sensitivity and specificity were at the lower end of the range reported. This same technique can be used if there are two studies that do not agree. We can check out both sets of test characteristics and ask ourselves if that would change medical decision making. All of this points to the fact that the interactive nomogram allows us to efficiently deal with the contingencies we encounter when evaluating and applying the medical research.

Of course the major contingency is to preview different clinical scenarios before you order the test and know whether it is positive or negative. If the test characteristics are poor and pre-test probability is mid-range, then doing the test probably has no value whether or not it is positive or negative. It would be good to check this out before ordering the test.

Another 'gem' buried inside this website is access to the TRIP (Turning Research into Practice) evidence based database. We have found this to be one of the easiest and relevant databases around. It draws from some of the other proprietary databases, so it is somewhat of a 'back-door' to information that otherwise requires a subscription fee. This feature replicates the more traditional EBM infrastructure that requires outside vendors to process information for the busy clinician who does not have time for EBM.[4] We of course perceive the situation to be totally different – a paradigm change – in the way EBM is practiced. But for now, it is important to know where to look for it within the Centre for Evidence Based Medicine's website. It is a useful tool for patient care when foraging gets tough.

Evidence Databases/Resources

Remember in the Preface we referred to a clinician who despaired of EBM ever being useful enough for clinicians to implement? Over the past decade, there has been a substantial change. Much effort has been put into synthesizing medical research and writing systematic reviews with graded evidence. Like any new business, there has been some 'shake-out', e.g. Info Retriever became part of Essential Evidence, etc. There are now about 10 major competitors, most all of whom are subscription based (they cost money). All have their advantages and disadvantages. Some of the major ones include:

➤ E-Medicine.
➤ Essential Evidence.
➤ Evidence Matters.
➤ Guideline Clearinghouse.
➤ Cochrane Library.

➤ Database of Abstracts of Reviews of Effects (DARE).
➤ Dynamed.
➤ OVID EBMR.
➤ ACP Journal Club.
➤ Bandolier.
➤ Clinical Evidence.

Remember that each of these resources originated with the concept that doctors required 'middlemen' to do the work of accessing and evaluating the quality of the medical literature. We fundamentally disagree with this assumption – doctors of the future need to be able to access research, evaluate it, and apply it at the site of care. This essentially cuts out the 'middlemen.' We acknowledge that this is unorthodox and some might say blasphemous position to take, but all of these services share the same Achilles heel. The research used as base material and the questions generated and answered are ALL from the doctor's perspective, many times using disease oriented evidence. This fundamental bias of giving pre-eminence to the questions doctors think are important replicates the 'Translational' flaw from research to practice within a social context. We foresee a future where clinicians are much more closely connected to the original research and are able to deploy it in the exam room. So, we suggest doctors subscribe to *one* of these services and interact with it on a consistent basis, building a knowledge base sufficient to do this type of work. We refer to this as a 'reading service.' We pay someone to scan, select, read, and report medical literature as *foundational knowledge* to practicing EBM. Our preferred reading service is Primary Care Medical Abstracts (www. ccme.org/PCMA/index-frame.html). We subscribe to the Audio CD version and listen during commuting time. Not only is the study data reported, but there is always a careful review of the research methodology and a perspective about how to apply the information to practice – the patient perspective is represented. Not surprisingly, we appreciate the social perspective that is also provided. We are all biased to some degree, but PCMA allows us to 'make up our own mind' about the literature because we feel free to disagree with the interpretation of the data. After a while, you will realize that the medical literature is like a soap opera. There are episodes where important questions get reported frequently and you build a sense of how the research story is structured. They even 'write characters out' of the medical literature, such as the IIb-IIIa inhibitors.

By saying that, we also imply that an EBM database will not transform your practice – you have to do that. Where we differ from orthodox approach to EBM is that the patient is part of the process. Technology was made for man; man was not made for technology.

STORY TIME

We once had a patient come in and ask for a shingles vaccine. We did not even know if a shingles vaccine existed (it was relatively new at the time). Using the foraging techniques reviewed in this book, we were able to find the one randomized controlled trial demonstrating efficacy. This was undoubtedly the trial that the Food and Drug Administration used to approve the vaccine for clinical use.

The point of the story is ... We can learn from our patients since they tell us what is important to them. Quickly re-educating ourselves in this fast paced world of changing medicine requires that we find and be able to analyze clinical information quickly.

NARRATIVE ASPECTS OF ACCESSING INFORMATION

The type of information that is or is not available creates the narrative choices for our patients. Remember, the patient's life story is not a finished work of art. There are still choices to be made. For many years we told our patients to 'ask me again next year,' about the value of PSA screening for prostate cancer. Now we share the PLCO trial[5] and the European trial[6] data. As the evidence changes, so does the story.

In a similar way, publication of the ACCORD trial[7] and the ADVANCE trial[8] changed daily conversations in the exam room. Even though our institution, the American Diabetic Association, and HEDIS monitors continue to emphasize and reward decreasing A1C levels, the evidence simply does not support this. This is a case where a surrogate marker and pathophysiologic evidence contradicts Patient Oriented Evidence. Patients really struggle with daily life when they live with diabetes. Rather than engage in a power struggle to force behaviors related to lowering blood sugars, we emphasize statins, metformin, healthy eating, physical activity, retinal exams, foot care and other common sense health measures. The publication of these two trials changed the way we perceived our own role in the co-constructed narratives of our patients with diabetes. Although we have changed our practice, we also perceive a lack of change in our colleagues who are not so attuned to the evidence.

APPLICATION TO OUR CLINICAL SCENARIO

Recall that the search terms come directly from the PICO question, 'In patients at risk for coronary artery disease, do statins reduce mortality?' Let us try the following search terms in Google Scholar: risk, coronary, artery, disease, statin, mortality reduction.

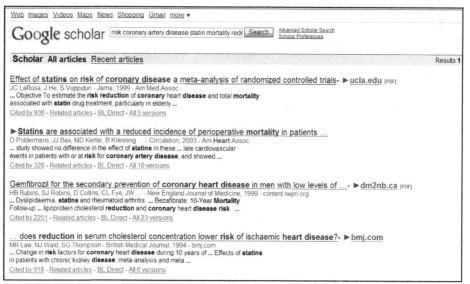

Figure 9.1 Foraging for Information on Statin Therapy.

The first article looks excellent. It is a large meta-analysis directly related to our clinical question. We may not have to look further; however, it might still be important to see if there is additional information published more recently. We can check this with advanced search by adjusting the search dates. We choose 2007–2009 and get the following results:

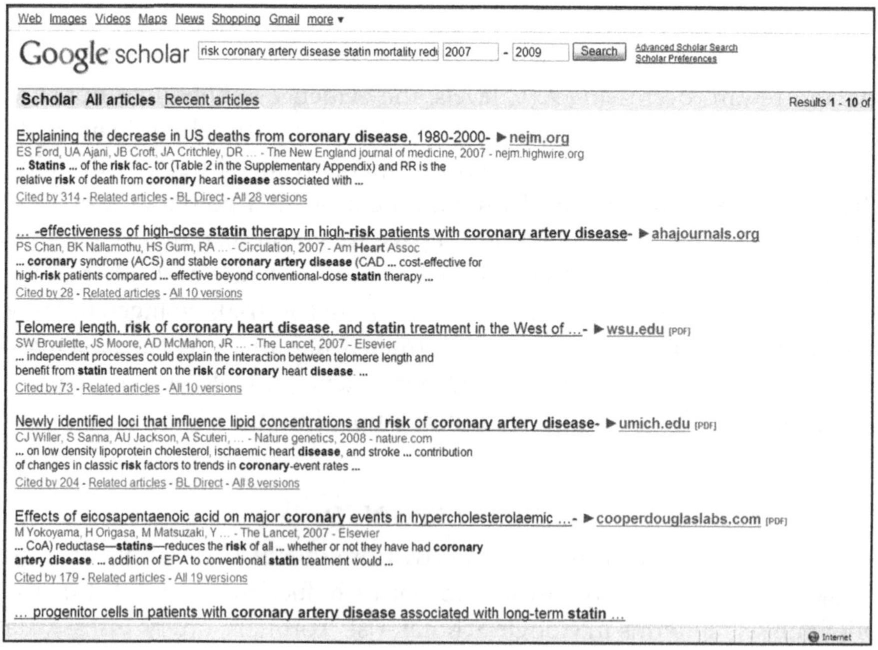

Figure 9.2 Foraging for Information on Statin Therapy Using Advanced Scholar.

Scanning these, it is pretty clear that this search yielded less relevant results and our original search has a low probability of being improved upon. With this additional search we felt confident that our original search returned the best results for our patient's concern. We decided that we did not need to look further. From our experience, the search is often this quick and easy; however, occasionally a more lengthy process as illustrated in Chapter 3 is required. The reason this example was so short is because high quality meta-analysis is available. When the development of the medical literature only includes multiple small, poorly designed studies a lengthier search is required to convince us that we have the most relevant information.

The study selection criteria for this meta-analysis were clearly identified in following abstract:

Effect of Statins on Risk of Coronary Disease
A Meta-analysis of Randomized Controlled Trials

John C. LaRosa, MD

Jiang He, MD, PhD

Suma Vupputuri, MPH

Context Lowering low-density lipoprotein cholesterol (LDL-C) is known to reduce risk of recurrent coronary heart disease in middle-aged men. However, this effect has been uncertain in elderly people and women.

Objective To estimate the risk reduction of coronary heart disease and total mortality associated with statin drug treatment, particularly in elderly individuals and women.

Data Sources Trials published in English-language journals were retrieved by searching MEDLINE (1966–December 1998), bibliographies, and authors' reference files.

Study Selection Studies in which participants were randomized to statin or control treatment for at least 4 years and clinical disease or death was the primary outcome were included in the meta-analysis (5 of 182 initially identified).

Data Extraction Information on sample size, study drug duration, type and dosage of statin drug, participant characteristics at baseline, reduction in lipids during intervention, and outcomes was abstracted independently by 2 authors (J.H. and S.V.) using a standardized protocol. Disagreements were resolved by consensus.

Data Synthesis Data from the 5 trials, with 30817 participants, were included in this meta-analysis. The mean duration of treatment was 5.4 years. Statin drug treatment was associated with a 20% reduction in total cholesterol, 28% reduction in LDL-C, 13% reduction in triglycerides, and 5% increase in high-density lipoprotein cholesterol. Overall, statin drug treatment reduced risk 31% in major coronary events (95% confidence interval [CI], 26%-36%) and 21% in all-cause mortality (95% CI, 14%-28%). The risk reduction in major coronary events was similar between women (29%; 95% CI, 13%-42%) and men (31%; 95% CI, 26%-35%), and between persons aged at least 65 years (32%; 95% CI, 23%-39%) and persons younger than 65 years (31%; 95% CI, 24%-36%).

Conclusions Our meta-analysis indicates that reduction in LDL-C associated with statin drug treatment decreases the risk of coronary heart disease and all-cause mortality. The risk reduction was similar for men and women and for elderly and middle-aged persons.

JAMA. 1999;282:2340-2346   www.jama.com

Figure 9.3 Statin Therapy Meta-Analysis Abstract. Reprinted from *JAMA*. **282**(24): 2340. LaRosa JC, He J, Vupputuri S, Effect of statins on risk of coronary disease: a meta-analysis of randomized controlled trials. Copyright (1999), American Medical Association. All rights reserved.

This meta-analysis is definitive evidence; it would be quite hard to accumulate more or better information than is presented here. This is essentially a distillation of all the major randomized controlled trials.

Note that only five of 182 trials were included. If these five trials had not been done, our search would have resulted in multiple small trials with variable methodological quality. As you gain more experience using Google Scholar, these patterns will become recognizable and you will learn to assess a 'body of literature' more quickly. It takes practice.

Assessing for Comprehensiveness in PubMed

Once again, we took the meta-analysis located in our Google Scholar search and re-located the paper in PubMed and followed the link to 'related citations.'

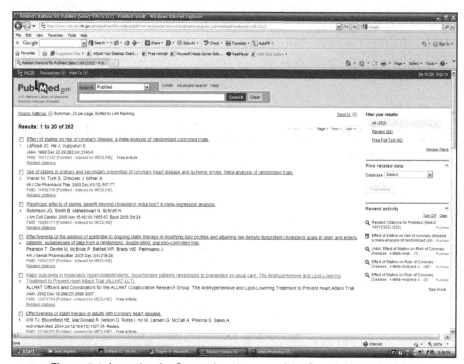

Figure 9.4 Assessing for Comprehensiveness of the Search Using PubMed.

After reviewing the first three pages of results, we found three more meta-analyses of statin therapy.[9-11] Notice that each contained a different number of original research trials (10, 62, 14 trials respectively). The additional studies were published later than the original trial. The results were all consistent with our original meta-analysis, so once again, we are confident that we have comprehensively searched the medical literature for relevant research.

Evaluating the quality of a meta-analysis is beyond the scope of this book. We would prefer to reinforce some of the concepts on how to evaluate and apply original research. For that reason, we are going to choose the first of the five large trials included in the meta-analysis for further discussion. It is significant that there are only five trials included in the meta-analysis from our original Google Scholar search. This means that the authors were careful to select high quality trials.

Table 1. Characteristics of 5 Randomized Controlled Cholesterol-Lowering Trials Using Statin Drugs*

Characteristics	4S[1] (1994)	WOSCOPS[3] (1995)	CARE[4,5] (1996)	AFCAPS/TexCAPS[7] (1998)	LIPID[8] (1998)
No. of participants	4444	6595	4159	6605	9014
Follow-up, mean, y	5.4	4.9	5.0	5.2	6.1
Study drug	Simvastatin	Pravastatin	Pravastatin	Lovastatin	Pravastatin
Baseline data					
Age, mean, y	59	55	59	58	62
Age ≥65 y, %	23	0	31	21	39
Women, %	19	0	14	15	17
History of myocardial infarction, %	79	0	100	0	64
Cholesterol level, mean, mmol/L†					
Total cholesterol	6.75	7.03	5.40	5.71	5.64
LDL-C	4.87	4.97	3.59	3.89	3.88
HDL-C	1.19	1.14	1.01	0.95	0.93
Triglycerides	1.50	1.84	1.76	1.78	1.58
Net change in lipid levels, mean, %					
Total cholesterol	−26	−20	−20	−19	−18
LDL-C	−36	−26	−28	−27	−25
HDL-C	+7	+5	+5	+5	+5
Triglycerides	−17	−12	−14	−13	−11

*4S indicates Scandinavian Simvastatin Survival Study; WOSCOPS, West of Scotland Coronary Prevention Study; CARE, Cholesterol and Recurrent Events trial; AFCAPS/TexCAPS, Air Force/Texas Coronary Atherosclerosis Prevention Study; LIPID, Long-term Intervention With Pravastatin in Ischaemic Disease trial; LDL-C, low-density lipoprotein cholesterol; and HDL-C, high-density lipoprotein cholesterol.
†To convert total cholesterol, HDL-C, and LDL-C from mmol/L to mg/dL, divide by 0.02586. To convert triglycerides from mmol/L to mg/dL, divide by 0.01129.

Figure 9.5 Table 1 from Meta-Analysis. Reprinted from *JAMA.* **282**(24): 2342. LaRosa JC, He J, Vupputuri S, Effect of statins on risk of coronary disease: a meta-analysis of randomized controlled trials. Copyright (1999), American Medical Association. All rights reserved.

Looking at the above table, there are five trials that we can take a closer look at. The study populations were generally similar and under-represented women. The subsequent meta-analyses found in the PubMed search all found similar 'size effect' that is larger than the study we will use as an example, but smaller than the largest effect in the original meta-analysis. For actual patient care, we would synthesize this information and try to use what we consider to be the best estimate for the 'real number.' However, let us select the Scandinavian Simvastatin Survival Study to use as an example only for the purposes of illustrating the lessons of EBM in this book. This particular clinical trial is also called 'the 4S trial' and it changed clinical practice in the 1990s. (Something we call 'seminal literature' – the ability to change clinical practice.) It provided some of the first patient oriented evidence. Prior to that, we knew that statins lowered cholesterol but we did not know they lowered mortality. This is the difference between DOE and POEM, a threshold that was crossed with the publication of this trial. Another reason we chose to proceed with the actual data from the 4S trial is that this research article is commonly used as a teaching example for learning EBM.

A CONTINGENT, EMERGENT, SITUATED, AND CONTEXTUAL MEDICAL KNOWLEDGE

Foraging for information is *contingent* because we do not know what we are going to find. The *contingency* remains until we choose what information to use.

The *emergent* nature of the information is a result of search strategies. We are continually filtering information, looking for relevant, high quality information. As the information is filtered, *information with specific characteristics emerges*.

This particular foraging journey shows how the information is **situated in time**, as subsequent meta-analyses confirmed the first and original POEM trial (the 4S trial). The information retrieved is also *situated within the patient's narrative dilemma* – should she take the pill or not?

The *context* is highlighted in this search by the variability seen in the meta-analyses, each choosing different randomized controlled trials to analyze. The criteria for choosing those particular trials were determined by the search criteria – the *context* of the author's intentions – within a building body of scientific research. It would probably no longer be ethical to do a trial of statin versus placebo, since we know that statins prevent death in this population. Thus the context of the studies has determined what can and cannot be done at this point and therefore the types of questions that can be researched. We have to accept what we have, with all the strengths and weaknesses of these trials, because we cannot go back to the early 1990s and change the study method designs.

REFERENCES

1 www.cebm.net/ (accessed December 10, 2010).
2 Ebell M, Siwik J, Weiss B, *et al.* Strength of recommendation taxonomy (SORT): a patient-centered approach to grading evidence in the medical literature. *Journal of American Board of Family Practice.* 2004; **17**: 59–67.
3 Fagan T. Nomogram for Bayes's Theorem. *New England Journal of Medicine.* 1975; **293**(5): 297.
4 Glasziou P, Haynes B. The paths from research to improved health outcomes. *ACP Journal Club.* 2005; **142**(2): A-8–A-10.
5 Andriole G, Crawford D, Grubb R, *et al.* Mortality results from a randomized prostate cancer screening trial. *New England Journal of Medicine.* 2009; **360**(13): 1310–19.
6 Schroder F, Hugosson J, Roobol M, *et al.* Screening and prostate-cancer mortality in a randomized European study. *New England Journal of Medicine.* 2009; **360**(13): 1320–8.
7 ACCORD SG. Effects of intensive glucose lowering in type 2 diabetes. *New England Journal of Medicine.* 2008; **358**(24): 2545–59.
8 ADVANCE SG. Intensive blood glucose control and vascular outcomes in patients with type 2 diabetes. *New England Journal of Medicine.* 2008; **358**(24): 2560–72.
9 Gould A, Davies G, Alemao E, *et al.* Cholesterol reduction yields clinical benefits: meta-analysis including recent trials. *Clin Ther.* 2007; **29**(5): 778–94.
10 Cheung B, Lauder I, Lau C, *et al.* Meta-analysis of large randomized controlled trials to evaluate the impact of statins on cardiovascular outcomes. *Br J Clin Pharmacol.* 2004; **57**(5): 640–51.
11 Baigent C, Keech A, Kearney P, *et al.* Efficacy and safety of cholesterol-lowering treatment: prospective mea-analysis of data from 90,056 participants in 14 randomized trials of statins. *The Lancet.* 2005; **366**(9493): 1267–78.

Assess the Quality of the Information

KEY CONCEPTS TO REMEMBER

➤ The influence of the pharmaceutical industry on research publications is vastly underestimated – beware.

➤ The research question should be stated clearly. Focus on how the study groups were defined, selected, and monitored; identify the main outcome measure. Ignore other data and results, because they are usually derived from subgroup analyses and therefore less valid.

➤ Be wary of combination endpoints.

➤ It is not necessary to be a statistician to evaluate research design, but knowing a few terms and what they mean can be helpful.

➤ There is a standard set of research methodology questions that should be answered when evaluating any article on therapy. If the quality of the study is so poor that you do not believe the conclusion, do not bother taking the time and effort to review it in detail. Cut your losses; time is precious.

LEARNING ABOUT ASSESSING THE QUALITY OF RESEARCH

We present a couple of topics that we believe to be important and then review the standard questions to evaluate research articles related to therapy.

Pharmaceutical Industry and the Medical Literature: A Cautionary Tale

Recently, ghost writing by the pharmaceutical industry with subsequent recruiting with honoraria of academic investigators to serve as principle 'authors' of clinical trials was documented.[1, 2] The practice is extended throughout the entire course of generating research, from study design to analysis and writing. This is done by an intermediary company that then recruits ghost authors.[3] We have already expressed some concerns about the validity of meta-analyses compared to how they are revered by EBM aficionados. There is evidence that these prestigious articles are heavily influenced by pharmaceutical funding.[4] The problem extends to peer reviewers and other aspects of producing medical literature. One study compared Cochrane Reviews to published meta-analyses and, not surprisingly, there was a difference in quality and recommendations, with Cochrane reviews more conservative and other published meta-analyses favorable to the experimental drug.[5] Additionally, journals get a financial 'kick-back' for large quantities of reprints that are then used by pharmaceutical companies and the drug representatives they hire.[6] These examples only deal with how the medical literature is produced. We need to be cautious about what we cite as 'evidence.'

Some Statistical Terms

Most doctors cringe when they hear the word statistics even more than when they hear the word research. Let us reassure you that however uncomfortable you are with statistics, you can still follow the process of care outlined in this book. That is because 95% of evaluating the validity of a research paper is being able to understand the design and magnitude of the bias. Statistics are helpful, but less important.[7] It is time for true confessions. One of the two authors has taken many courses in statistics and is a real 'geek,' while the other hasn't, but we both teach evidence based medicine and use the processes in this book with equal success. For busy practitioners, we recommend the two books by Katz on statistics for clinicians.[8, 9]

Research is About Measuring Things

Variables are things that are measured. We measure things by counting them, ranking them, or assigning a number to them. These three different types of measurements describe three types of variables. The three ways of measuring variables are used for three types of data – nominal, ordinal, and ratio data.

Nominal (Also Called Categorical) Data are Counted

What we are counting is the number of items in each category. Let us count the numbers of people with red hair. We hope you see the problem – how red does the hair have to be before we call it red hair? If we use two categories, then it is red hair or not red hair. If it is flame red; tinted red; or brown, black, blond and all others, there are more categories. So, with the type of data and measurement a research study is using, the most important thing is how the researchers defined their categories. Often we take this for granted, but do not be fooled. Categories such as 'has coronary artery disease' are devilishly difficult to define.

Ordinal Data are Ranked

The most common ranked data are from surveys that use a Likert scale such as none, some, less than half, about half, more than half, many, almost all, etc. The intervals cannot be equally spaced and the importance of knowing that when using such data is to verify that the appropriate statistic is used to interpret the data. The biggest mistake is to add the numbers up from each of the questions and pretend they are ratio data. This is common practice, but theoretically wrong.

Ratio Data are Numbers

Where $1 + 1 = 2$ and $4 \div 2 = 2$ is the most informative type of data. We should note that you can always collapse the data from ratio to ordinal or nominal, but you can never go the other way.

What is a Statistic?

Most studies use two different types of statistics – *descriptive statistics and inferential statistics.* Let us explore descriptive statistics first. Like the name says, descriptive statistics use numbers to describe a data set. To describe nominal data, researchers report how many cases were counted in each category. This describes the distribution of the data. For ratio data, the description involves not only how many cases there were, but reports the mean (median, mode) and standard deviation. The standard deviation again describes the dispersion or distribution (the shape of) the data set. We all know this as the bell shaped curve. The standard deviation is simply an algebraic equation that converts the data into a central tendency (mean) and distribution (how spread out the data looks on a graph). Again, descriptive statistics describe – they describe data sets and are a standardized way of reporting them. It is a description by convention.

Inferential statistics use (surprisingly) *statistics,* which are simple equations that describe an expected distribution of data. By comparing the actual distribution to the expected distribution, you can infer that they are different [or not]. Different equations are used to compare the two groups depending on the types of variable (nominal, ordinal, or ratio data) of each of the two (or more) groups. Notice that you can compare the height (ratio data) between boys and girls (nominal data). This would be done with the typical Student's T-test (assuming that boys and girls were randomly sampled from the larger group called human beings.)

So far we have been talking about inferring difference between two groups at a particular moment in time. Often, we observe treatment groups over time (time series) and these data sets are recorded differently and use different statistics (equations) to compare the treatment group to the comparator group.

In order to choose the correct statistic (equation), you have to know the type of data (categorical/nominal, ordinal, ratio) of the independent and the dependent variable. In experimental research designs, the variable you change is the independent variable and it comes earlier in time than the dependent variable, which is the one that you measure later. We like to call the dependent variable the outcome variable. Again, the most important thing (which is brought out in the research methodology questions) is how well the researchers define what the outcome being measured actually is.

Probability

Because *statistics are used to describe probabilities* that the data distribution occurred by chance alone (compared to the predicted distribution described by the statistical equation), you can never say for sure that two groups are the same. You can say that it would be very rare, or improbable that they are the same. If the comparison is so unlikely to be the same, we reject the (null) hypothesis that they are the same and call them different – because the probability of them being the same is so unlikely that it is unbelievable. A p value is the probability that the distributions of the two data sets are the same – so an incredibly small p value means there is an incredibly small chance that the two data sets are sampling from the same group. We just do not believe it. We usually set the level of unbelievability at 5% or less ($p <= 0.05$), but the smaller the p value lower the probability that the two groups are similar. When the p value shows a very small probability that the two data sets are samples of the same set, we call it 'statistically significant.' These are almost like magic words in research, but do not overestimate their utility – clinically significant differences are more important than statistically significant differences.

We know that all these numbers are in relationship to each other. If there are a very small number of cases, it is difficulty to show a difference. Any data set can show a difference if there are enough cases, but the difference is going to be incredibly small, so small that nobody cares. Always check the real difference in size between the groups and decide if it would change decisions.

Again, we are not trying to make you into statisticians; it is helpful to understand what researchers are counting and what they are using to compare different groups. Remember, the study design tells you more about the quality of the study than the statistics, which are only used to compare the groups.

Therapeutic Article Research Questions

In Chapter 4, we discussed universal questions that can be used to discuss the quality of the article being analyzed. The questions in Chapter 4 were for diagnostic studies. A similar set of questions can be used for therapeutic studies. These questions assist the clinician in determining the quality of the research articles generated by the search. The questions for a therapeutic study are as follows:

1. Was the Assignment of Patients to Treatments really Randomized?

The importance of randomization can easily be understood by thinking about a research study where patients are not randomized. Examples of this include open labeled trials where clinicians may unconsciously steer sicker patients towards the treatment group hoping for a better outcome for their patient. This is just being a good doctor, but does not lead to good quality research.

Adequate randomization is the most important methodological feature in a therapeutic study as it equally distributes the confounding factors among the study groups thereby isolating the therapy as the single differentiation between the two groups, resulting in an adequate assessment of the therapy itself. The equalization of confounding factors is important because there could be many reasons for a response to an individual therapy. If confounding factors are not controlled for by randomization, the strength of the evidence to infer cause and effect (treatment and outcome) is impaired.

There are multiple standard, acceptable methods for randomization. In many multi-centered studies, block randomization is used to eliminate between-center biases. (Each center enrolls proportionately similar number of patients into each group.) Generally though, assignment to the groups is considered random if each an every patient has an equal probability of being assigned to any one of the groups. The process of randomization should be described in the methods section. To demonstrate that randomization occurred appropriately, multiple demographic descriptors are always described in 'Table 1.' The assumption here is that if gender, age, co-morbidities, etc. are equal in the two groups, then other potential biases are also equally distributed and randomization worked. It is important to evaluate Table 1. The authors are not required to report all relevant baseline demographics. For example, in a study that examines coronary artery disease treatment, are there more smokers in the control group? How do the authors define 'smokers?' The experimental group might look better because the smokers are a sicker population of patients – not because the experimental intervention conferred benefit.

2. Were All Clinically Relevant Outcomes Reported?

To determine whether or not a specific therapy worked, the researchers have to specifically mention outcome measures. Usually these are divided into primary outcome measure and a series of secondary outcome measures. In family medicine, we are very careful to distinguish patient orientated outcomes and disease oriented outcomes (as discussed in Chapter 2).

Another important concept highlighted by this question is combination endpoints. A combination endpoint is defined as multiple different outcomes that are aggregated to determine if the therapy worked. In the article, 'Benazepril plus amlodipine or hydrochlorothiazide for hypertension in high-risk patients'[10] the researchers compared the combination of benazepril with amlodipine to benazepril with hydrochlorothiazide to determine if the amlodipine combination pill was better. They used the combination endpoint of death from cardiovascular causes, nonfatal myocardial infarction, nonfatal stroke, hospitalization for angina, resuscitation after sudden cardiac arrest, and coronary revascularization. The authors claimed that the amlodipine combination pill was 'superior.' Statistically, that may be true when all of these endpoints are added together, but only one endpoint, myocardial infarction, was statistically significant by itself. Also, a statistical purist would suggest that because multiple outcomes were measured, the appropriate p value to determine 'statistically significant' should be adjusted (Bonferroni correction). Myocardial infarction reduction is certainly a patient oriented outcome; however, the authors did not provide any data for that outcome so that we could independently determine how significant it was. In other words, was there a big difference in MI or just a small difference? The authors were able to manipulate the numbers to make their claim, and sell more drugs. The literature is saturated with such articles. It is important that you are able to recognize this so that you can help your patient make a decision that meets their needs.

Another frequent study design flaw has been called the 'straw-man analysis.' This is when a new or experimental drug is not compared to the standard of care, but to an alternative treatment that is known to be inferior to the standard of care. In the 'Comparison of carvedilol and metoprolol on clinical outcomes in patients with chronic heart failure in the Carvedilol Or Metoprolol European Trial (COMET): randomized controlled trial'[11] the authors compared carvedilol 25 mg twice daily to metoprolol 50 mg twice daily and found a very small difference in mortality favoring carvedilol in congestive heart failure patients. The authors concluded, 'Our results suggest that carvedilol extends survival compared with metoprolol.' However, the metoprolol dose used was not the maximal dose used for congestive heart failure patients. Their conclusion was based on a straw man analysis. Would the results have been the same if the proper dose of metoprolol was used? Well, we will never know. There are actually physicians in our academic center that prescribe carvedilol instead of metoprolol based on this biased study .

3. Were the Study Patients Recognizably Similar to Your Own?

We are trying to determine if the therapy is appropriate for our patient. If the study patients are different than our own patient then we might not be able to use the results of the study to help our patient make a decision. In the 'Secondary stroke prevention with low-dose aspirin, sustained release dipyridamole alone and in combination' trial, the authors concluded that aspirin is beneficial for the secondary prevention stroke.[12] However, it cannot be inferred that it is beneficial for primary prevention. The secondary prevention patients are sicker as they have more advanced atherosclerotic disease.

Selection bias also is produced by the way the medical research literature has been produced. Most of the studies are done in tertiary care hospitals which causes a selection bias so that, in fact the patient in the study has a low probability of being similar to your patient in primary care practice. In recent years, this problem has been addressed by the advent of primary care based research networks (PBRN), for example OKPRN, RIOS NET, PEARL NETWORK, SNO-CAP, IMPLICIT NETWORK, etc. A practice based research network is built on the fundamental concept that 'A primary care physician's research laboratory is his/her clinical practice.' This directly addresses the selection bias inherent in referral to academic settings where the population demographics characteristics and similarities of the study population are more closely aligned for practicing physicians. The types of questions asked and answered also have the potential to be more relevant to the practicing physicians. The United States government Agency on Healthcare Research and Quality (AHRQ) has emphasized developments of new knowledge at this level. As with the rest of clinical practice, we certainly expect this to continually evolve. This source of information is emphasized as a reminder of the importance of, 'Were the study patients similar to your own?'

4. Were Both Clinical and Statistical Significance Considered?

The relevance to this question is best illustrated with an example. We once casually reviewed a research article from NEJM where the outcome variable was a score on a questionnaire containing more than 40 questions, but the psychometric reliability and validity of the questionnaire had never been demonstrated. The authors claimed efficacy based on a two- or three-point spread that was 'statistically significant'. We immediately recognized that the *clinical significance* was never addressed. This concept is closely related to patient oriented evidence that matters, described in Chapter 2. The opposite is also true. A trend that does not reach statistical significance may be important, particularly in the early stages in exploring knowledge. This problem is exacerbated by underpowered studies. Unfortunately, there is a severe publication bias against studies that lack 'statistical significance.' This means that those studies are never published.

5. Is the Therapeutic Maneuver Feasible in Your Practice?

In our practice a typical example is immediate angioplasty in the setting of myocardial damage. It is available at large hospitals, but not in the community hospitals in the surrounding area. This produces a clinical dilemma because patients in different geographic locations do not have access to identical therapeutic choices. If you are a treating physician in one of these community hospitals, a study about the benefits of immediate angioplasty is not feasible in your practice.

6. Were All the Patients who Entered the Study Accounted for at its Conclusion?

This question addresses the drop-out rate in the study. It is the researcher's responsibility to design a study that patient's can adhere to. If the study is vigorous, then patients who find the drug ineffective or harmful are more likely to drop out of the study than patients who find the drug beneficial. This creates a bias that favors the experimental drug. If the percentage of cases that are unaccounted for is large relative to the effect size of the outcome measurement, this makes the results un-interpretable. For example, in 'A comparison of cilostazol and pentoxifylline for treating intermittent claudication,' study, 17% dropped out of the study.[13] One can see that the effect size can be totally obscured by the drop out rate. A good rule of thumb is to always check and make sure the numbers add up between enrollment and cases with reported results. That is a measure of drop-out rate which should then be compared to the effect size between the two outcome groups.

7. Were Patients Analyzed in the Groups to Which They Were Randomized?

This is known as intention-to-treat analysis. When reviewing the methods section of a study there should be an explicit statement saying that an intention-to-treat analysis was used. In an intention-to-treat analysis, patients that start in each group need to remain in that group for analysis regardless of adherence to the study protocol. For example, if a patient was in an experimental drug group and they had an adverse reaction, thus stopped taking the experimental drug, then they still need to be counted in the experimental drug group at the time of analysis. This makes sense because when clinicians and patients are trying to decide about a particular therapy, they cannot foresee whether the drug or therapy will be tolerated. By using this type of analysis, the information in the study closely mirrors information relevant to the physician during the time of decision making.

In many studies, this term is used incorrectly. In the above example, 'A comparison of cilostazol and pentoxifylline for treating intermittent claudication,' the authors used a 'run-in' period in which the study subjects were given the study drugs prior to randomization. If the patient could not tolerate the medication, then they were eliminated from the study. Patients who found the experimental medicine intolerable or ineffective were selected out, creating a severe bias favoring the experimental drug.

8. Were All Patients, Health Workers, and Study Personnel Blinded?

The reason a randomized double blind controlled trial is held in such esteem is because it best able to infer cause and effect. Most research attempts to minimize bias or confounding factors that may explain the outcome. In addition to randomization, 'blinding' is an essential part of the study design. Clinicians and investigators are only human and subconsciously or otherwise have preferences about the hypothesis being studied. The researcher wants to see their hypothesis validated. This often has implications for funding, social prestige, or financial incentives. It is also very difficult to invest time and energy which results in a lack of efficacy. Typical sources of bias in non-blinded studies occur during chart reviews, or any result that must be interpreted such as a radiograph outcome. Even assignment to categories can be subjective. Good research minimizes as many types of biases as possible. Blinding allows results to be observed and interpreted by people without invested interest in the outcome.

In addition to the health care workers being blinded, the patients need to be blinded so that the placebo effect can be accounted for. Expectation of improvement can physiologically result in self reported benefit. We encourage our readers to think of placebo as an alternative treatment rather than participants finding benefits in their 'head.'

9. Aside from the Experimental Intervention, Were the Groups Treated Equally?

This is particularly important because of behavioral components of the therapy that might effect outcomes. Simply participating in a research program will have a beneficial effect and if the number of visits or frequency of testing differs then the social variables of receiving 'care' can become a confounding factor. For example, when comparing low molecular weight heparin to unfractionated heparin for the treatment of acute DVT, the nursing staff evaluated the unfractionated heparin group every four hours to check their coags while only evaluating the low molecular weight heparin group every eight hours to check their vitals.[14] If an unfractionated heparin patient was getting sicker, the nurse will recognize it earlier. Thus, affecting the potential adverse outcome rate between the two groups.

STORY TIME

I recently saw a man who came in for a 'yearly check up who requested a screening PSA. I asked him more about his request and he said, 'I'm supposed to get that test at my age.' We have trained our patients to ask for this test without any evidence to support the recommendation. I did our usual routine of explaining what we know, what we do not know, how we know it, and the tradeoffs of getting the test or not getting it. He interrupted me and said, 'To tell you the truth, doctor, it is my wife that wants me to get the test.' It turns out that the whole story involves a new small business venture, pre-conceptual counseling, etc. I realized that the patient's wife needed to have information, as well as the patient, so I printed the PLCO trial[15] and the European Randomized PSA screening trial.[16] I highlighted information in the abstract for the patient to take home, but had to cross out the relative risk reduction on the European trial, because it claimed, 'PSA-based screening reduced the rate of death from prostate cancer by 20%' which is very deceptive because relative risk reduction overstates the benefits. Also, I made an important distinction between the quality of the methodology in the two research trials. I pointed out that neither article addressed the adverse effects of treatment, so there is no way to fairly compare risk of harm versus risk of benefit. I asked him if he was inclined to get the test and he said no. I gave him the lab slip and told him to discuss it with his wife. We then discussed the possible options and choices for screening (none of which meet United States Preventative Services Task Force (USPSTF) standards. He chose to

---

have a digital rectal exam. After I told him the exam was normal he said, 'Thank you.' I replied, 'I don't think I've ever had a guy thank me after that exam.' He said, 'Now I have something to give my wife.'

The point of the story is … that sometimes patients need a narrative answer in order to have the right answer.

NARRATIVE ASPECTS OF ASSESSING THE QUALITY OF THE INFORMATION

As we mentioned in Part I of the book, being able to assess the quality of the research methods allows you to answer the question, 'Do you believe the results? When we ask this question at Journal Club, it is surprising how many times the group disagrees with the claims made by the authors of the articles. If we do not believe the conclusions, why should our patients? It is important to recognize that 'science' is given a pre-eminent position in society and the patient's story is undervalued. When you really scrutinize the evidence, you realize that researchers make up stories too. The story that matters is the one the patient chooses to claim as his/her own. We need to be honest and forthright with what we know, what we pretend to know, and what we 'know.' Remember, 'science' has a fair amount of subjectivity built into the process. Any researcher has to make difficult decisions about the trade-offs in choosing methodological strategies.

APPLICATION TO OUR CLINICAL SCENARIO

Part of our goals for our readers is to encourage them to look at original research literature. For this reason, we are including the complete text of the randomized trial of cholesterol lowering in 4444 patients with coronary heart disease: the Scandinavian Simvastatin Survival Study (4S). When trying to teach others this process, it is important for the reader to understand where to find specific types of information. A standard research article is divided into five sections: abstract, introduction, methods, results, and discussion. Many of the topics we talked about in reviewing methodology are embedded in the methods section. This is where you check for the study type and quality. The results section usually puts most of the relevant information in tables and figures. This requires very careful reading of the titles, headings, groups, types of comparisons, and specific outcomes listed. This is where you screen for the patient orientated evidence and try to ignore subgroup analyses. A good example would be our selections from the diagnostic article where we made the selection for you. This article is reproduced in its entirety. You should practice finding the information in the publication as we discuss it below.

Randomised trial of cholesterol lowering in 4444 patients with coronary heart disease: the Scandinavian Simvastatin Survival Study (4S)

Scandinavian Simvastatin Survival Study Group*

Summary

Drug therapy for hypercholesterolaemia has remained controversial mainly because of insufficient clinical trial evidence for improved survival. The present trial was designed to evaluate the effect of cholesterol lowering with simvastatin on mortality and morbidity in patients with coronary heart disease (CHD). 4444 patients with angina pectoris or previous myocardial infarction and serum cholesterol 5·5–8·0 mmol/L on a lipid-lowering diet were randomised to double-blind treatment with simvastatin or placebo.

Over the 5·4 years median follow-up period, simvastatin produced mean changes in total cholesterol, low-density-lipoprotein cholesterol, and high-density-lipoprotein cholesterol of −25%, −35%, and +8%, respectively, with few adverse effects. 256 patients (12%) in the placebo group died, compared with 182 (8%) in the simvastatin group. The relative risk of death in the simvastatin group was 0·70 (95% CI 0·58–0·85, p=0·0003). The 6-year probabilities of survival in the placebo and simvastatin groups were 87·6% and 91·3%, respectively. There were 189 coronary deaths in the placebo group and 111 in the simvastatin group (relative risk 0·58, 95% CI 0·46–0·73), while noncardiovascular causes accounted for 49 and 46 deaths, respectively. 622 patients (28%) in the placebo group and 431 (19%) in the simvastatin group had one or more major coronary events. The relative risk was 0·66 (95% CI 0·59–0·75, p<0·00001), and the respective probabilities of escaping such events were 70·5% and 79·6%. This risk was also significantly reduced in subgroups consisting of women and patients of both sexes aged 60 or more. Other benefits of treatment included a 37% reduction (p<0·00001) in the risk of undergoing myocardial revascularisation procedures.

This study shows that long-term treatment with simvastatin is safe and improves survival in CHD patients.

Lancet 1994; **344**: 1383–89

*Collaborators and participating centres are listed at the end of the report.

Correspondence to: Dr Terje R Pedersen, Cardiology Section, Medical Department, Aker Hospital, N 0514 Oslo, Norway

Introduction

High serum cholesterol is regarded by many as the main cause of coronary atherosclerosis.[1] Several cholesterol-lowering interventions have reduced coronary heart disease (CHD) events in primary and secondary prevention clinical trials.[2-9] Expert panels in Europe and the USA have therefore recommended dietary changes and, if necessary, addition of drugs to reduce high cholesterol concentrations—specifically low-density-lipoprotein (LDL) cholesterol[10-13]—especially in patients with CHD. However, these recommendations have been questioned,[14,15] mainly because no clinical trial has convincingly shown that lowering of cholesterol prolongs life. Furthermore, overviews of these trials have suggested that survival is not improved, particularly in the absence of established CHD, because the observed reduction of CHD deaths is offset by an apparent increase in non-cardiac mortality, including cancer and violent deaths.[14-18]

Simvastatin is an inhibitor of hydroxy-methylglutaryl coenzyme A (HMG-CoA) reductase, which reduces LDL cholesterol[19,20] to a greater extent than that achieved in previous diet and drug intervention trials. The Scandinavian Simvastatin Survival Study (4S) was conceived in April, 1987, to test the hypothesis that lowering of cholesterol with simvastatin would improve survival of patients with CHD. Other objectives were to study the effect of simvastatin on the incidence of coronary and other atherosclerotic events, and its long-term safety.

Patients and methods

Organisation

The study design has been published previously.[21] Patients were recruited at 94 clinical centres in Scandinavia. A steering committee made up of cardiologists, lipidologists, and epidemiologists had scientific responsibility for the study and all reports of the results. One member was the scientific coordinator who worked closely with the study monitors in the Scandinavian subsidiaries of Merck Research Laboratories. Major study events were classified by an independent endpoint classification committee (two experienced cardiologists) without knowledge of treatment allocation. A data and safety monitoring committee performed independent interim analyses of total mortality at prespecified numbers of deaths. The statistician of this committee received information on all deaths directly from the investigators. The study protocol was approved by regional or, if applicable, national ethics committees and by the regulatory agencies in each of the participating Scandinavian countries.

Figure 10.1a The 4S Trial. Reprinted from *The Lancet.* **344**/8934: 1383–89. Scandinavian Simvastatin Survival Study Group, Randomized trial of cholesterol lowering in 4444 patients with coronary heart disease: The Scandinavian Simvastatin Survival Study (4S). Copyright (1994), with permission from Elsevier.

THE LANCET

Recruitment and randomisation

Patient records of men and women aged 35–70 years with a history of angina pectoris or acute myocardial infarction (MI) were systematically screened for study eligibility. The exclusion criteria were: premenopausal women of childbearing potential, secondary hypercholesterolaemia, unstable or Prinzmetal angina, tendon xanthomata, planned coronary artery surgery or angioplasty, MI during the preceding 6 months, antiarrhythmic therapy, congestive heart failure requiring treatment with digitalis, diuretics, or vasodilators, persistent atrial fibrillation, cardiomegaly, haemodynamically important valvular heart disease, history of completed stroke, impaired hepatic function, partial ileal bypass, history of drug or alcohol abuse, poor mental function, other serious disease, current treatment with another investigational drug, or hypersensitivity to HMG-CoA reductase inhibitors. Potentially eligible patients were invited to the clinic for a briefing about the study. If none of the exclusion criteria applied and the patient consented, fasting serum cholesterol and triglyceride were determined by a local laboratory. If serum total cholesterol was >5·5 mmol/L, patients were invited to participate in the study and were given dietary advice.[11] After 8 weeks blood was drawn and serum was sent to the central laboratory for analysis of lipid concentrations and a 2-week placebo run-in phase was initiated. If serum cholesterol was 5·5 to 8·0 mmol/L, serum triglyceride was ≤2·5 mmol/L, and the patient was compliant and still eligible, final informed consent was obtained and the patient was randomly assigned to treatment with simvastatin 20 mg or placebo, to be taken before the evening meal. Randomisation was stratified for clinical site and previous MI.

Laboratory measurements

The patients visited the clinics every 6 weeks during the first 18 months and every 6 months thereafter for determination of serum aspartate aminotransferase, alanine aminotransferase, and creatine kinase in the local laboratories. Routine haematology and urine examinations were done at baseline and at the final visit. Lipids were measured[21] at the central laboratory every 6 weeks during the first 6 months and half yearly thereafter. Patients were queried for adverse experiences after 6 weeks, 12 weeks, and 6 months, and every 6 months thereafter. A clinical examination with resting electrocardiogram was performed annually.

Dosage titration

Dosage was adjusted, if necessary, at the 12-week and 6-month visits, on the basis of serum total cholesterol at 6 and 18 weeks. The goal of treatment was to reduce serum total cholesterol to 3·0–5·2 mmol/L. A computer program at the central laboratory issued dosage adjustment messages without revealing lipid levels or treatment allocation. Patients in the simvastatin group whose serum cholesterol was out of range had their dose increased to 40 mg daily, as two 20 mg tablets, or reduced to one 10 mg tablet. To maintain the double-blind, patients in the placebo group were randomly assigned to take matching placebo tablets.

Endpoint definition, ascertainment, and analysis

The primary endpoint of the study was total mortality. The secondary endpoint, analysed by time of first event, was "major coronary events", which comprised coronary deaths, definite or probable hospital-verified non-fatal acute MI, resuscitated cardiac arrest, and definite silent MI verified by electrocardiogram. The tertiary endpoints, also analysed by time of first event, were: (1) any coronary event, ie, the secondary endpoint events plus myocardial revascularisation procedures and hospital admission for acute CHD events without a diagnosis of MI (mainly prolonged chest pain); (2) death or any atherosclerotic event (coronary, cerebrovascular, and peripheral), ie, death from any cause and events included under the first tertiary endpoint, plus hospital-verified non-fatal non-coronary atherosclerotic events; (3) incidence of myocardial

revascularisaton procedures, either coronary artery bypass grafting or percutaneous transluminal coronary angioplasty; (4) incidence of hospital admission for acute CHD events without a diagnosis of MI. The fifth and final tertiary endpoint, which relates to health economics, will be addressed in a subsequent report. The protocol specified subgroup analyses of females and of patients aged ≥60 years, with recognition that these analyses had less statistical power than those based on the whole population. Whether the patients were alive or not was ascertained half-yearly and at the end of the study by contact with each patient or another member of the household. Cause of death was ascertained from hospital records and death certificates, as well as interviews with physicians and relatives. A summary of these records, and of hospital records of patients with suspected nonfatal endpoint events, was provided to the endpoint classification committee, who then determined and categorised each event for use in the analysis.

Hospital-verified cardiovascular events were classified according to a modification of the WHO MONICA method.[22,23] Annual electrocardiograms were coded for major Q-wave pattern changes,[24] with confirmation by visual overreading. When such a change appeared without a corresponding hospital-verified acute MI, a silent MI was recorded and dated as the midpoint between the two corresponding visits.

The study was planned to have 95% power to detect a 30% reduction in total mortality at $\alpha=0.05$ (two-sided, adjusted for three preplanned interim analyses and one final analysis). To achieve this power the protocol specified 4400 patients to be followed until the occurrence of 440 deaths, unless the trial was stopped early on the basis of an interim analysis. Vital status was monitored throughout the study. Treatment group differences were assessed by the logrank test. Relative risk and 95% confidence intervals were calculated with the Cox regression model.[25] Mortality data were also analysed with the same model, with baseline variables that were significantly related to outcome. Two-sided p values ≤0·05 were regarded as significant and only in the case of the primary endpoint was the significance level adjusted for the three interim analyses. All data were analysed by intention-to-treat.

Results

Of the 7027 patients recruited for the diet period 4444 fulfilled the entry criteria and were randomised between May 19, 1988, and Aug 16, 1989. The main reasons for exclusion were serum total cholesterol after diet outside the 5·5–8·0 mmol/L range (n=1300), serum triglyceride >2·5 mmol/L (n=864), and unwillingness to participate (n=396).

Having completed the third (and final) interim analysis of available endpoint reports, the data safety and monitoring committee advised (on May 27, 1994) that the study should be stopped as soon as was possible. At this analysis the p value crossed the boundary of the predefined statistical guideline. After discussion with the chairman of the steering committee, Aug 1, 1994 was selected as the cut-off date at which it was anticipated that the protocol-specified target of 440 deaths would be approximated.

Median follow-up time was 5·4 years (range of those surviving was 4·9–6·3). Confirmation of whether the patients were alive or dead was obtained in every case at the end of the study. The two treatment groups were well matched at baseline (table 1). 288/2223 (13%) patients in the placebo group and 231/2221 (10%) in the simvastatin group stopped taking their tablets. Adverse events were the reason for discontinuing therapy in 129 patients in the placebo group and 126 in the simvastatin group, and patient reluctance to continue accounted for most of the remainder.

Figure 10.1b The 4S Trial.

	Placebo (n=2223)	Simvastatin (n=2221)
No (%) of patients		
Male	1803 (81)	1814 (82)
Female	420 (19)	407 (18)
Age ≥60 yr	1126 (51)	1156 (52)
Qualifying diagnosis		
Angina only	456 (21)	462 (21)
Infarction only	1385 (62)	1399 (63)
Both angina and infarction	381 (17)	360 (16)
Time since first diagnosis of angina or infarction		
−1 yr	589 (26)	602 (27)
≥1–5 yr	961 (43)	929 (42)
≥5 yr	673 (30)	690 (31)
Major ECG Q-wave	782 (35)	724 (33)
Secondary diagnoses		
Hypertension	584 (26)	570 (26)
Claudication	123 (6)	130 (6)
Diabetes mellitus	96 (4)	105 (5)
Previous CABG or angioplasty	151 (7)	189 (9)
Non-smokers	562 (25)	558 (25)
Ex-smokers	1065 (48)	1121 (50)
Smokers	596 (27)	542 (24)
Other therapy		
Aspirin	815 (37)	822 (37)
Beta-blockers	1266 (57)	1258 (57)
Calcium antagonists	668 (30)	712 (32)
Isosorbide mono/dinitrate	727 (33)	684 (31)
Thiazides	138 (6)	151 (7)
Warfarin	51 (2)	29 (1)
Fish oil	293 (13)	283 (13)
Mean (SD)		
Age (yr) men	58·1 (7·2)	58·2 (7·3)
Age (yr) women	60·51 (5·7)	60·5 (6·4)
Body mass index (kg/m²)	26·0 (3·3)	26·0 (3·4)
Heart rate	64·2 (10·1)	63·8 (10·1)
Blood pressure (mm Hg)		
Systolic	139·1 (19·6)	138·5 (19·6)
Diastolic	83·7 (9·5)	83·2 (9·5)
Cholesterol (mmol/L)		
Total	6·75 (0·66)	6·74 (0·67)
HDL	1·19 (0·29)	1·18 (0·30)
LDL	4·87 (0·65)	4·87 (0·66)
Triglycerides (mmol/L)	1·51 (0·52)	1·49 (0·49)

CABG=coronary artery bypass grafr; HDL=high-density lipoprotein; LDL=low-density lipoprotein.

Table 1: **Baseline characteristics of randomised patients**

Changes in serum lipid concentrations

37% of the patients taking simvastatin had their dose raised to 40 mg during the first 6 months after randomisation, while the rest continued to take 20 mg daily, except for 2 patients whose dosage was reduced to 10 mg daily, according to protocol.

Lipid concentrations showed little change in the placebo group, except for an upward drift in serum triglycerides. After 6 weeks of therapy with simvastatin, at which point all patients were still taking 20 mg daily, total cholesterol was reduced on average by 28%, LDL cholesterol by 38%, and triglycerides by 15%, whereas high-density-lipoprotein (HDL) cholesterol rose by 8%. After 1 year, 72% of the simvastatin-treated patients had achieved the total-cholesterol goal (<5·2 mmol/L). In subsequent years there was a small increase in mean total and LDL cholesterol, while HDL cholesterol and triglycerides tended to move in parallel with changes in the placebo group. Over the whole course of the study, in the simvastatin group the mean changes from baseline in total, LDL, and HDL cholesterol, and serum triglycerides, were −25%, −35%, +8% and −10%, respectively. The corresponding values in the placebo group were +1%, +1%, +1%, and +7%, respectively. 35 patients in the placebo group were switched to lipid-

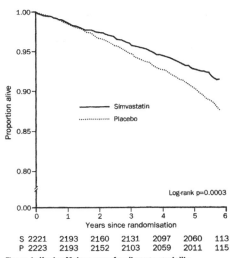

Figure 1: **Kaplan-Meier curves for all-cause mortality**
Number of patients at risk at the beginning of each year is shown below the horizontal axis.

S	2221	2193	2160	2131	2097	2060	113
P	2223	2193	2152	2103	2059	2011	115

lowering drugs, either because serum cholesterol rose above the protocol-specified limit of 9·0 mmol/L (16 patients) or because such therapy was initiated by non-study physicians (19 patients).

Mortality

The primary endpoint was total mortality. During the double-blind study period 438 patients died, 256 (12%) in the placebo group and 182 (8%) in the simvastatin group (table 2); the relative risk was 0·70 (95% CI 0·58–0·85, p=0·0003) with simvastatin. The Kaplan-Meier 6-year (70 months) probability of survival (figure 1) was 87·7% in the placebo group and 91·3% in the simvastatin group. Adjustment for the baseline covariates made no material difference to the results for survival or the other endpoints. There were 189 coronary deaths in the placebo group (74% of all deaths in this group), compared with 111 in the simvastatin group. The relative risk of coronary death was 0·58 (95% CI 0·46–0·73) with simvastatin. This 42% reduction in the risk of coronary death accounts for the improvement in survival. There was no statistically significant difference between the two groups in the number of deaths from non-cardiovascular causes. There were similar numbers of violent deaths (suicide plus trauma) in the two groups, 7 versus 6. Of the fatal cancers, 12/35 in the placebo group and 9/33 in the simvastatin group arose in the gastrointestinal system. There were similar numbers of cerebrovascular deaths in the two groups, and the difference (6 vs 11) in deaths from other cardiovascular diseases is not significant.

Nonfatal and combined endpoints

The secondary study endpoint was major coronary events: coronary death (table 2), nonfatal definite or probable MI, silent MI, or resuscitated cardiac arrest (table 3). 622 (28%) patients in the placebo group and 431 (19%) in the simvastatin group had one or more secondary endpoint events. The relative risk of a major coronary event in the simvastatin group was 0·66 (95% CI 0·59–0·75, p<0·00001). The Kaplan-Meier 6-year

Figure 10.1c The 4S Trial.

THE LANCET

Causes of death	No (%) of patients		
	Placebo (n=2223)	Simvastatin (n=2221)	Relative risk (95% CI)
Definite acute MI	63	30	
Probable acute MI	5	5	
Acute MI not confirmed			
Instantaneous death	39	29	
Death within 1 h*	24	8	
Death within 1–24 h	15	9	
Death >24 h after onset of event	11	10	
Non-witnessed death†	23	13	
Intervention-associated‡	9	7	
All coronary	189 (8·5)	111 (5·0)	0·58 (0·46–0·73)
Cerebrovascular	12	14	
Other cardiovascular	6	11	
All cardiovascular	207 (9·3)	136 (6·1)	0·65 (0·52–0·80)
Cancer	35	33	
Suicide	4	5	
Trauma	3	1	
Other	7	7	
All noncardiovascular	49 (2·2)	46 (2·1)	
All deaths	256 (11·5)	182 (8·2)	0·70 (0·58–0·85)

Relative risk, calculated by Cox regression analysis. MI=myocardial infarction.
*Following acute chest pain, syncope, pulmonary oedema, or cardiogenic shock.
†With no likely non-coronary cause. ‡Coronary death within 28 days of any invasive procedure.

Table 2: **Mortality and causes of death**

Event	No (%) of patients*		
	Placebo (n=2223)	Simvastatin (n=2221)	
Major coronary			
Definite acute MI	270 (12·1)	164 (7·4)	
Definite or probable acute MI	418 (18·8)	279 (12·6)	
Silent MI	110 (4·9)	88 (4·0)	
Resuscitated cardiac arrest	0	1	
Acute MI, intervention-associated	25	12	
Any major coronary*	502 (22·6)	353 (15·9)	
Coronary surgery or angioplasty	383 (17·2)	252 (11·3)	
Non-MI acute CHD	331 (14·9)	295 (13·3)	
Acute non-CHD cardiac	109 (4·9)	109 (4·9)	
Cerebrovascular			
Stroke, non-embolic	33	16	
Stroke, embolic	16	13	
Stroke, haemorrhagic	2	0	
Stroke, unclassified	13	15	
Stroke, intervention-associated	10	3	
Transient ischaemic attack	29	19	
Any cerebrovascular*	95 (4·3)	61 (2·7)	
Other cardiovascular	33 (1·5)	24 (1·1)	

*A patient with 2 or more events of different types will appear more than once in a column but only once in a row.

Table 3: **Patients with nonfatal cardiovascular events during follow-up**

probability of escaping such events was 70·5% in the placebo group and 79·6% in the simvastatin group (figure 2A). The relative risk of hospital-verified non-fatal definite or probable acute myocardial infarction was 0·63 (95% CI 0·54–0·73).

Results for the four tertiary endpoints are presented below. The relative risk of having any coronary event in the simvastatin group was 0·73 (95% CI 0·66–0·80, p<0·00001). The 6-year Kaplan-Meier probability of

escaping any coronary event was 56·7% in the placebo group and 66·6% in the simvastatin group (figure 2B). The relative risk of death or having any atherosclerotic cardiovascular event was 0·74 (95% CI 0·67–0·81, p<0·00001). The probability of escaping such events was 53·0% in the placebo group and 62·9% in the simvastatin group (figure 2C). Simvastatin also reduced the patient's risk of undergoing coronary artery bypass surgery or angioplasty (table 3 and figure 2D): the relative risk was 0·63 (95% CI 0·54–0·74, p<0·00001). There was no significant difference between treatment groups with regard to non-MI acute CHD events. A post-hoc analysis was performed on fatal plus nonfatal cerebrovascular events: there were 98 patients with such events in the placebo group and 70 in the simvastatin group, relative risk 0·70 (95% CI 0·52–0·96, p=0·024).

Results in women and patients aged ≥60

The results in the protocol-specified subgroups are presented in table 4. Only 52 of the 827 women died in the trial, 25 (6%) in the placebo group and 27 (7%) in the simvastatin group. Of these deaths 17 and 13, respectively, were the result of CHD. The probability that a woman would escape a major coronary event was 77·7% in the placebo group and 85·1% in the simvastatin group: relative risk was 0·65 (95% CI 0·47–0·90, p=0·010). For both the primary and secondary endpoints, there were no

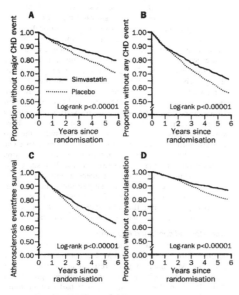

Figure 2: **Kaplan-Meier curves for secondary and tertiary endpoints**
(A) major coronary events; (B) any coronary event; (C) survival free of any atherosclerotic event; (D) myocardial revascularisation procedures.

	No (%) of patients		
	Placebo	Simvastatin	Relative risk* (95% CI)
Death			
Women	25 (6·0)	27 (6·6)	1·12 (0·65–1·93)
Men	231 (12·8)	155 (8·5)	0·66 (0·53–0·80)
Age <60 yr	89 (8·1)	55 (5·2)	0·63 (0·45–0·88)
Age ≥60 yr	167 (14·8)	127 (11·0)	0·73 (0·58–0·92)
Major coronary event			
Women	91 (21·7)	59 (14·5)	0·65 (0·47–0·91)
Men	531 (29·4)	372 (20·5)	0·66 (0·58–0·76)
Age <60 yr	303 (27·6)	188 (17·6)	0·61 (0·51–0·73)
Age ≥60 yr	319 (28·3)	243 (21·0)	0·71 (0·60–0·86)

*Calculated by Cox regression analysis.

Table 4: **Endpoints in predefined subgroups**

Figure 10.1d The 4S Trial.

significant interactions between treatment and either sex or age. Although the observed relative risk reductions produced by simvastatin were somewhat less in the patients aged ⩾60, they were statistically significant (p<0·01 in both age groups for mortality and p<0·0001 for major coronary events) and the absolute differences between treatment groups were similar in the two age groups.

Adverse experiences

The overall frequency of adverse events was similar in the two groups. As previously noted, 6% of patients in both groups discontinued the study drug because of adverse events. In addition to the cancer deaths reported in table 2, there were 61 nonfatal cases of cancer in the placebo group and 57 in the simvastatin group, of which 14 and 12, respectively, arose in the gastrointestinal system. These totals exclude cases of non-melanoma skin cancer, of which there were 6 in the placebo group and 13 in the simvastatin group. There were no significant differences between the treatment groups for fatal plus nonfatal cancer as a whole or at any particular site. A single case of rhabdomyolysis occurred in a woman taking simvastatin 20 mg daily; she recovered when treatment was stopped. An increase of creatine kinase to more than ten times the upper limit of normal occurred in 1 and 6 patients in the placebo and simvastatin groups, respectively, but in none of the latter was this high level maintained in a repeat sample or accompanied by muscle pain or weakness. Increases of aspartate aminotransferase to more than three times the upper limit of normal occurred in 23 patients in the placebo group and 20 in the simvastatin group. For alanine aminotransferase the corresponding numbers were 33 and 49.

Discussion

As expected in a large study, the groups were well matched at baseline. 79% of patients had a history of MI. Patients were excluded if they had a history of complicated MI with significant myocardial dysfunction, or required drug therapy for heart failure. This was done to avoid excess early mortality from congestive heart failure or arrhythmias, which might dilute the postulated effect of simvastatin on deaths caused by progression of coronary atherosclerosis. These factors resulted in a selection of patients with a lower risk of death in the placebo group than has usually been seen in postinfarction populations.[13]

The effect of simvastatin on lipids was similar to that observed in other long-term controlled trials with this drug.[26,27] As often happens in long-term studies analysed by intention-to-treat, there was a slight attenuation of the mean drug effect over time, due at least in part to dilution by patients who stopped treatment but continued to provide blood samples.

Simvastatin produced highly significant reductions in the risk of death and morbidity in patients with CHD followed for a median of 5·4 years, relative to patients receiving standard care. The results in CHD endpoints and in subgroups are internally consistent and very robust. They indicate that addition of simvastatin 20–40 mg daily to the treatment regimens of 100 CHD patients, with characteristics similar to those of our patients, can be expected, on the basis of the corresponding Kaplan-Meier curves, to yield the following approximate benefits over the first 6 years: preservation of the lives of 4 of the 9

patients who otherwise would die from CHD, prevention of nonfatal MI in 7 of an expected 21 patients, and avoidance of myocardial revascularisation procedures in 6 of the 19 anticipated patients.

No previous unifactorial trial of any lipid-lowering therapy has demonstrated reduction of total or even coronary mortality during the planned follow-up period. In the extended follow-up of the first Oslo Diet-Heart study[2] there was a significant reduction after 11 years in fatal MI. In the niacin arm of the Coronary Drug Project trial there was a significant 11% reduction in total mortality over 15 years.[28] Except for the POSCH study,[9] in which patients with a history of MI underwent partial ileal bypass to reduce mean LDL cholesterol by 38%, none of these trials achieved changes in LDL cholesterol comparable with the 35% average reduction observed in this trial; the reductions in these earlier trials averaged about 10%. The POSCH trial was not large enough to show an effect on total or coronary mortality, but there was a significant 35% reduction over 5 years in CHD deaths plus nonfatal myocardial infarctions, which is in good agreement with our results. Combining the results from twenty-eight cholesterol-lowering trials, Law et al[29] estimated that the risk of coronary death plus nonfatal MI was reduced by 7% (95% CI 0–14%) per 0·6 mmol/L reduction in serum total cholesterol concentration in the first 2 years of treatment, and 22% (95% CI 15–28%) in years 3–5. In our study a mean reduction of serum cholesterol of 1·8 mmol/L (25%) was achieved. With the exclusion of silent MI, the risk of coronary death plus nonfatal MI was reduced by 37% over the whole study, by 26% in the first 2 years, and by 46% thereafter. Thus our results are consistent with the estimates of Law et al.

Our study also provided evidence for a beneficial effect of simvastatin on fatal plus nonfatal cerebrovascular events. This finding is consistent with a report[30] that lovastatin, a closely related inhibitor of HMG-CoA reductase, can reverse the progression of carotid atherosclerosis. Since it is based on a data-driven post-hoc analysis, prospective trials are needed to confirm this possible additional benefit.

Patient compliance with the demands of the study protocol was generally good and doubtless contributed substantially to the clearcut outcome. Under 1% of placebo patients discontinued study drug to receive open-label cholesterol lowering therapy—an indication that treatment allocation was seldom unblinded by measurement of serum cholesterol outside the study. This reflects in part the contemporary conservative attitude of Scandinavian physicians towards drug treatment of hypercholesterolaemia.

The impact of simvastatin on CHD seems to begin after about 1 year of therapy and increases steadily thereafter. This is consistent with several angiographic studies showing beneficial effects on coronary atherosclerosis within 2 years of effective lipid-lowering therapy.[31,32] Progression of coronary atherosclerotic lesions clearly predicts subsequent coronary events.[33] Lately the Multicentre Anti-Atheroma Study (MAAS) investigators[27] showed by quantitative angiography a retardation of the progression of coronary atheromatous lesions, compared with standard care, at 2 and 4 years after starting treatment with simvastatin in patients similar to those studied in 4S. Significantly fewer new lesions and total occlusions developed in the simvastatin group. Coronary lesions may stabilise as their lipid core shrinks or at least

Figure 10.1e The 4S Trial.

THE LANCET

does not further enlarge; there is thus a drop in risk of plaque rupture, which triggers intramural haemorrhage and intraluminal thrombosis, which in turn may cause coronary events.[31-35] Stabilisation of coronary lesions is most likely the main reason for the improved survival observed in our trial.

Only 19% of the study population were women. In the placebo group mortality rate for women was less than half that for men. With only 52 deaths among women, demonstration of improved survival in women as a separate subgroup was unlikely. Nevertheless, simvastatin did reduce the risk of major coronary events in women to about the same extent as it did in men. It also improved survival in patients aged 60 or more. This is the first trial to show that cholesterol-lowering reduces major coronary events in women and the first to show that it improves survival in older patients.

The improvement in survival produced by simvastatin was achieved without any suggestion of an increase in non-CHD mortality, including deaths due to violence and cancer, which have raised concern in some overviews of cholesterol-lowering trials.[14-18] The overall incidence of fatal plus nonfatal cancer was also similar in the two groups. Simvastatin therapy was well tolerated and the frequencies of adverse events in general, and those associated with drug discontinuation in particular, were similar in the two groups. Rhabdomyolysis, the most important adverse effect of inhibitors of HMG-CoA reductase, occurred in 1 patient who recovered when treatment was stopped. No previously unknown adverse effects were apparent in this trial. Thus the substantial and sustained reduction of total and LDL cholesterol in the simvastatin group was not associated with any serious hazard. The results of the 4S are consistent with the idea that raised LDL cholesterol is an important factor in pathogenesis of CHD.

We thank the monitoring personnel, the many doctors, nurses, and hospital management staff who made this study possible, and above all the patients for their participation.

The study was supported by a grant from Merck Research Laboratories, Rahway, New Jersey, USA.

Writing committee. T R Pedersen, J Kjekshus, K Berg, T Haghfelt, O Færgeman, G Thorgeirsson, K Pyörälä, T Miettinen, L Wilhelmsen, A G Olsson, H Wedel.

Steering committee. J Kjekshus (Chairman), K Berg, T R Pedersen, T Haghfelt, O Færgeman, G Thorgeirsson, K Pyörälä, T Miettinen. L Wilhelmsen, A G Olsson (Co-chairman), H Wedel, K Kristianson (Merck Research Laboratories Scandinavia) (non-voting).

Investigators. Denmark (713 randomised patients), H Thomsen, E Norderø, B Thomsen, Dr Alexandrines Sygehus, Faeroe Islands; K Lyngborg, G Steen Andersen, F Nielsen, U Talleruphuus, A McNair, Frederiksberg Hospital, Copenhagen; K Egstrup, E Hertel Simonsen, I Simonsen, Haderslev Sygehys; H Vejby-Christensen, L Sommer, P O Eidner, E Klarholt, A Henriksen, Herning Sygehus; K Mellemgaard, J Launbjerg, P Freuergaard, L Nielsen, Hillerød Sygehus; E Birk Madsen, H Ibsen, U Andersen, H Enemark, J Haarbo, B Martinsen, C G Dahlstrøm, L Thyrring, K Thomassen, Holbæk Sygehus; G Jensen, S Lind Rasmussen, N Skov, Hvidovre Hospital Copenhagen; T Haghfelt, K Nørregaard Hansen, M Lytken Larsen, B Haastrup, I Hjære, A Thurøe, Odense Sygehus; A Leth, M Munch, R Worck, B Nielsen, A G Thorn, K A S Glostrup, Copenhagen; O Pedersen-Bjergaard, B Fournaise, Nyborg Sygehus; B Sigurd, B Enk, H Nielsen, L Jacobsen, Nykøbing Falster Sygehus; T Lysbo Svendsen, A Høegholm, H Münter, P Kaufmann, Næstved Sygehus; S Haunsø, P Grande, C Eriksen, H Høegh Nielsen, B Jurlander, Rigshospitalet, Copenhagen; T Pinborg, J Pindborg, H Tost, Svendborg Sygehus; B Dorff Christiansen, M Oppenhagen, Varde Sygehus; F Egede, S Hvidt, T Kjærby, Vejle Sygehus; O Færgeman, L Lemming, I Klausen, Århus Amstssygehus.

Finland (868 randomised patients) T A Miettinen, H Vanhanen, T E Strandberg, K Hölttä, H Luomanmäki, T Pekuri, A Vuorinen, Helsinki University Hospital; A Pasternack, H Oksa, L Siitonen, R Rimpi, Tampere University Hospital; Y A Kesàniemi, M Lilja, T Korhonen, A Rantala, M Rantala, M Savolainen, O Ukkola, L Laine, L Virkkala, Oulu University Hospital; K Pyörälä, S Lehto, A Rantala, H Miettinen, A Salokannel, R Räisänen, Kuopio University Hospital.

Iceland (157 randomised patients), G Thorgeirsson, J Högnason, H Kristjansdottir, G Thorvaldsdottir, Landspitalinn University Hospital, Reykjavik; G Sigurdsson, Reykjavik City Hospital; J T Sverrisson, Sjukrahusid Akureyri.

Norway (1025 randomised patients), T R Pedersen, V Hansteen, F Kjelsberg, K Berget, R Pettersen, E R Balto, T Holm, Aker Sykehus, Oslo; T Gundersen, B Aslaksen, E Hauge Andersen, Aust-Agder Sentralsjukehus, Arendal; H Torsvik, R Pettersen, J Kjekshus, A Faber, Bærum Sykehus, Sandvika; T Indrebø, A Ose, T Roterud, Gjøvik Fylkessykehus; L Holst-Larsen, K Waage, E Holst-Larsen, Fylkessjukehuset i Haugesund; J W Hærem, P Aukrust, R Torp, K Risberg, K Mauseth, Hamar Sykehus; E Gerdts, O Nygård, A Hallaråker, G Gradek, E Moberg Vangen, Haukeland Sykehus, Bergen; H Schartum-Hansen, A M Refsum, S Listerud, B Gundersrud, A M Stene, Hedmark Sentralsykehus, Elverum; B Klykken, O Aakervik, A Loraas, P O Foss, A Haga, L Thoresen, Innherred Sykehus, Levanger; A Drivenes, P Lem, F Gabrielsen, S Hestad, Moss Sykehus; R Røde, B Kvamme Haug, G Skjelvan, E Eldorsen, Norland Sentralsykehus, Bodø; K Ytre-Arne, K Rasmussen, E S P Myhre, I Nermoen, L Christiansen, A S Karlsen, K Walberg, Regionsykehuset i Tromsø; H A Tjønndal, B Kulseng, R Rokseth, T Vigeland Nergård, M Olstad Røe, Regionsykehuset i Trondheim; O Tenstad, I L Løfsnes, U Bergsrud, Ringerike Sykehus, Hønefoss; T H Melberg, C von Brandis, S Barvik, L Woie, A M Abrahamsen, T Aarsland, H Svanes, Rogaland Sentralsjukehus, Stavanger; G Noer, K E Nordlie, A E Hanedalen, Sandefjord Sykehus; T Johansen, T Holm, C B Larsen, E Østholm, Østfold Sentralsykehus, avd Fredrikstad; K Overskeid, P Sandvei, Aa Johansen, Østfold Sentralsykehus, avd Sarpsborg; E Søgnen, D Aarskog, A Dale, S Hegrestad, Å Reikvam, L Hawkes, Sogn og Fjordane Sentralsjukehus, Førde; S Hoff, T Torjussen, R Norvik, C Jørgensen, Spesialistsenteret, Kristiansand; I Hjermann, P Leren, A Narvestad, Ullevål Sykehus, Oslo; D Fausa F T Gjestvang, B Nordland, Vest-Agder Sentralsykehus, Kristiansand.

Sweden (1681 randomised patients) P Brunmark, H Biöklund, B Biöklund, Arvika Sjukhus; H Forsberg, B Bergström, I Laaksonen, M B Vestermark, Boden/Luleå Sjukhus; G Mascher, E Hammarström, K Trosell, Bollnäs Sjukhus; L Karlsson, L Hallström, Enköping Lasarett; A Stjerna, M K Slette, E Diderholm, K P-Berglund, Eskilstuna, Mälarsjukhuset; B Linde, G Ahlmark, H Sætre, G Ahlberg, K Sundkvist, Falun Lasarett; P E Gustafsson, E Gustafsson, Gävle Sjukhus; A Norrby, B Jaup, L Svensson, Göteborg, GLF Lundby Sjukhus; O Wiklund, T Lindén, C H Bergh, K Jonsteg, B Bonnier, Y Lundin, K Romanus, Göteborg, Sahlgrenska Sjukhuset; G Ulvenstam, S Johansson, I Wallin, K Dudas, M Andreasson, G Torelund, Göteborg, Östra Sjukhuset; E Skarfors, G Rüter, L Åkesson, Halmstads Länssjukhus; F Wagner, L Ljungdahl, V Wagner, Helsingborg Lasarett; G Rasmanis, O Edhag, D Vourisalo, H Hjelmseil, G Wesley, Huddinge Sjukhus; Hudiksvalls Sjukhus (L Lundkvist, K Ångman, A Olsson); O Svenson, J Kuylenstierna, K Frisenette-Fich, E Bergman, Jönköping, Länssjukhuset Ryhov; H Strömblad, S Jensen, E Jönsson, C Levin, Karlshamn Länslasarett; H Odeberg, P O Bengtsson, E Holmesson, Karlskrona Centrallasarett; H Hedstrand, L Bojö, S Öberg, Karlstad Centralsjukhus; H Leksell, P Werner, S Persson, M Simonsson, U B Wirenstam, Kristianstads Centralsjukhus; B Moberg, A B Ekstrand, Kristinehamn Sjukhus; P Nicol, B Malmros, J Saaw, N Arcini, J Kobosko, I G Ånevik, S Johansson, Köping Lasarett; F Gyland, B Lundh, M Wennerholm, C Olsson, Landskrona Lasarett, J Kjellberg, K Fabianson, Lidköping Bassjukhus; T Fraser, I Bergkvist, Lindesberg Lasarett; A G Olsson, B Bergdahl, C Fluur, S Wärjerstam, Linköping Universitetssjukhus; K A Svensson, L Ekholm, E Torebo, A Ryberg, Ljungby Lasarett; J E Frisell, A Hedman, L Wallrup, G Andersen, M Sandström, K Alberg, Ludvika Lasarett; B Fagher, T Thulin, I Svenstam, Lund, Universitetssjukhuset; A Bjurman, E Skoglund, G Dahl, Lycksele Lasarett; T Kjellström, M Sjöö-Boquist, Malmö Allmänna Sjukhus; A Sjögren, E Loogna, T Jansson, Nacka Sjukhus; J Fridén, O Nilsson, P O Andersson, C Henriksson, Norrköping Lasarett; J Ellström, H Brodersson, L Lundquist, M Åslund, Sandviken Lasarett; K Boman, J H Jansson, B Norrfors, Skellefteå Lasarett; C Höglund, M Lundblad, Stockholm Heart Center; I Liljefors, L Wennerström, I Petz, Stockholm, Sabbatsberg Sjukhus; B Leijd, C Falkenberg, L Bergsten, S Ström, A C Engström, Stockholm, St Göran Sjukhus; J Ejdebäck, K Malmberg, S Hogström, L Ståhl, Skövde Kärnsjukhus; B H Möller, M Lycksell, M Söderström, Sundsvalls Sjukhus; E Hansson, C Hallén, Säffle Sjukhus; H Stakeberg, J Börretzen, B Hedén, K Andersson, Trollhättan NÄL; O Johnson, L Slunga Birgander, S Jensen, B Elander, Umeå Universitetssjukhus; C Lidell, P E Andersson, E Marklund, Uppsala Akademiska Sjukhus; M Dahlen, F Rücker, M Löfqvist, B Wannberg, Visby Lasarett; B H Lim, O Larsson, G Andersson, A Hansson, M Uchto, M Gowenius, I Uggeldahl, Växjö Lasarett; D Ursing, P Hammarlund, P Nyman, E Tsuppuka, Ängelholm Sjukhus; L Malmberg, K Göransson, P Hasselgren, C M Insberg, S Petterson, A Åhrlin, Örebro Regionsjukhus; O Lövheim, L O Andersson, I Grundström, Örnsköldsvik Sjukhus.

Figure 10.1f The 4S Trial.

Coordinator. R Pedersen.

Data and safety monitoring committee. D G Julian (chairman),
S G Thompson, W McFate Smith, C D Furberg, J Huttunen, J Lubsen.

Endpoint classification committee. M Romo, K Thygesen.

Clinical events ECG coding centre. S Lehto, H Miettinen.

Annual ECG Coding Centre. R Crow.

Central lipid laboratory. B Kristoffersen, Marie Buchman, Toril Gran.

Data analysis. T Cook (Merck Research Laboratories).

Monitoring offices, Merck Sharp & Dohme. G Renström Moen,
J Hylerstedt; V Larsen; S Lillsjö, R Nyberg; C Eriksen, D Fogh Nielsen,
T Musliner, R Greguski.

References

1 Gotto AM Jr, LaRosa JC, Hunninghake D, et al. The cholesterol facts. A summary of the evidence relating dietary fats, serum cholesterol, and coronary heart disease. *Circulation* 1990; 81: 1721–33.

2 Leren P. The Oslo Diet Heart Study: eleven-year report. *Circulation* 1970; 42: 935–42.

3 Coronary Drug Project Research Group. Clofibrate and niacin in coronary heart disease. *JAMA* 1975; 231: 360–81.

4 Carlson LA, Danielson M, Ekberg I, Klintemar B, Rosenhamer G. Reduction of myocardial reinfarction by the combined treatment with clofibrate and nicotinic acid. *Atherosclerosis* 1977; 28: 81–86.

5 Committee of Principal Investigators. A co-operative trial in the primary prevention of ischaemic heart disease using clofibrate. *Br Heart J* 1978; 40: 1069–118.

6 Lipid Research Clinics Program. The Lipid Research Clinics coronary primary prevention trial results. *JAMA* 1984; 251: 351–74.

7 Frick MH, Elo O, Happa K, et al. Helsinki Heart Study: primary-prevention with gemfibrozil in middle-aged men with dyslipemia. *N Engl J Med* 1987; 317: 1237–45.

8 Dorr AE, Gundersen K, Schneider JC Jr, Spencer TW, Martin WB Colestipol hydrochloride in hypercholesterolemic patients—effect on serum cholesterol and mortality. *J Chron Dis* 1978; 31: 5–14.

9 Buchwald H, Varco RL, Matts JP, et al. Effect of partial ileal bypass on mortality and morbidity from coronary heart disease in patients with hypercholesterolemia—report of the Program on the Surgical Control of Hyperlipidemias (POSCH). *N Engl J Med* 1990; 323: 946–55.

10 Lowering blood cholesterol to prevent heart disease: consensus conference. *JAMA* 1985; 253: 2080–90.

11 Study Group, European Atherosclerosis Society. Strategies for the prevention of coronary heart disease: a policy statement of the European Atherosclerosis Society. *Eur Heart J* 1987; 8: 77–88.

12 Expert Panel on Detection, Evaluation, and Treatment of High Blood Cholesterol in Adults. Summary of the second report of the National Cholesterol Education Program (NCEP) Expert Panel on Detection, Evaluation, and Treatment of High Blood Cholesterol in Adults (adult treatment panel II). *JAMA* 1993; 269: 3015–23.

13 Pyörälä K, De Backer G, Graham I, on behalf of the Task Force. Prevention of coronary heart disease in clinical practice. Recommendations of the Task Force of the European Society of Cardiology, European Atherosclerosis Society and European Society of Hypertension. *Eur Heart J* 1994; 15: 1300–31.

14 Oliver MF. Doubts about preventing coronary heart disease. Multiple interventions in middle aged men may do more harm than good. *BMJ* 1992; 304: 393–94.

15 Davey Smith G, Pekkanen J. Should there be a moratorium on the use of cholesterol lowering drugs? *BMJ* 1992; 304: 431–34.

16 Muldoon MF, Manuck SB, Matthews KA. Lowering cholesterol concentrations and mortality: a quantitative review of primary prevention trials. *BMJ* 1990; 301: 309–14.

17 Rossouw JE, Lewis B, Rifkind BM. The value of lowering cholesterol after myocardial infarction. *N Engl J Med* 1990; 323: 1112–19.

18 Ravnskov U. Cholesterol lowering trials in coronary heart disease: frequency of citation and outcome. *BMJ* 1992; 305: 15–19.

19 Todd PA, Goa KL. Simvastatin, a review of its pharmacological properties and therapeutic potential in hypercholesterolemia. *Drugs* 1990; 40: 583–607.

20 Illingworth DR, Erkelens DW, Keller U, Thompson G, Tikkanen MJ. Defined daily doses in relation to hypolipidaemic efficacy of lovastatin, pravastatin, and simvastatin. *Lancet* 1994; 343: 1554–55.

21 The Scandinavian Simvastatin Survival Study Group. Design and baseline results of the Scandinavian Simvastatin Survival Study of patients with stable angina and/or previous myocardial infarction. *Am J Cardiol* 1993; 71: 393–400.

22 WHO MONICA Project. MONICA manual, revised edition. Geneva: Cardiovascular Diseases Unit, WHO: 1990.

23 Tuomilehto J, Arstila M, Kaarsalo E, et al. Acute myocardial infarction in Finland: baseline data from the FINMONICA AMI register in 1983–85. *Eur Heart J* 1992; 13: 577–87.

24 Crow RS, Prineas RJ, Jacobs DR Jr, Blackburn H. A new epidemiologic classification system for interim myocardial infarction from serial electrocardiographic changes. *Am J Cardiol* 1989; 64: 454–61.

25 Cox DR. Regression methods of life tables (with discussion). *J R Stat Soc* 1972; B34: 187–220.

26 Keech A, Collins R, MacMahon S, et al. Three-year follow-up of the Oxford Cholesterol Study: assessment of the efficacy and safety of simvastatin in preparation for a large mortality study. *Eur Heart J* 1994; 15: 255–69.

27 MAAS investigators. Effect of simvastatin on coronary atheroma: the Multicentre Anti-Atheroma Study (MAAS). *Lancet* 1994; 344: 633–38.

28 Canner PJ, Berge KG, Wenger NK, et al, for the Coronary Drug Project Group. Fifteen year mortality in coronary drug project patients: long-term benefit with niacin. *J Am Coll Cardiol* 1986; 8: 1245–55.

29 Law MR, Wald NJ, Thompson SG. By how much and how quickly does reduction in serum cholesterol concentration lower risk of ischaemic heart disease? *BMJ* 1994; 308: 367–72.

30 Furberg CD, Adams HP Jr, Applegate WB, et al. Effect of lovastatin on early carotid atherosclerosis and cardiovascular events. *Circulation* 1994; 90: 1679–87.

31 Brown BG, Zhao X-Q, Sacco DE, Albers JJ. Lipid lowering and plaque regression. New insights into prevention of plaque disruption and clinical events in coronary disease. *Circulation* 1993; 87: 1781–91.

32 Vos J, deFeyter J, Simoons ML, Tijssen JGP, Deckers JW. Retardation and arrest of progression or regression of coronary artery disease: a review. *Prog Cardiovasc Dis* 1993; 35: 435–54.

33 Waters D, Craven T, Lesperance J. Prognostic significance of progression of coronary atherosclerosis. *Circulation* 1993; 87: 1067–75.

34 Davies MJ, Krikler DM, Katz D. Atherosclerosis: inhibition or regression as therapeutic possibilities. *Br Heart J* 1991; 65: 302–10.

35 Fuster V, Badimon L, Badimon JJ, Chesebro JH. The pathogenesis of coronary artery disease and acute coronary syndromes. *N Engl J Med* 1992; 326: 242–50, 310–18.

Figure 10.1g The 4S Trial.

1. Was the Assignment of Patients to Treatments Really Randomized?

In this trial, patients were legitimately randomized to placebo versus active treatment. There was a two week run-in phase to determine if the patient was 'compliant.' This reflects the highly controlled environment of a clinical trial and points out the difference between efficacy trials and effectiveness trials. Remember, efficacy means that the drug works under ideal circumstances and effectiveness means how the drug works under 'real-world' circumstances. The authors do not reveal how many patients were dropped from the study because of 'lack of compliance.' In general, we prefer full disclosure so that we can make up our own mind how it affects the interpretation of the results. On the positive side, it was a placebo run-in, not an active drug run-in phase. Thus, they did not skew the results by selecting patients that can tolerate the medicine. In general, we consider this to be an acceptable method and conclude that it has a minimal effect on the interpretation of the trial in general. This question, is really asking whether or not the study subjects were randomized appropriately. The study group did stratify the patients for clinical site and previous myocardial infarction, which is a very appropriate process when multiple different sites for a single clinical trial are used. In summary, we are confident that randomization occurred appropriately.

2. Were All Clinically Relevant Outcomes Reported?

As seen in Figure 10.1d, the primary clinical outcome was mortality, which is clearly a patient oriented outcome and probably the most important endpoint considered. The study reported all-cause mortality, which is important because this accounts for unknown and unexpected side effects. For example, the study drug may cause unforeseen side effects such as decreased night vision, which could result in increased motor vehicle accidents and traumatic deaths. If only cardiac deaths were counted, then these traumatic deaths would go unnoticed. All-cause mortality accounts for these unanticipated events, preventing bias in reporting outcomes. Indeed, there are many examples where 'cardiac events' show a discrepancy with all-cause mortality. In the end, the patient does care how he died, he just cares that he died.

The authors also present many other relevant clinically orientated outcomes which can be seen in Figure 10.1d, including coronary deaths, major coronary events (definite acute MI, definite or probable MI, silent MI, resuscitated cardiac arrest, acute MI with intervention), coronary surgery or angioplasty, congestive heart failure, stroke. Notice that these outcomes are also patient oriented outcomes since they severely impact the quality of life and functioning of our patient. However, the long term consequences of 'silent MI' may not be important as a patient orientated outcome. In general, we believe the authors were thorough and complete in giving us all clinically relevant outcomes as well as some disease orientated information.

3. Were the Study Patients Recognizably Similar to Your Own?

This question needs to be answered in two ways. We need to be able to convince ourselves that our patient's concern is addressed by the research data presented, but in a more general way. Do the inclusion and exclusion criteria match our patient population in our own clinical practice? The authors do a good job of delineating the inclusion and exclusion criteria. They studied men and women aged 35–70 years with a history of angina pectoris or acute myocardial infarction. There was also a very long list of exclusion criteria seen in the Recruitment and Randomization section under the Patients and Methods heading. In general, a long list of exclusion criteria is used to focus the study group on one specific trait and patients in real practice typically have more than one problem. In this particular case chest pain in otherwise healthy people is such a common complaint that the exclusion criteria do not eliminate a significant portion of our practice population. Although our patient has no definitive angina pectoris, she does have atypical chest pain with multiple risk factors. Because our patient is female, we can consider these roughly equivalent circumstances. In summary, we think the study patients are similar to our patients and our clinic practice population.

4. Were Both Clinical and Statistical significance Considered?

Because the authors used patient oriented outcomes, this study is easily applicable in a clinical setting. As we worked through the process there is enough information presented in an appropriate way to incorporate these results into a conversation with the patient. This is in contrast to some studies that only report relative risks and therefore have limited utility. In addition, the authors used appropriate statistical measures (Kaplan-Meier curves) which measure the number of events over time. Since the proposed treatment is not a single event, we really need to understand the cumulative affect of taking this medication. The median follow up was 5.4 years, with a range of 4.9–6.3 years. Our patient is probably going to be asked to make a lifetime commitment, but this particular trial had a long enough duration to provide good evidence. Indeed, it would be hard to continue the trial for a longer duration and still meet the ethical requirements of the data and safety monitoring committee. In summary, we believe that both clinical and statistical significance was addressed.

5. Is the Therapeutic Maneuver Feasible in Your Practice?

Historically, when this trial was performed there was a lot of controversy about the use of statins. Statin use now is widely available in part because of this hallmark study. This treatment modality is readily available, accepted by patients, and affordable for our patients.

6. Were All the Patients who Entered the Study Accounted For?

This question again has two parts. We need to verify that the specified outcomes were measured correctly and that every patient was evaluated for every outcome. Mortality was determined every six months and at the end of the study by contact with the patient or another member of the household. Cause of death was obtained from hospital records, death certificates, and interviews with physicians and relatives. The fact that the study did not use only death certificate diagnoses, as the death certificate diagnosis is often invalid, but used a multi-method process to determine the cause of death creates a high validity or truth value in the actual cause of death. This type of follow up and measurement is typical of studies done in Scandinavia and serves as a model of superior methodology. Since they contacted every single patient who entered the study, we are confident that all the patients were accounted for. The secondary end points were done in a comparable manner.

7. Were Patients Analyzed in the Groups to Which They Were Randomized?

In the abstract, the authors state that 256 patients (12%) in the placebo group died. From Table 10.1, we know that 2223 patients were randomized to the placebo group. In the results section, the authors report that 129 patients in the placebo group discontinued therapy. This question is actually asking about intention-to-treat, which means even the patients that discontinued therapy need to be included in the analysis.[17] Note that 256/2223 equals 11.51%, which would be the intention-to-treat result. However, if the dropouts are excluded, then only 2094 (2223 – 129 dropouts) patients would be left to analyze in the placebo group, resulting in 256/(2223 – 129 dropouts) equals 12.22%. The authors reported 12%.

Using a parallel analysis for the treatment group, in the abstract, the authors state that 182 patients (8%) in the statin group died. From Table 10.1, in the study we know that 2221 patients were randomized to the statin group. In the results section, the authors report that 126 patients in the statin group discontinued therapy. Note that 182/2221 equals 8.19%, which would be the intention- to-treat result. However, if the dropouts are excluded, then only 2095 (2221–126 dropouts) patients would be left to analyze in the statin group, resulting in 182/(2221 – 126 dropouts) equals 8.68%. The authors reported 8%. We outlined this in Table 10.1 below.

Table 10.1 Table with data to calculate number-needed-to-treat.

		Placebo	Simvastatin
Intention-to-treat analysis	Entered study	2223	2221
	Dropouts excluded	0	0
	Number used for analysis	2223	2221
	Deaths	256	182
	Mortality rate	11.51%	8.19%
Analyzed with dropouts excluded	Entered study	2221	2221
	Dropouts excluded	129	126
	Number used for analysis	2223–129=2094	2221–126=2095
	Deaths	256	182
	Mortality rate	12.22%	8.68%

These minor differences may be important because eventually we need to calculate the absolute risk reduction and the number-needed-to-treat. These rounding errors may change the story when it is eventually told. This level of analysis points out the importance of re-checking the results reported by the authors. In this case, it does not make a significant difference in how we will eventually use the information, but for other, less well done and reported studies, we need to always check for whether all the patients were analyzed in the group to which they were randomized. *The most important criterion to perform an intention-to-treat analysis is that even patients who stopped treatment or sought alternate treatment need to have the outcome measured.* If too many patients were 'lost to follow up' (and the outcome unable to be determined), an intention-to-treat analysis cannot be performed; although other types of analyses could be performed.[17]

8. Were All Patients, Health Workers, and Study Personnel Blinded?

This article that we are reviewing does not directly answer this question. In this paper the authors state, 'The study design has been published previously.' Unfortunately, that means to answer this question, we need to do more work. The good news is that they referenced the full methods in a previous publication in the American Journal of Cardiology. As described above, the reference wasn't immediately available, so that we had to use our university subscription. After reviewing the article, we found the follow excerpt:

> The Scandinavian Simvastatin Survival Study (4s) is a multicenter, double-blind [in fact the design is 'triple-blind' because patients, investigators and study administration are unaware of patients' drug assignment], randomized, placebo-controlled trial with simvastatin in 4444 men and women aged between 35 and 70 years with established CAD and serum total cholesterol levels between 5.5 and 8.0 mmol/liter (212 to 309 mg/dl).[18]
>
> Since the patients, investigators, and study administrators were unaware of the patient's drug assignments, this study was indeed blinded to patients, health care workers, and all study personnel.

9. Aside From the Experimental Intervention, Were the Groups Treated Equally?

All patients underwent blood sampling, interviews for adverse reactions, full clinical examination, and electrocardiogram at the same intervals. The researchers did treat the two groups identically. Additionally, the 4S trial states, 'A computer program at the central laboratory issued dosage adjustment messages without reviewing lipid levels or treatment allocation.' – 'to maintain the double-blind, patients in the placebo group were randomly assigned matching placebo tablets.' Because the study design insured elegant blinding, we can be confident that the two groups were treated equally.

Application of SORT criteria

Because it is a high quality randomized controlled trial with patient oriented evidence, we categorized the level of evidence as level 1 according to the SORT criteria.

A CONTINGENT, EMERGENT, SITUATED, AND CONTEXTUAL MEDICAL KNOWLEDGE

Patients go to doctors with the belief that doctors have a specialized knowledge that gives them power. In our society that belief is created with the image of doctor as scientist. What the doctor knows is dependent upon the sources of information he/she uses to acquire that knowledge. Pharmaceutical companies with a profit motive have a heavy influence on the 'science' upon which doctors depend. Good doctors re-create a *contingency of suspended belief* until they evaluate the evidence as presented.

As the doctor evaluates the quality of the evidence, an opinion *emerges* about whether or not to believe the claims of the authors of the medical literature. A healthy skepticism is recommended. As the process of care emerges, new sets of contingencies result; the emergent nature of knowledge is a result of the processual nature of decision making in an ongoing process over time.

Whether or not the clinical research agrees with the pre-formed opinions of the doctor depends on how it is interpreted within the *situated* position in the web of belief of the clinician scientist. Remember poor Galileo and his defense of the heliocentric theory of planetary motion.

Pharmaceutical companies are part of the *context* of medical literature and therefore a constituent part of EBM.

REFERENCES

1 Ross J. Guest authorship and ghostwriting in publications related to refocoxib: a case study of industry documents from refecoxib litigation. *JAMA.* 2008; 299(15).
2 Fugh-Berman A. The corporate coauthor. *J Gen Intern Med.* 2005; 20(6).
3 Sismondo S. Ghost management: how much of the medical literature is shaped behind the scenes by the pharmaceutical industry? *PLoS Medicine.* 2007; 4(9): e286.
4 Yank V. Financial ties and concordance between results and conclusions in meta-analyses: retrospective cohort study. *BMJ.* 2007; 335.
5 Jorgensen A. Cochrane Reviews compared with industry supported meta-analyses and other meta-analyses of the same drugs: systematic review. *BMJ.* 2006; 333.
6 Smith R. Medical journals are an extension of the marketing arm of pharmaceutical companies. *PLoS Medicine.* 2005; 2(5): e1382(5).

7   Stang A. The ongoing tyranny of statistical significance testing in biomedical research. *European Journal of Epidemiology.* 2010; **25**(4): 225–30.

8   Katz MH. *Study Design and Statistical Analysis: a practical guide for clinicians.* Cambridge: Cambridge University Press; 2006.

9   Katz MH. *Multivariable Analysis: a practical guide for clinicians.* 2nd ed. Cambridge: Cambridge University Press; 2006.

10 Jamerson K, Weber M, Bakris G, *et al.* Benzapril plus amlodipine or hydrochlorothiazide for hypertension in high risk patients. *New England Journal of Medicine.* 2008; 359(23): 2417.

11 Poole-Wilson P, Swedberg K, Cleland J, *et al.* Comparison of carvedilol and metoprolol on clinical outcomes in patients with chronic heart failure in the Carvedilil Or Metoprolol European Trial (Comet): randomised controlled trial. *The Lancet.* 2003; 362: 7–13.

12 Forbes C. Secondary stroke prevention with low-dose aspirin, sustained release dipyridamole alone and in combination. *Thrombosis Research.* 1998; 92(1): S1–S6.

13 Dawson D, Cutler B, Hiatt W, *et al.* A comparison of cilostazol and pentoxifylline for treating intermittent claudication. *American Journal of Medicine.* 2000: **109**(7): 523–31.

14 Harenberg J, Schmidt J, Koppenhagen K, *et al.* Fixed-dose, body weight-independent subcutaneous LMW heparin versus adjusted dose unfractionated intravenous heparin in the initial treatment of proximal venous thrombosis. *Thromb Haemost.* 2000; 83: 652–6.

15 Andriole G, Crawford D, Grubb R, *et al.* Mortality results from a randomized prostate cancer screening trial. *New England Journal of Medicine.* 2009; 360(13): 1310–19.

16 Schroder F, Hugosson J, Roobol M, *et al.* Screening and prostate-cancer mortality in a randomized European study. *New England Journal of Medicine.* 2009; 360(13): 1320–8.

17 Montori VM, Guyatt G. Intention to treat principle. *Canadian Medical Association Journal.* 2001; **165**(10): 1339–1341.

18 4S Group. Design and baseline results of the Scandinavian simvastatin survival study of patients with stable angina and/or previous myocardial infarction. *Am J Cardiol.* 1993; **71**: 393–400.

CHAPTER 11

Apply the Information to the Clinical Question

KEY CONCEPTS TO REMEMBER

➤ Make sure you select the most relevant outcomes to calculate Number Needed to Treat.

➤ Avoid Relative Risk Reductions since they are misleading

➤ Don't forget to calculate number needed to harm for the most important side effects of therapy so you can give both sides of the benefit-harm discussion.

LEARNING ABOUT APPLYING INFORMATION TO CLINICAL QUESTIONS

Number Needed to Treat

During the Google Scholar search, it is important to scan the results looking for information with the highest validity as described in Chapter 9. After selecting a link, then the next step is to scan the abstract looking for the components of the PICO question. In this chapter, we introduce a concept called *number needed to treat*, abbreviated NNT, which is calculated from the data related to I, C, and O of the PICO question. In summary, we are verifying that the research article has the components that we are going to need for the next step in the process, which is calculating NNT.

Finding the Numbers for Number Needed to Treat

Many studies report multiple different outcomes. Some of the outcomes reported are patient oriented evidence that matters, while many of them are usually disease oriented evidence. Sometimes you have to choose the most relevant outcomes from a series of reported outcomes. It is important before beginning the application of the data to the patient's problem because the eventual explanation shared with the patient must reflect this difference.

In order to move forward, we need to clearly delineate the intervention group and the comparator group and verify at the outset how these two groups are defined. Remember, as explained in Chapter 10, the intervention group needs to be compared to the standard of care, which should be the C in your PICO question. We often find that a 'straw man analysis' is used. This means the new pharmaceutical is compared to an obviously inadequate or inappropriate comparator group to ensure 'perceived' efficacy.

We also have to be as careful with the researcher's choice of outcome measures. This is particularly important because during the analysis the researchers often report results of subgroups and secondary outcomes which can make for a lot of numbers, charts, tables, all of which can be confusing. Our advice is to select only the predefined treatment and comparative groups as well as the predefined patient oriented outcomes; it is reasonable to completely ignore all other results. There is evidence that research reports that are published 'cheat' by changing the primary outcome after the data are collected.[1] Preventing this is part of the reason for the National Register of Clinical Trials. This is an efficient way to select only the most appropriate information. Researchers sometimes present it as percentages or total number of cases with a specific outcome. The typical outcome reported is an adverse event such as death or myocardial infarction. These four numbers – 1. total number of patients in the treatment group; 2. total number of patients in the comparator (control) group; 3. the number of patients in the treatment group with the measured event; 4. the number of patients in the comparator (control) group with the measured event) – are used to arithmetically compute the number needed to treat. Again, finding these four numbers will allow you to proceed. The rest can be ignored!

For example, in the Carvedilol and Morbidity and Mortality in Chronic Heart Failure study:

> In the intention-to-treat analysis, there were 31 deaths (7.8%) in the placebo group and 22 deaths (3.2%) in the carvedilol group; this difference represents a 65% decrease in the risk of death (95% confidence interval, 39 to 80%; $p < 0.001$) in patients assigned to carvedilol.[2]

Table 11.1 Data needed to calculate the number needed to treat (NNT).

1	Total number of patients in treatment group	696
2	Total number of patients in control group	398
3	The number of patients in the treatment group with the measured event (death)	22
4	The number of patients in the control group with the measured event (death)	31

Calculating Number Needed to Treat

Now that we have our four numbers, we can begin to calculate the number needed to treat. The formula is fairly simple, one divided by the *absolute risk reduction* as illustrated below.

$$NNT = \frac{1}{arr}$$

So what is an absolute risk reduction? The absolute risk reduction is the difference in the event rate between the two groups. At this point, it is important to point out that you will be dividing an integer by another integer, which creates a ratio. This will yield a number less than one and should be expressed as a decimal, NOT a percentage. The same process needs to be done in the comparator (control) group. Divide the number of patients with the measured event in the comparator group by the total number of patients in the comparator group, which creates another ratio. Calculate a similar ratio for the treatment group. Again, it needs to be expressed as a decimal. Note that you have to calculate the ratio for each group independently because there are different total numbers of subjects in each of the groups.

Usually authors present the events both as the number of events and a percentage. However, occasionally, only a percentage will be reported. In that situation, multiply the percentage by the total number in the group to get the number of events in that group.

The formula to calculate the absolute risk reduction (arr) is:

$$\text{arr} = \frac{\text{Patients in the control group with the measured event}}{\text{Total number of patients in control group}} - \frac{\text{Patients in the treatment group with the measured event}}{\text{Total number of patients in treatment group}}$$

$$\text{arr} = \frac{31}{398} - \frac{22}{696}$$

$$\text{arr} = .078 - .032$$

$$\text{arr} = .046$$

In simpler terms, assuming the therapy group worked better; subtract the smaller number from the bigger number. The absolute risk reduction represents the ratio of events in the comparator (control) group minus the ratio of events in the treatment group. In other words, how much smaller was the event rate smaller in the treatment group (fewer deaths)?

Now that we have calculated the absolute risk reduction, we are ready to calculate the number needed to treat using the initial formula. Thus:

$$\text{NNT} = \frac{1}{\text{arr}}$$

$$\text{NNT} = \frac{1}{.046}$$

$$\text{NNT} = 22$$

So, what does this mean? We need to treat 22 people who have angina, with carvedilol to prevent one death. But, the next question is, for how long? To answer this, we need to look back to the original research study and we find that the length of treatment was 12 months. *Therefore, 22 people with systolic heart failure would need to take carvedilol for 12 months before one death will be prevented.* Notice, that this only pertains to people with systolic heart failure and does not tell us how many people we would need to treat over a longer period of time. The number needed to treat is closely related to the context of the original study (inclusion criteria, exclusion criteria, duration of treatment, dose of medicine, etc.).

Number Needed to Harm

Of course, medications have side effects. In order to compare the benefit of the treatment group, we should also try and quantify the risk of side-effects. Using a similar process we could calculate a number needed to harm (NNH) for specific adverse events. The formula for number needed to harm is as follows:

$$NNH = \frac{1}{ari}$$

(Where 'ari' stands for absolute risk increase.) Just like absolute risk reduction, the absolute risk increase is the difference in event rate between the treatment group and the control group. However, with absolute risk increase, the treatment group has an unwanted event, such as headache, nausea, or even death.

Finding the Numbers for Number Needed to Harm

Continuing with the example discussed in the above section, in the Carvedilol and Morbidity and Mortality in Chronic Heart Failure study, six patients in the carvedilol group suffered from bradycardia. The bradycardia was significant enough to cause discontinuation of the study drug. Zero patients in the placebo group experienced this.

Table 11.2 Data needed to calculate the number needed to harm (NNH).

1	Total number of patients in treatment group	696
2	Total number of patients in control group	398
3	The number of patients in the treatment group with the measured event (bradycardia)	6
4	The number of patients in the control group with the measured event (bradycardia)	0

Calculating Number Needed to Harm

In order to calculate number needed to harm, we must first calculate the absolute risk increase (ari), by:

$$\text{ari} = \frac{\begin{array}{c}\text{Patients in the treatment group}\\ \text{with the measured event}\end{array}}{\begin{array}{c}\text{Total number of patients in}\\ \text{treatment group}\end{array}} - \frac{\begin{array}{c}\text{Patients in the control group}\\ \text{with the measured event}\end{array}}{\begin{array}{c}\text{Total number of patients in}\\ \text{control group}\end{array}}$$

Notice that this equation is nearly identical to the absolute risk reduction equation above. The idea is that you need to find the difference of the event rate between the treatment and control group. We never think about these equations. We simply subtract the event rates, the ratios, from each other. If we are looking at a beneficial event, like mortality rate reduction for the study drug, then it is an absolute rate reduction. If it is an unwanted event, like symptomatic bradycardia for the study drug, then we label an absolute rate increase.

Plugging the numbers into our example below:

$$\text{ari} = \frac{6}{696} - \frac{0}{398}$$

$$\text{ari} = .009 - 0$$

$$\text{ari} = .009$$

Now that we have calculated the absolute risk increase, we are ready to calculate the Number Needed to Harm using the initial formula. Thus:

$$\text{NNH} = \frac{1}{\text{ari}}$$

$$\text{NNH} = \frac{1}{.009}$$

$$\text{NNH} = 111$$

This means, that we need to treat 111 people that have systolic heart failure, with carvedilol to cause one patient to have bradycardia significant enough to cause discontinuation. Just as with number needed to treat, since the study length was 12 months, 111 people with systolic heart failure would need to take carvedilol for 12 months in order to cause one person to have bradycardia.

We cannot directly compare number needed to treat with number needed to harm. It is like comparing apples to oranges. There is a big difference between bradycardia significant enough to cause discontinuation of a drug and death. These numbers need to remain in their context when discussing it with patients.

Relative Risk

In this section, we were working with absolute risk reduction as one of the variables to calculate number needed to treat. Earlier in this book, we discussed actual clinical practice when patients bring in newspaper articles or information from the internet. A typical claim will be 30% improvement with treatment X. This is a RELATIVE risk reduction. It is vital to recognize the difference relative risk reduction and absolute risk reduction. The classic example is if a treatment decreases an adverse event from 3/1000 to 2/1000, the relative risk reduction is 33% – which seems like a large reduction. However, compare that to the absolute reduction, which is .001 (.1%), which seems like a very small number. The number needed to treat would be 1000. That is a lot of people. Newspapers and advertisements use relative risk reduction to create the perception of a large benefit.

We recommend never using relative risk reductions as they are misleading. Always be cautious when anyone makes this type of claim. Unfortunately relative risk reduction is sometimes used in the medical literature, such as in the Screening and Prostate-Cancer Mortality in a Randomized European Study, where the authors report, 'PSA-based screening reduced the rate of death from prostate cancer by 20%...' Reporting in this format is deceptive and should be avoided. Be cautious if you encounter it while reading the medical literature.

STORY TIME

Many people just do not like taking pills. Even after reviewing all of the information, showing them where it comes from and telling them how reliable it is, they simply refuse medication. This is a very common scenario. The important thing is to be patient. The patient needs to be ready to act on the information. We usually say, 'We'll talk about it again next year.' If you try to insist that they take a pill, the adherence rate would most assuredly be low. We have had many patients that go over the same information several years in a row. The stories they tell us are about how they tried to manage the problem with diet, exercise, or some alternative therapy. With patience, many of these patients will one day ask us to review the information again and then say, 'OK, I'll take the pill this time.'

The point of the story is ... It has to make sense to the patient and this often takes more time than we as doctors believe is necessary.

NARRATIVE ASPECTS OF APPLYING THE EVIDENCE

Being able to find the evidence and being able to understand it from the doctor's perspective still does not benefit the patient. We are taking research results and converting it into a format to prepare for re-integrating evidence into the lives and life stories of our patients. By using standardized protocols, we are getting ready to begin the work of the co-constructed narrative. This gives us a language not only to talk with other physicians about the relative benefits of the treatment, but we have to remember it is the patient who will eventually need to decide the relative importance of the evidence. By calculating a NNT and a NNH, we will be prepared to answer some basic questions most of our patients will want to know.

APPLICATION TO OUR CLINICAL SCENARIO

Our patient is interested in preventing her cardiac death. One of the endpoints in the 4S trial is cardiovascular mortality. It is important that when multiple relevant clinical endpoints are reported in an article, we use the numbers in the endpoint most relevant to our patients concern. Our patient does not want to die from a heart attack; however, it is also reasonable to assume that our patient does not want to die from anything. Even though the author's report cardiovascular death, we are going to use all-cause mortality as the endpoint to answer our patients concern.

In the explanation above, we showed how to calculate the percentage of deaths in each group. Often, the authors provide these numbers in a table as they did in this case, Table 2 from the 4S trial. We can make our table as shown above:

Table 11.3 Data needed to calculate the number needed to treat (NNT).

1	Total number of patients in treatment group	2221
2	Total number of patients in control group	2223
3	The number of patients in the treatment group with the measured event (total death)	182
4	The number of patients in the control group with the measured event (total death)	256

In order to calculate the number needed to treat, we need to calculate the absolute risk reduction, which is the percentage of all cause mortality in the treatment group subtracted from the all cause mortality in the placebo group, by:

$$\text{arr} = \frac{\text{Patients in the control group with the measured event}}{\text{Total number of patients in control group}} - \frac{\text{Patients in the treatment group with the measured event}}{\text{Total number of patients in treatment group}}$$

$$\text{arr} = \frac{256}{2223} - \frac{182}{2221}$$

$$\text{arr} = .115 - .082$$

$$\text{arr} = .033$$

Notice that the .115 and .082 are provided for us in Table 2 of the 4S Trial. These numbers are in parenthesis and formatted as a percentage. Most studies provide the event ratio, but it is almost always as a percentage. In order to use the absolute risk reduction equation, the decimal format must be used. Repeat, the DECIMAL format must be used. So we have to convert 11.5 (%) to .115 and 8.2 (%) to .082 for this equation.

We can now calculate the number needed to treat with the absolute risk reduction by the following equation:

$$\text{NNT} = \frac{1}{\text{arr}}$$

$$\text{NNT} = \frac{1}{.033}$$

$$\text{NNT} = 30$$

This trial included patients who were at relatively high risk for coronary artery disease and the length of the median length of this trial was 5.4 years.

Thus, 30 similarly high risk patients would have to be treated with simvastatin for 5.4 years to prevent one death. That also means that 29 people will take the medication and be exposed to the side effects without ever receiving benefit with regard to mortality. Also, this research trial was limited to 5.4 years and our patient might reasonably be expected to be treated for five, 10, or even 20 years. We can only extrapolate how many patients need to be treated for 20 years to prevent one death. The next section is how we need to present this to the patient.

Of course, medications have side effects. In order to compare the benefit of the treatment group, we should also try and quantify the risk of side-effects. Using a similar process we could calculate a number needed to harm (NNH) for specific adverse events. In this particular trial, there was no statistically significant increase in side effects reported. However, your effort to fully inform you patient, you must carefully scan the article for these events as well. We will illustrate this in the example in Chapter 12.

A CONTINGENT, EMERGENT, SITUATED, AND CONTEXTUAL MEDICAL KNOWLEDGE

Although many patients hear about therapies on direct to consumer advertisements, those television commercials also have 'the fine print,' when the voice-over rattles off a list of potential adverse events and then says, 'consult your doctor.' The *contingency* involved is the size of the risk of benefit versus the risk of harm, the acceptability of the potential adverse events, and how desperate the patient is to risk taking the pill to get the potential benefit. All this remains *contingent* until that conversation occurs with 'your doctor.'

The *emergent* nature of this step in the process is that the magnitude of benefit versus harm emerges from the calculations. These numbers are often a surprise, which verifies that the understanding emerges; by actually doing the math, we destroy our naive assumptions that every patient will experience benefit – that notion just seems like so much common sense, despite being wrong. The information we use in the co-constructed narrative is *situated* within a matrix of thousands of decisions that have occurred during the office visit and the continuity relationship. Most of those decisions remain unconscious, but when examined closely, create the history of how we got there and set up the future expressed as the management plan.

The *context* of applying the information is to whom it was and will be applied.

REFERENCES

1 Ewart R, Lausen H, Millian N. Undisclosed changes in outcomes in randomized controlled trials: an observational study. *Annals of Family Medicine.* 2009; 7(6): 542–6.
2 Packer M, Bristow MR, Cohn JN, *et al.* The effect of carvedilol on morbidity and mortality in patients with chronic heart failure. *New England Journal of Medicine.* 1996; 334: 1349–55.

Assist the Patient In Making a Decision

KEY CONCEPTS TO REMEMBER

➤ Communicating uncertainty to patients is difficult; there is no agreement or consistent best method.

➤ Different people may have different preferences for receiving information; we suggest multi-method attempts to see if you can find one that works for that particular patient.

➤ Using hand motions and body motions can create 'cognitive artifacts' or spatial representations that can persist within the context of a conversation. Body language is a great tool for communication.

➤ The way the evidence is presented becomes a moral enterprise because it can sway the patient's decision about life, life's experiences, and death.

➤ Numeracy (the ability to comprehend the meaning of numbers) varies widely.

➤ Narrative reasoning has equal influence when making clinical decisions.

LEARNING ABOUT MAKING DECISIONS

Introduction

One of the things that is most confusing in the literature is how to convey risk information to patients. The problem revolves around explaining uncertainty to patients. We explored this issue in patient communication literature and found some of the following discussions of the problem.

Despite the summary of an extensive body of literature regarding patient physician communication, we are left with little understanding of how this is accomplished in the social setting of the office visit.[1] Roter et al. described six key variables: (1) information giving; (2) information seeking; (3) social talk; (4) positive talk; (5) negative talk; and (6) partnership building. What these authors do highlight is that the flow of information between the patient and the physician is an integral and necessary part of the therapeutic nature of the doctor–patient relationship. In a separate meta-analysis of provider behaviors, satisfaction was predicted by the amount of information given by the providers.[1] Studies have shown that patients place a high value on receiving information.[2, 3] The communication literature specific to conveying health risks has changed little in terms of definitive, evidenced based recommendations from 1988 until 2007.[3] Content analysis of office visits show that physicians typically spend less than one minute out of a 20 minute visit discussing treatment and planning.[4]

Uncertainty

One of the inherent difficulties in the therapeutic conversation introduces the concept of understanding uncertainty. Spiegelhalter describes two contributing factors to this uncertainty. *Epistemological* uncertainty talks about our lack of knowledge about the topic being discussed. We have encountered this in our discussions of validity and truth value of the medical literature. Although we can approximate truth through science, it can never be fully known. *Aleatory* uncertainty refers to random chance of a future phenomenon.[5] We have also encountered this as statistical concepts such as 95% confidence intervals or p values, expressions of probability (a closely related concept).

Epistemological uncertainty talks about what we know and what we are still ignorant of. Research studies have a varying degree of cause and effect 'truth value'. This is illustrated when higher quality evidence supplants and reverses recommendations based on less valid studies. The problem is that information from research studies will only give us the probability of a future event in a population – that is the nature of a research trial.

Making Uncertainty Personal

Our patient does not care anything about what happens to a group of people, and in fact, all that they're interested in is what is going to happen to them.[6-8] From the patient's perspective, it is a guessing game. This refers to the *aleatory* uncertainty or the random chance that they might be the one to be lucky enough to benefit from therapy or have the test accurately reflect the presence or absence of disease. This aleatory uncertainty is constituent of likelihood ratios and NNT/NNH. We believe that the only way to understand these risks and uncertainty is within a narrative context

The perception of these uncertainties varies. A person may acknowledge the population likelihood yet believe his or her individual probability is different.[3] The difficulty is illustrated when a doctor says, 'There is a one in 10 chance that you will develop X' and the patient hears 'I'm sure I will be one of the nine who will not get it.' Basically, people perceive their own risks different than the general population. Despite our efforts to define the 'patient population' back when we started with the PICO question, patients don't relate to being part of that group. Spiegelhalter says, 'My personal feeling is to acknowledge there is no correct answer and to pursue multiple representations, telling multiple stories, each with their own capacity to influence.'

Using Man's First and Best Tool: The Body

This subheading comes from a quotation from Marcel Mauss. There is a good evidence of using the body as a 'cognitive artifact' is a paralinguistic tool and patients can maintain three dimensional imaginative model in space during a conversation with ease.[6] This has the advantage of maintaining the conversational flow simultaneously using visual graphic aids and integrating a discussion of risk magnitude into the narrative, sort of like a 'picture book.' When we continue our case discussion, we provide a visual example using the body to represent abstract numbers and circumvent the problem of poor numeracy. Most literature says that patients prefer relative risk (which inflates differences or benefits) to absolute risk information. EBM physicians axiomatically condemn relative risk as misleading. Using the hand gestures and the doctor's body as symbols for numbers, we convey magnitude of benefit (or magnitude of harm) with a shared cognitive representation without resorting to abstract numbers. *This body language as symbol conveys both relative risk and absolute risk concurrently, sidestepping the problem of poor numeracy in patients.* All we can say is that it seems to work.

The mindful doctor will recognize that not only the patient must deal with uncertainty – so must the doctor. Like emotions, it requires a highly reflective doctor to be aware of whose uncertainty affects the clinical decision the most. We found an interesting article describing how doctors can use the hand (a body part) as a mnemonic to lessen their own anxiety with uncertainty.[7]

Narrative Portrayal of Risk

Another way to convey risk in a narrative format is to share information and then create a visual spectrum anchored by two imaginary patients with diametrically opposed values and beliefs. A common scenario prior to the recent publication of the PLCO and the European Prostate Screening Trial was to explain the clinical dilemma of finding cancer but not knowing how it would affect the patient's future health. Spreading the arms apart as far as possible and using body motions to represent a teeter-totter, we say, 'on this side you have a guy that says, "I'm terrified of cancer. I understand that there are surgical risks with potential problems, but if I have a single cancer cell in my body, then I want you to find it and take it out."' Then tilting our whole body and using the other hand we would say, 'You just told me that you are not even sure screening and treatment will prolong my life and I am terrified of leaking urine and even the possibility of impotence. Unless you can convince me that this really going to help, there is no way I want to even take the chance of those kinds of side effects.' After returning to a neutral position, we then say, 'Of course these are extremes and all you need to decide is that if you are more like the person (leaning toward to the arm to the left) or if you are more like the person to the right (leaning toward to the arm to the right teetering like a teeter totter) to see if you would want the screening PSA drawn during today's office visit.' This technique uses verbal and visual anchors on a three dimensional analog scale and integrates it with conversational transmission of information. It also highlights the 'decision balance' and tipping point that summarizes the inherent ambiguity of any decision. It preserves the story telling format and like the example above, patients are quite capable of understanding 'three dimensional, bodily, cognitive artifacts' while thinking about future decisions.

Organ Age as a Communication Tool

Intuitively people understand that you die when you are old. There are multiple attempts in the medical literature that use 'lung age' or 'artery age'[8] as a way of describing risk. These methods allow the patient to compare their chronological age to their lung age and figure out the state of their health. This technique isn't adaptable enough to discuss treatments and little information is available of how to link it to the medical literature, but it might be a helpful tool for talking with your patients.

These examples demonstrate that conveying risks during office visits do not necessarily be numerical or deductive. The literature does support trying to match your patients' cognitive style and discusses something called numeracy which implies understanding the meaning of probabilities expressed as numbers.

Discussing NNT with the Patient

Another way to share the information we discovered as outlined above is to use the concept of number needed to treat. We should caution our readers that we always do this in conversational style trying to avoid a terse technically correct statement. For example, this requires that you create a setting for the patient usually by saying, 'If there were a hundred patients just like you and *none of them took this medication,* over the next five years, 25 of them would wind up having a heart attack. Unfortunately we would have no way of determining if you would be one of those 25 people or not. Again, let us imagine if there were 100 people just like you and *all of the patients took the medicine.* Then 75 of the patients would have taken the medicine and have been exposed to the side effects but would not have benefited from the medicine. Of the 25 people who would have had a heart attack and decided to take the medicine, the medicine would have only worked for 9 of the people. Which means that 16 people would have taken the medicine and had a heart attack anyway. You might ask why would anyone take a pill like this. The answer is that nine of those 100 the pill prevented the heart attack. There is no way to know if you would be one of the lucky patients to fall into this group.' (We will use this same example with our case demonstration, except we will use different numbers.) This type of verbal description is almost always accompanied by a drawing with labels and numbers and creating a graph with the patient as you talk, allowing them to ask clarifying questions as you share the risk information. This combination of verbal description of numbers and graphical representation demonstrates one of the recommendations of using one of the multiple different modalities to convey risk information.

These conversations might be difficult or confusing to patients and we always pause frequently to allow for questions, re-explanations, or clarification. The goal here is to give the patient 'new narrative tools' because we always bring the conversation back to 'but this decision is really about how you want to handle the problem we spoke of earlier.' A co-constructive narrative is a social process and we strongly believe that the authority and the power of the physician created by the specialized knowledge and scientific authority needs to be shared with the patient during the process of decision making. Again, we believe that relationship centered care is the highest ideal for the doctor–patient therapeutic relationship and this means the doctor has to be willing to be vulnerable enough to allow the patient to disagree and prevail, sometimes against the 'technically correct' doctor's recommendation. We find that there is always another chapter in the patient's story and, more often than not, we continue conversation, discussion, and shared decision making, and both the doctor and the patient feel more comfortable with the decision making. One of our favorite phrases, 'I want us to work hard at this moment so that no matter what happens in the future you can say that I have made the best decision at the time.' Sometimes this requires repeated attempts at shared decision making until we get it right.

Uncertainty of Discussing Therapeutic Options

Politi *et al* also talk about communicating uncertainty of medical interventions.[9] Although sharing similar concerns with Spiegelhalter they highlight a few added burdens, including uncertainty arising from the complexity of risk information (the multiple interactions of risk factors) and the instability of risks and benefits over time. They also point out another source of uncertainty: ignorance. This is simply a statement that the medical literature fails to address most of our patients' real concerns.[10] This more recent article confirms that the medical literature has not progressed significantly in our understanding of ways to present scientific uncertainty to health care consumers. They state there are many recommendations for communicating uncertainty but few of these recommendations are supported by evidence.

The burden of uncertainty in our patients has the capacity to evoke emotional responses, which can be stressful for the patient. In fact, patients who negatively appraise uncertainty might experience fear, anxiety, or panic.[9] They acknowledged that there is no clear best practice for presenting uncertainty. From our perspective, this drive to decrease uncertainty is the reason why patients go to the doctor in the first place – we called it the 'narrative dilemma.' Patients are looking for information specifically to make decisions about what they should do next. Both from the patient's perspective and from the doctor's perspective, the task is to embrace the uncertainty, knowing that a decision has to be made about how to proceed. By following the process outlined in this book we teach doctors to embrace the uncertainty but strive for 'active decision making,' instead of passive decisions. Passive decisions are simply an avoidance of the problem. Avoiding the problem has the same risks and benefits as choosing management. The difference is that active decisions allow the doctor and patient to incorporate values, culture, and personal meaning into the medical management. Uncertainty is part of both diagnostic testing and therapy, and we believe that it is the moral obligation of physicians to be truthful with our patients up until the point that it no longer becomes beneficial, but harmful.[9]

Numeracy

This next section addresses another underlying dilemma which is called numeracy, analogous to literacy.[11] In fact, patients probably rely on heuristics and other cognitive strategies rather than numbers to make decisions. These mental representations get to the bottom line meaning, or gist, of a choice option.[9] Although researchers and some physicians are comfortable and skilled with manipulating numbers and interpreting their significance, the same is not necessarily true for all doctors or all patients. In fact, the literature suggests that patients have multiple different ways of understanding what 'makes sense.' Our own bias is that this deeply cultural and part of going to the doctor demonstrates a faith in technology and science and a desire to decrease uncertainty. Aleszewski and Jones[12] present the following contextual influences of responses to risk information:

➤ The extent to which the source of the information is trusted.
➤ The relevance of the information for everyday life and decision making.
➤ The relation to other perceived risks.
➤ The fit with previous knowledge and experience.
➤ The difficulty and importance of the choices and decisions.

Translating the language of technology and science for the patient is challenging.

There is a fair body of literature that talks about shared decision making. We will discuss evidence that relates the process of taking the medical literature and explaining it to the patient. Specifically, choices include decision aides (standardized shared decision making modules – typically done by video using a computer)[4, 13] where the patient explores their personal values in light of the literature. This has the advantage of no time constraints for the physician and standardization, but depersonalizes the care provided. The literature has also examined closely patient preferences for receiving numerical information as relative risk, absolute risk, subjective verbal methods using words such as 'highly uncertain',[3] number needed to treat,[14] pictures of populations at risk, and epidemiological graphs and charts. Multiple authors state that patients prefer relative risk reduction.[9, 11] Covey performed a meta-analysis of the effects of presenting treatment benefits in different formats, confirming that patients prefer relative risk rather than absolute risk or number needed to treat.[15] There is conflicting evidence for graphic discrete-frequency using highlighted human figures.[4, 13] The way the risk is presented influences patient's health care decisions.[12, 23, 24] A meta-analysis that showed treatments were more favorably evaluated when the information was presented as relative risk compare to absolute risk or number needed to treat.[15] A specific example of this is that 57% of patients chose the medication whose benefit was presented in relative terms and only 15% chose the same medication when the benefit was presented in absolute terms. Patients assume (incorrectly) that the risk of disease was one (100%), which highlights the problem of numeracy.[16] Skolbekkan reports that this finding has been repeatedly demonstrated and Covey confirms this in his meta-analysis of 24 studies.[16, 17] Sixteen to 20% of patients could not correctly answer basic risk questions such as, 'What constitutes a higher risk: 1%, 5%, or 10%.'[18]

Goodyear-Smith *et al* present data indicating that the majority of patients prefer graphical information (even more so than relative risk).[19] Few patients preferred absolute risk and none preferred number needed to treat. Difficulty understanding NNT was documented by Epstein and Sheridan. Halvorsen acknowledges the limitations of the number needed to treat, but then goes on to demonstrate its benefit over 'equivalent postponement' strategies similar to 'cardiovascular risk adjusted age' calculator.[20, 21] Sheridan states that 'NNT is often misinterpreted by patients and should not be used alone to communicate risk to patients.'[11] This summary illustrates how contradictory the literature is on conveying risk information to patients.

Many authors highlight the need for using the patient–physician relationship to accomplish the task of communicating health risk.[18, 22] There is a need for doctors to become effective risk communicators.[18] Pantilat makes several suggestions on phrases that are easier for patients to hear.[23] Makoul *et al* reviewed 'shared decision making' in the literature.[24] Despite a 750% relative increase (a 22% absolute increase) in the number of articles in MEDLINE from 1980 until 2003 mentioning 'shared decision making,' there is no shared definition of shared decision making. Oi! We note there is a very different process for shared decision making: the co-constructed narrative.

Narrative Reasoning

The above review of the literature is fairly convincing that patients are often unable to use numerical or technical data when they make important life decisions. Mattingly and Engel both discuss 'narrative reasoning.'[25, 26] Narrative reasoning is a type of cognitive process deeply embedded in human thinking that allows meaning to be generated from 'dramatic moments or narrative twists.' As the story unfolds most of us do not know the end and the drama is heightened because choices need to be made that will affect the way the story ends. This is the entire basis of the 'co-constructive narrative.' We tried to demonstrate how the doctor brings his/her specialized knowledge in numeracy and the patient contributes the 'meaning making' of their life story to face the challenges of writing the next chapter in the patient's story. Because we do this in an imaginative way considering alternate possibilities simultaneously in the exam room, we highlight the fact that these are actually choices. As mentioned above, we strongly encourage active choices instead of passive choices by imaginatively exploring different possibilities in the next episode of the patient's life story. This is the contingent part of the co-constructed narrative. The patient can begin to deal with the uncertainties of life and the practices of medicine. Mattingly calls this 'as if retrospection.'[27] Narrative as a cognitive process then becomes complementary to reductionist science. This is a case where the whole is more than the sum of the parts. The truly complete doctor is able to integrate this multiplicity of cognitive processes which we believe serves the patient better than either one individually.

Context and Framing Affects Patients' Understanding

There is no generally accepted 'best practice' for communicating risk.[28, 29] Therefore, this becomes one of the ethical and moral dimensions of medicine and why we consider integrating narrative and evidence based medicine one of the best options. The 'frame' becomes the patient's story. How the evidence is framed affects the patient's life choices. We struggle *to give them information within the framework that they can understand.* By integrating the techniques mentioned above into the story, the moral burden on the doctor is shared. The alternative would be more paternalistic or authoritarian and influencing the patient in their decisions without accepting responsibility for their consequences. Unfortunately, these influences are pervasive in medical care but at least this process acknowledges their existence and becomes a responsibility between the patient and the physician while preserving the expertise of the physician.

Medicine is a Moral Practice

There is a robust body of literature about physician self-reflection and how necessary it is to do this type of work. The fundamental problem addresses the question of 'Whose story is this?' Because narrative and medicine both deal with value systems and human lives there is an inescapable moral component to the practice of medicine. Relationship centered care openly acknowledges that both the patient and the physician influence each other and the ultimate decisions arising out of this relationship (co-constructive narrative) have moral dimensions.

STORY TIME

Seven years ago we were beginning to use these concepts and processes while teaching residents. We had a particularly brilliant young man who was destined to become an ophthalmologist. We were rounding in the hospital and had to decide whether or not to discharge a patient with pneumococcal bacteremia. We argued to keep her on IV antibiotics for another day and the resident wanted to send her home. He claimed to have 'evidence' that he was right. We eagerly took up the challenge and asked him to produce the article on afternoon rounds. The research trial turned out to have a very small number of subjects and claimed '100%' success. There is no such thing as 100%, so in such very small trials, we typically imagine the very next patient was a treatment failure and then recalculate the statistics. It turned out that the NNH with the harm being death was 1%. We asked him if he still wanted to discharge the patient. Being somewhat stubborn and unwilling to admit that he had been bested, he replied, 'Yes.' We looked at him and said we did not want him to be our doctor. This illustrates that the magnitude of the outcome has to be considered along with the frequency of the outcome. This helps determine the 'decision threshold.'

The point of the story is ... the decision threshold can be used as a test of uncertainty tolerance. 'Are you willing to accept a 1 in 100 chance that your patient will die if you discharge him today?'

THE NARRATIVE ASPECTS OF ASSISTING THE PATIENT TO MAKE A DECISION

Uncertainty is part of life. Our future is uncertain. We can always ask ourselves what type of story we are willing to tell. We had a 95-year-old woman tell us that she was ready to die (even though there was nothing wrong with her health.) We asked her how did she figure out she was ready? She said that, 'This body is just the preparation for eternal life. If this body will not do for me what I want it to do, then I'm ready to turn it in for another one. That's just the way it is.' She did not say anything about having lived a full life or about how worthless life was and how it wasn't worth living. She was looking to the future – to the next part of her life story. She was writing the story of her eternal life and that is what made sense to her. So now we know; our patient taught us about expectations and narrative dying and living.

Mattingly makes a provocative argument about narrative reasoning in clinical practice. This harkens back to what is a story, who it belongs to, the self perception of the physician as a scientist, and the need for a positivist, scientific basis for practice. What Mattingly suggests, however, is that clinicians also 'think' narratively.[26] If we admit that to ourselves, the barriers between the EBM and the patient's story diminish. Re-consider the following thought experiment: each research article is really a story about a particular test or drug – what are the narrative elements of scientific journal-writing genre as a literary text? This usually comes in the introduction – how the need to know is presented, in the methods – how we learn what we need to know, and in the conclusion – what we learned means and how it should be applied in practice. 'This is a story of a newly discovered pill that solves our patient's problems ...' Really?

APPLICATION TO OUR CLINICAL SCENARIO

1   *Doctor:*   Two weeks ago you were telling me about having shoulder
2   pains and we talked about some of your life experiences.
3   Ideally, we'd like to keep you healthy so you can help raise
4   your great grandchildren. We left off whether or not it would
5   make sense for you to take a cholesterol pill. You keep telling
6   me about foreign chemicals in your body. Could you help me
7   understand a little bit more about that?
8   *Patient:* I just want to be healthy. If I have to take a pill, it means that
9   there is something wrong with me. I was always too scared to
10   even think that there might be something wrong with me and
11   I didn't know about it. Taking pills reminds me that I am just
12   as vulnerable as my daddy. I'd like to think that would never
13   happen to me. If I have to take a pill, it is like admitting that I
14   have the same problem he did.
15 *Doctor:*   But you also told me about how hard it was for you to
16   lose your parents and the fact that you had to take such
17   responsibility at an early age. Maybe this is a way that you can
18   be different than your dad – different in a healthy way.
19   Silence
20   Silence
21   Silence
22 *Patient:* Ok, we've come this far. I appreciate your time and effort
23   looking up all of the medical information. I've never really
24   had a doctor that took such interest in being up to date in
25   all of the research. Whether or not I take the pill, I would be
26   interested to learn more about it.

27	*Doctor:*	Just like the test, there is nothing that is perfect. Some of
28		the side effects of this pill include muscle aches. These are
29		usually minor and go away if you stop the pill. The only other
30		thing you need to watch is if there is any irritation on your
31		liver. We do that by checking occasional blood tests. I have
32		only heard of one person that had a serious reaction to this
33		medicine, but my practice is filled with people that have had
34		heart problems from hardening of the arteries. I think that
35		the risks of the medicine is fairly low, your insurance covers
36		the medicine so I think that the cost would be something you
37		could handle, even though the cost would be about 10 dollars
38		a month. What we should do is talk about whether or not this
39		pill would do you any good. The research article we looked
40		at talked about heart attacks and death. Which one are you
41		mostly concerned about?
42	*Patient:*	I guess from the beginning it has been about dying, so maybe
43		we can talk about that.
44	*Doctor:*	OK. This conversation can get a little confusing so interrupt
45		me if there is anything you don't understand. I'd rather start
46		from the beginning than leave you confused. I do think this
47		is an important decision for you and I want to respect your
48		option to not take the pill. In fact, after you hear what I am
49		going to tell you either taking it or not taking it would both
50		be reasonable choices. Are you ready?
51	*Patient*	Go for it.
52	*Doctor:*	Let's start by pretending there are one hundred people
53		exactly like you with the same risk factors and in your
54		general state of health.

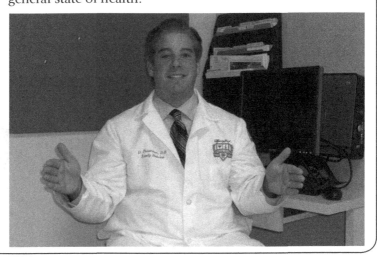

55
56
57

If you didn't do anything and none of those hundred patients took this pill, only a few of them would die in the next five years.

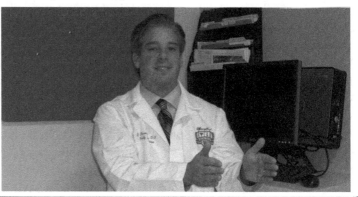

58
59
60

The unfortunate part is that we have no way to predict whether or not you would be in the group of people who would never have a problem,

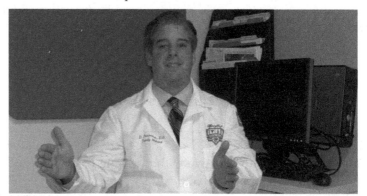

61
62

or whether you would be in the group of people that would die.

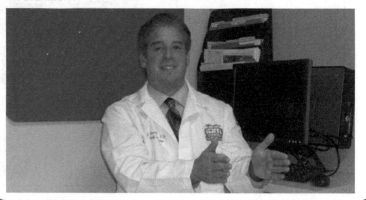

63   (Putting his hands down before continuing ...)
64   If you didn't take the pill and you were in the group that never
65   had a problem, you would probably say something like, 'See,
66   I didn't want all those chemicals and I didn't take them and
67   nothing happened to me.' You would be happy with that. But if
68   you were in the group that died, you'd probably haunt me from
69   the grave and say, 'Why didn't you try harder to convince me to
70   take that pill ... now Jason is alone and doesn't have anyone to
71   help him. You would regret having not taken the pill.

72

73   Now let's start over, but this time let's pretend that *everybody*
74   took the pill. Over here, is the group of people that never
75   would have had the problem anyway and wound up taking
76   the pill but never got any benefit. They still had to risk the
77   side effects and pay for the medicine, but it didn't make any
78   difference. If you knew that you were in that group, you'd be
79   mad that you put those chemicals in you body for nothing.

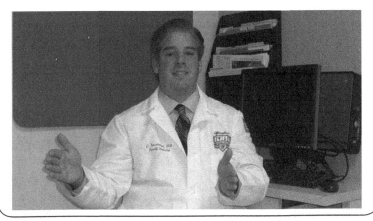

80   But remember over here is the group of people that would
81   have died in the next five years.

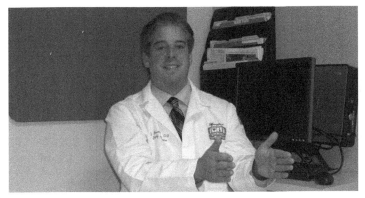

82   Unfortunately, most of those people would take the pill
83   but still die. In other words the pill isn't perfect and won't
84   prevent every death. You'd probably haunt me from the
85   grave and say something like, 'I did what you wanted me to
86   and it didn't do me any good.'

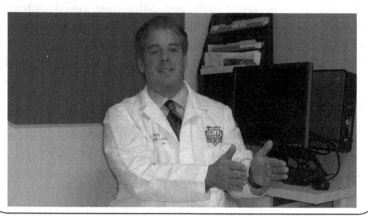

87   But right here in the middle is a small group, who took the
88   pill and the pill saved their life. They are the lucky people. If
89   you were in that group, you'd be thanking me that we had
90   this conversation and we prevented you from an early and
91   sudden death.

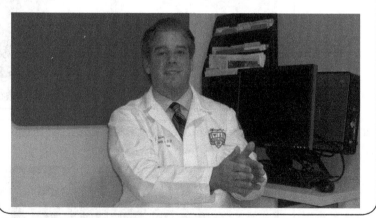

92   (Putting hands down before continuing...)
93   But remember, if you take the pill, we'll never know whether
94   the pill saved you life or you never would have had a problem
95   anyway. There's over a ninety percent chance you'll never have
96   a problem. Who knows, I might get some credit for doing
97   nothing.

98		But I want you to have a fairly good understanding of how
99		much this pill might help you. So, *for every 30 people who*
100		*took the pill there will be one person who took the pill and it saved*
101		*their life. That's what you really were concerned about. The only*
102		*way to give yourself a better chance is to try it.* This study only
103		lasted five years and my common sense as a doctor says that
104		you will probably take this pill for the next 25 years. So, the
105		real chance that this pill might save your life is probably
106		much greater than that, but there is no way for us to put a
107		specific amount of benefit because we just don't have enough
108		information. It might also be true that most of the benefit
109		occurs in the first five years anyway and the lives saved as
110		demonstrated in this study are about as much benefit as you
111		could expect.
112		So if I had to sum it up for you, I think that the side
113		effects of the pill are manageable and taking this pill merely
114		improves your chances of avoiding death, like your daddy.
115		Most doctors just tell their patients to take the pill. But I want
116		you to know approximately how much benefit you're really
117		going to get. Because we can't predict the future and we don't
118		know which specific group you're in, all we can do is tell you
119		the risk or odds just as you were going to the casino and play
120		roulette. But, if you could imagine looking back on your life
121		and you happen to be one of those lucky people where the
122		pill saved your life, you would certainly be happy you decided
123		to take it. If you take your chances and skip the pill, you have
124		to hope you will be in that group that never needed it anyway.
125		So there is no right or wrong answer. It is all about what you
126		are more comfortable with.
127		I think your choice is going to boil down to accepting
128		another 'chemical' in your body that might improve your
129		chances to avoid repeating your family's tragedy. Why don't
130		you tell me what you think?
131	*Patient:*	I am disappointed because I thought those pills worked much
132		better than that. *I appreciate your honesty doctor, but when you*
133		*said that thing about my great grandchildren I had already made*
134		*up my mind I was going to take that pill.*

NARRATIVE INTERPRETATION OF CLINICAL CASE

Lines 1–7: The conversation resumes after an exploration of the medical literature and creates an 'anticipatory retrospection' by saying, 'We'd like to keep you healthy so that you can raise your great grandchildren.' This combines the theme of the relationship contrasting sudden death with longevity, parenting, raising children, but extends the horizon of the end of the story by including another generation by using the word 'great grandchildren.' The very next sentence talks about cholesterol pills. The narrative creates meaning by metonymically associating longevity with cholesterol pills. After teasing the patient with one possible outcome, the physician returns and asks for a further explanation of the patient's concept of foreign chemicals in the body.

Lines 8–18: The patient responds with her definition of health and reveals that medication is a marker for undiagnosed disease, vulnerability, and the trauma of her father's death. The entire diagnostic and therapeutic conversation revolves around the plotline of this patient's index traumatic event, namely the sudden death of her father. The doctor responds by forcing the patient to imagine a possible alternative ending to her life story stating, 'Maybe this is a way you can be different than your dad-different in a healthy way.'

Lines 19–51: The following silence heightens the tension of the story and the doctor wisely maintains the silence as the patient decides whether or not to embark on this discussion at this time. Recall that this topic has arisen earlier in the narrative, but this time the story heads off in a different direction as the patient is willing to accept an explanation of medical information. The doctor then provides a fairly long explanation about the risks and benefits of this particular therapy. At one point, the doctor creates a personalized POEM by asking the patient to identify which outcome she would like further information. The doctor then gives permission for the patient to interrupt and validation of multiple possible patient choices endorsing the patient decision even before the explanation starts. The patient invites the doctor to continue.

Lines 52–97: At this point, the doctor uses props to facilitate the story telling, in this case, body language and the 'cognitive artifacts' mentioned above. The doctor personalizes the medical literature by saying there are saying 'there are one hundred people exactly like you ...' He then embarks on an explanation of contingent outcomes as well as narratively incorporating the concept of uncertainty. After explaining the uncertainty and the potential different outcomes, the doctor personalizes the uncertainty by using the patient's own story and language and assigns them to each of the study groups. In an anticipatory fashion the patient is able to explore various different outcomes and attaches her own personal story to each of the research groups.

In a similar way, the doctor explains the choice and ultimate decision by breaking it into two groups: nobody took the pill verses everybody took the pill. This is a way to narratively address the problem of population science and applying it to an individual. Again, he incorporates the patient story and the major theme of this narrative by stating, 'If you were in that group, you'd be thanking me we had that conversation and we prevented you from an early and sudden death.'

Lines 98–130: The doctor reviews all of the evidence using the concept of number needed to treat and explains that a true difference in outcomes occurs in only one in 30 people. Again, in an effort to take population science to the level of the individual, the doctor states, 'The only way to give yourself a better chance is to try it.' The doctor continues with explanation within the frame of the above narrative and uses the metaphor of a casino for taking chances or probability. Acknowledging the only correct answer is what the patient is comfortable with, the doctor distills the medical conversation down to 'chemicals in the body' versus 'repeating the family tragedy.' After a very long explanation, the doctor invites the patient to resume the role of story teller. As mentioned above, individuals can cognitively process information in different ways.

Lines 131–134: The doctor made every possible effort to assist the patient with 'numeracy,' but the patient uses narrative reasoning in making her choice stating, '... when you said that thing about my great grandchildren I had already made up mind I was going to take that pill.' Thus, the story struggles for a happy ending by using narrative methods the co-constructive narrative embodies shared responsibilities and ethical or moral dimensions to care. Ultimately, both the evidence based medicine and narrativity support the doctor–patient relationship, an example of relationship centered care.

A CONTINGENT, EMERGENT, SITUATED, AND CONTEXTUAL MEDICAL KNOWLEDGE

The *contingent* nature of communicating evidence is most graphically demonstrated by considering all the options of whether or not to take the pill or not and the different potential outcomes in each group. These contingencies are not only described verbally, but also with body language.

The *emergent* nature of the discussion comes from the narrative – the patient is making clinical decisions based on the words, 'great grandchildren.' Although the doctor probably understood that using such a word related to the thematic nature of the narrative, he also probably thought the patient might have been more interested in the evidence. In this case, the evidence did not lead to the *emergence* of a decision; that sub-plot led nowhere in the overall narrative.

The *situational nature* of the medical knowledge is created by the narrative elements of 'chemicals,' 'sudden death,' 'primary prevention,' 'statins,' and how sudden death interrupts a life story not yet complete.

The *contextual* nature of this medical knowledge is the patient's disappointment that the medicine isn't a magic cure coupled with willingness to take risks defined by the medical literature to complete the story that the patient wants. In a strange way, the original study participants in Scandinavia are the context for a life in southeastern Michigan.

REFERENCES

1   Roter DL, Hall JA, Katz N. Patient-physician communication: a descriptive summary of the literature. *Patient Education and Counseling.* 1988; **12**: 99–119.

2   Waitzkin H. Information giving in medical care. *Journal of Health and Social Behavior.* 1985; **26**(2): 81–101.

3   Lipkus IM. Numeric, verbal, and visual formats of conveying health risks: suggested best practices and future recommendations. *Medical Decision Making.* 2007; **27**: 696–713.

4   Epstein RM, Alper BS, Quill TE. Communicating evidence for participatory decision making. *JAMA.* 2004; **291**(19): 2359–66.

5   Spiegelhalter DJ. Understanding uncertainty. *Annals of Family Medicine.* 2008; **6**(3): 196–7.

6   Enfield NJ. The body as a cognitive artifact in kinship representations: hand gesture diagrams by speakers of Lao. *Current Anthropology.* 2005; **46**(1): 51–81.

7   Brill JR. 'Handling uncertainty. *Family Medicine.* 2010; **42**(7): 471–2.

8   Winslow R. Your risk of heart disease. *Wall Street Journal.* June 1, 2010.

9   Politi MC, Han PKJ, Col NF. Communicating the uncertainty of harms and benefits of medical interventions. *Medical Decision Making.* 2007; **27**: 681–95.

10 Winslow R. Study questions evidence behind heart therapies. *The Wall Street Journal.* August 6, 2008: D1–D2.

11 Sheridan SL, Pignone MP, Lewis CL. A randomized comparison of patients' understanding of number needed to treat and other common risk reduction formats. *J Gen Intern Med.* 2003; **18**: 884–92.

12 Alaszewski A, Horlick-Jones T. How can doctors communicate information about risk more effectively? *BMJ.* 2003; **327**: 728–31.

13 Cohen DJ, Crabtree B. Evaluative criteria for qualitative research in health care. *Annals of Family Medicine.* 2008; **6**: 331–9.

14 Mangset M. ' Two percent isn't a lot, but when it comes to death it seems quite a lot anyway': patients' perception of risk and willingness to accept risks associated with thrombolytic drug treatment for acute stroke. *J Med Ethics.* 2009; **35**: 42.

15 Covey J. A meta-analysis of the effects of presenting treatment benefits in different formats. *Medical Decision Making.* 2007; **27**: 638–54.

16 Malenka DJ, Baron JA, Johansen S, *et al.* The framing effect of relative and absolute risk. *J Gen Intern Med.* 1993; **8**: 543–8.

17 Skolbekken J-A. Communicating the risk reduction achieved by cholesterol reducing drugs. *BMJ.* 1998; **316**:1956–8.

18 Ghosh AK, Ghosh K. Translating evidence-based information into effective risk communication: current challenges and opportunities. *J Lab Clin Med.* 2005; **145**(4): 171–80.

19 Goodyear-Smith F, Arroll B, Chan L, *et al.* Patients prefer pictures to numbers to express cardiovascular benefit from treatment. *Annals of Family Medicine.* 2008; 6(3): 213–17.

20 Halvorsen P, Selmer R, Kristiansen IS. Different ways to describe the benefits of risk-reducing treatments. *Ann Intern Med.* 2007; **146**(12): 848–56.

21 Goldman RE, Parker DR, Eaton CB, *et al.* Patients' perceptions of cholesterol, cardio-vascular disease risk, and risk communication strategies. *Annals of Family Medicine.* 2006; 4(3): 205–12.

22 Alaszewski A. A person centered approach to communicating risk. *PLoS Medicine.* 2005; 2(2): e41.

23 Pantilat S. Communicating with seriously ill patients: better words to say. *JAMA.* 2009; **301**(12).

24 Makoul G, Clayman ML. An integrative model of shared decision making in medical encounters. *Patient Education and Counseling.* 2006; 60: 301–12.

25 Engel JD, Zarconi J, Pethtel LL, *et al. Narrative in Healthcare: healing patients, practitioners, profession and community.* Oxford: Radcliffe Publishing; 2008.

26 Mattingly C. In search of the good: narrative reasoning in clinical practice. *Medical Anthropology Quarterly.* 1998; **12**(3): 273–97.

27 Mattingly C. *Healing Dramas and Clinical Plots: the narrative structure of experience.* Cambridge: Cambridge University Press; 1998.

28 Halvorsen P. Different ways to describe the benefits of risk-reducing treatments. *Annals of Internal Medicine.* 2007; **146**(12).

29 Timmermans D. Presenting health risk information in different formats: the effect on participants' cognitive and emotional evaluation and decisions. *Patient Education & Counselling.* 2008; **73**: 443–7.

PART III

Theoretical Considerations

James P Meza

THE SOCIAL PRACTICE OF HEALING

When doctors listen to patients' stories, they merge the individual's narrative with the cultural power of the medical profession and produce a co-constructed narrative within the context of an institutionalized social framework, creating coherence between the 'inner experience' of the individual and the socially authorized version of the same story. This practice harmonizes two stories, creating personal meaning and reinforcing social norms.

Introduction

Several years ago, I attended a lecture at Wayne State University School of Medicine given by Gordon Guyatt, a pre-eminent and foundational thinker in the realm of evidence based medicine. I remember the lecture like I had heard it yesterday. The topic was thrombolytic therapy for acute myocardial infarction. His Powerpoint® slides portrayed a chronology of each major randomized controlled trial with the date of publication. His composite slide gave the odds ratio with 95% confidence intervals for each trial that graphically displayed a convincing argument that thrombolytic therapy was beneficial for survival (a Patient Oriented Outcome). He asked a penetrating question and made a wise proclamation.

The penetrating question was, 'Why did it take 10 years after the evidence was crystal clear for clinicians to begin to put the evidence into practice?' That question has subsequently become known as 'Translational Science.' The question implies a frustration of lost opportunities and has provoked the NIH Roadmap for translational research. Because this is articulated in the documents and structure of a governmental agency that oversees billions of dollars of societal investment in an activity that consumes 14% of the Gross Domestic Product, I am going to say that this is a pretty good example of the body politic, a term that I will define later in this section. Alternatively, it could be called a social narrative. In fact, the range of terminology in use implies that we are dealing with a topic that is poorly understood. An example of this occurred recently when I was talking about EBM and someone responded, 'Oh, you mean Translational Medicine.' Are these terms really synonymous? How do we improve the translation of evidence into practice? I'm going to suggest that in order to truly understand that question, we require a cultural analysis. What cultural framework do physicians practicing in institutions use to facilitate change in practice such as this? There are reasons why it took 10 years after the evidence was available to begin using thrombolytic therapy for acute myocardial infarction. An anthropologist would seek understanding sufficient to identify what those reasons are.

Gordon Guyatt's wise proclamation was, 'Evidence doesn't make decisions.' Evidence guides decision making, acknowledging that there are multiple other factors and contextual information required to make medical decisions. I would like to think that he was referring to the patient and the patient's values, beliefs, and preferences. This is of course what we are seeking when we explore the patients' narrative, or the 'Illness Story.' Each patient is unique and it would be foolish to think that the proper use of the same research evidence would result in identical decisions in every case. I'm concerned that the focus on guidelines and pay for performance will obscure the voice of the patient in medicine. Rather, the task of Translational Research should be to understand how to translate the evidence into the Illness Story. We use the patient's narrative as a proxy for the *individual body* (a theoretical term to be defined later in this section). Again, there is a multiplicity of terms, but one of the most frequent in the literature is *narrative embodiment*. The Illness Story is about experiences told from the perspective of the *mind-body*.

I've been advised by many senior scholars to stop using the word 'healing' because it is so ambiguous and non-scientific. Somewhat stubbornly I've continued to use it because I think it is real and does exist. It is something experienced by the individual, acted out in social spaces, and related to cultural and societal norms. Translational Medicine, Translational Science, narrative evidence based medicine, and 'healing' are all trying to describe the same thing. In this section, I will (stubbornly) continue to use the word healing because healing highlights the cultural perspectives which address the fundamental questions of Translational Research and narrative evidence based medicine. Healing is a process of translating and harmonizing the needs of the body politic and the needs of the individual body. Every society has this need and its own unique cultural solution to getting this need met. Narrative evidence based medicine is simply one of the prominent ways we do it in Western medicine. In order to scientifically study 'healing' or any of its synonyms described above, there needs to be a theoretical framework. By using a single example, this book is about describing that theory and suggesting that there is a scientific method for studying the *social practice of healing* that addresses some of the most perplexing questions in medicine today.

The task in this section of the book is to explore the theoretical foundation of the social practice of healing. We hope that the previous two sections were recognizable as something that occurs in clinical practice. Instead of simply repeating that medicine is both an art and a science, I hope to show how both art and science are cultural resources and both are part of the cultural practice of clinical medicine. It is the juxtaposition of method and theory that allow us to envision a research agenda. Narrative evidence based medicine as a method results in Translational Practice. The cultural theory underlying the practice allows for exploration of Translational Science. It is the broader understanding of how theory and method are interrelated that leads me to believe both belong in the same book. For those of you not interested in 'the bench science of healing,' simply consider Part III as interesting essays and reflections on what doctors might actually be doing when they work in clinical settings.

CHAPTER 13

Theoretical Issues Regarding the Everyday Social Practice of Healing

James P Meza

ANTHROPOLOGICAL THEORY

In the Volume 1, No.1 issue of *Medical Anthropology Quarterly*, Nancy Scheper Hughes and Margaret Lock wrote an article entitled *Mindful body: a prolegomenon for [studies] in medical anthropology*.[1] In this paper, they outlined a systematic model for anthropological analysis based on the range of perspectives of the anthropological endeavor from micro-level perspective, through mid-level perspective, to macro level perspectives. They stated that, 'The body is good to think with.' This is consistent with their opening quotation by Marcel Mauss: 'The body is the first and most useful tool of man.' They explicate this range of analysis using the following three categories:

1. Individual Body.
2. Social Body.
3. Body Politic.

This 'trope' of 'the three bodies' has been widely used within the anthropological literature to describe data and analytic strategies. I will describe the individual body, the social body, finishing with a description of body politic and how they were represented in this book.

Healing as Illustrated by our Case Scenario

In a very general sense, the trope of the 'three bodies' mentioned above maps onto the terms we have been using in the following way:

➤ The individual body: *Illness narrative*
➤ The social body: *Relationship centered care*
➤ The body politic: *Evidence based medicine*

This book is a case example of the social practice of healing. The previous chapters provide the methodology of healing, while this chapter attempts to explain some of the underlying theoretical structure of why the method works. It is not necessary to teach doctors theory, but the theory challenges what method we ought to be teaching in medical schools. Review the case in your mind and ask yourself *who defined reality?* Since it was a co-constructed narrative, the power to define reality was shared between the patient and the physician.

The Individual Body

The individual body includes the experiences and inner world of the patient. Narrative is a proxy for that experience. Remember the mirror neurons – humans can understand the experience of other humans. Our patient experienced (re-experienced) the loss of her mother only after struggling to deal with the emotions of losing her father. Her story externalizes her experience and presents it into the social arena. She does this in a culturally appropriate way – going to the doctor and telling an illness story.

The Social Body

It is the ritual of the office visit that reveals the structure of the 'social body' in action.

The social body is manifest when the doctor listens, trying to hear both illness and disease in the story. Is the patient suffering from heart disease or heart ache? Both types of suffering are real and become part of the medical ritual. The doctor uses his/her cultural authority to mediate between the individual illness story and the dominant cultural beliefs of biomedicine. Relationship Centered Care is a name for the ritual of doctoring in Western medicine. The doctor allows advanced technology to be used to explore the illness story when the 64-slice CT coronary angiography is ordered; the scan is not helpful to treat vulnerable plaque. By traveling the journey of the illness storyline, the doctor is able to eventually prescribe a statin in a way that the patient can accept. When the doctor prescribed a statin to prevent heart attacks, he /she reinforced the dominant social ideology of the 'cholesterol hypothesis.'[2] Multiple cultural factors structure this relationship, for the patient and the doctor.

The Body Politic

Another term for the body politic is the 'social narrative.' The body politic is reflected when the public health needs to decrease incidence of heart disease and avert lost productivity are accomplished. The institution of medicine itself is a way of controlling the random suffering that would otherwise be disruptive to society. This type of institutional control of bodies is strictly a Foucauldian argument. The political economy of referral hospitals and distribution of resources through the health care system is a reflection of the body politic. The doctor responds to these societal needs by making judgments about resource allocation within the context of the clinical case. How is our technology to be used properly? Who writes the prescription? Who fills out the level of service to initiate the monetary transaction of reimbursement? Who decides what constitutes heart disease? Who decides how heart disease is to be treated? In our case scenario, the doctor initiated primary prevention of coronary artery disease by creating that part of the co-constructed narrative which started statin therapy for the treatment of risk factors. All these decisions reflect the dominant ideology of our society. Reflect back on the case when the doctor ritualistically goes through the process of informed consent – this is a reflection of our societal value placed on individualism and the logic of choice. It was only part of the clinical scenario because it reinforces social values. The body politic by definition is omnipresent and powerful; the body politic is the social environment in which we live.

The Three Bodies

In our case scenario, the patient experienced the creation of personal meaning, the doctor engaged in the moral practice of a healing relationship, and society's need to stabilize the health of the population and distribute resources were met. Thus the individual body, the social body, and the body politic were all very much present throughout the entire case scenario. Through the social practice of healing, all three 'bodies' were brought into harmony with the others. The case scenario is an idealized case. Most of the time social actors are unaware of the dominant culture within which they exist. True 'healing' may be a rare thing; learning how to be better healers, however, should be the norm. On some level, survival of the society and benefit to the individual depend on it.

THE INDIVIDUAL BODY AND NARRATIVE EMBODIMENT

Narrative studies are almost ubiquitous across disciplines. Within that wide range of theoretical and methodological scholarship is a narrower focus on 'narrative embodiment.' These are stories about health, one's own body, how the body functions, and the choices one makes about what goes into one's own body and to what we are willing or unwilling to subject our bodies.[9-25] The answers to these questions comprise the illness story. The illness story belongs to the patient; it is a reflection of each patient's 'inner experience.' I am suggesting that these *stories have social power to define reality*.

The Individual and the Self in Narrative

It is almost impossible to read a text on 'narrative' theory without stumbling across the word 'healing' and the word 'self.' These three words are so closely connected that they are linguistic cultural artifacts indicating that there is a large overlap in meaning. The anthropology of the self is too vast to attempt to cover here, but for simplicity, I will refer to the self as a sentient body. But let us go back to the basics of narrative theory. A story must have a storyteller and a listener, the basis of a healing relationship. If the doctor and the patient can easily agree upon the self-medical story, then that is a quick office visit. But what if there is disagreement? What if the patient refused to get well? What if the patient does not accept the burden of suffering that accompanies chronic illness? What if a life remains disrupted? All too often, doctors rhetorically dismiss such patients as 'cranks', 'malingerers', non-compliant', etc. This is where the real work of healing begins. It requires a suspension of judgment by the doctor and a careful listening to the story. It requires a temporary sharing of power to the patient to be 'in charge' and to be the storyteller, while the doctor must submit to the 'power-down' position of the listener. Remember, stories have power in the social realm.[3] Within the context of care – *relationship centered care* – the story gets re-written to everyone's satisfaction. That becomes an example of healing.

Healing the 'Self'

Doctors who practice narrative medicine are drawing on this type of cultural authority based on deep-seated and longstanding cultural values that are embedded in the healing ritual. The personal relationship and bearing witness to suffering are historically part of the role of the healer.[4] Consider the following excerpt from the Hippocratic Oath: 'I do solemnly swear ... That whatsoever I shall see or hear of the lives of patients which is not fitting to be spoken, I will keep inviolably secret.' Doctors are given special cultural legitimacy to hear stories of patients' lives in a relationship of trust and safety. The individual self is reflected in the individual's story; the story is how we discover the self. Individuals have a need to create meaning; in Western society, this is manifest as creating meaning for an individual 'self.' One of the attributes frequently associated with *healing is 'being whole.'* I take this to mean *someone has been able to hear my whole story,* even if it takes time for me to discover it myself. By listening, the doctor validates the story and facilitates the transition to 're-incorporation into society' by blending the illness story with the medical story. Re-incorporation into society is a common attribute of healing rituals.

THE SOCIAL BODY
How Healing Stories are Created

Mattingly notes that in order for the emergent story to change toward a story imbued with meaning, both the patient and the healer must participate and there has to be a development of desire toward an imagined outcome. Mattingly's desire – born of dramatic moments in the narrative – and motivation – defined as a cognitive schema – are the place where stories are born, a place shared by narrative embodiment and socially embedded schemata.[5] Cognitive anthropologists have examined this concept of motivation and demonstrate how it is a dominate schema created within a cultural context.[6-11] Thus, the desire is shared by the patient and healer acting as the agent of society. In addition to desire and motivation, dramatic moments are born of emotion and feeling-thoughts. Again, narrative theory and cognitive anthropology reinforce each other synergistically. Culture has been described as shared cognitive structures.[12] Emotions help to create social structure and social structures are experienced with an emotional valence.[13-18] Thought feelings and cognitions are embodied in individuals. Scheper-Hughes and Lock identify emotions as the 'missing link ... capable of bridging mind and body, individual and society.'[1] This recognition of thought feelings as closely bound to the body as experienced by the individual and bridging to social structures reinforces the central thesis of this analysis.

My theoretical area of interest within the topic of healing has been the interface between the individual and society. The above work in cognitive anthropology and narrative theory suggest that the phenomenon is a dynamic relationship and that the process is a complex, interdependent cycle of culture creating individuals and individuals affecting culture (emotions, schemas, social actors) through the healing relationship, the Western medicine version of the healing ritual.

Although I believe this is an area of great theoretical interest, I can't explicate it in a scholarly way in this context, so I'll have to convey the concept with a metaphor. The relationship of the individual's genetic make-up is to the population gene pool as the sentient body experience is to culture. Genetics implies chromosomes, genes, gonads, meiosis, copulation, and reproduction resulting in a new and unique member of a population. That individual has the potential to add or subtract from the future gene pool through the processes of mutation, genetic drift, founder effect, differential mating behaviors, and gene flow. Similarly, although the individual has been equipped with a wide variety of culturally determined tools embodied as schemata and emotions, thought-feelings, all of these inner experiences also have an effect on culture, cultural reproduction, and social structure. You can't have one without the other. Both the individual and society are part of a larger, interactive, dynamic system. Notice the similarities between what I just described and a folk description of 'healing.'[19, 20] I believe that this ebb and flow from the individual and culture is the explanation that social narratives share a concordance with personal narratives of the social actors.[21]

The clinician–patient relationship intensely condenses, in a microcosm, powerful forces referred to as the body politic and patient agency in the form of narrative embodiment. My model of healing capitalizes on the realization that these two diverse levels of theoretical analysis intersect and co-exist within the clinician–patient relationship. *The interactions and performances of both the patient and the physician are the social body in action.* Both patient and physician are drawing on cultural resources to represent two vastly different levels of analytic perspective, based on their unequal ability to draw on different ends of the spectrum of analysis described above.

Complex societies have a need to control bodies (the docile body mentioned above). Biomedicine must make diagnoses and prescribe treatments or cures. This entire process is supported by a research paradigm based on diagnosing and treating disease. 'Healing' is a process where both the needs of individuals and society are met. The mediating interaction between the individual and society is *the social body, as manifested in the doctor–patient relationship.* The doctor–patient relationship is imbued with many layers of cultural norms and follows a ritualized pattern. I am suggesting that we need to re-capture the essential components of that ritual to prevent it from disappearing under the pressure of increasing commodification; it is the balance that is important.

Michael Balint was a Hungarian-born psychoanalyst who worked with General Practitioners at the Tavistock Clinic in London. He noticed that doctors struggled with certain patients and developed a methodology to explore these doctor–patient relationships. He is credited with coining the term 'patient-centered care.'[22] I think he would have also appreciated the term relationship centered care. Balint groups are case discussions where doctors explore three domains: (1) What is it like to be the physician? (2) Who is this patient? (3) What type of doctor–patient relationship does this patient need? The process is an intensively self reflective experience. He was adamant about needing to explore a research agenda on this topic.[23] In the following description, notice the elements of narrative and culture.

> Culture is an ensemble of stories we tell ourselves. One of the best ways to understand others is by telling and re-telling stories. The tale well told gives us the capacity to imagine ourselves anew, and to revisit experience with fresh eyes. The stuff of narratives lies in the gap between what ought to be and what is, how these dissonances are read and variously dealt with. Hovering between realism and fantasy, they have the power to reveal deep truths about ourselves and the times we live in.
>
> Stories about what are too easily called emotions are simultaneously stories about society. Even as they address individual uniqueness, the cornerstone of Balint teaching, narratives are encoded deep in the cultural values of a particular time and place. They make sense of experience because they already produce it in culturally specific ways, anticipating as much as making sense of action already taken. They are therefore conservative as well as liberating. Stripped of such context, however, narratives may lose depth, and become simply biographical solutions to systemic problems: the finger points – in one direction only.
>
> Hence the emphasis here is not on whether the stories doctors tell about themselves and their patients unravel the inner self. Ultimately the self remains

unknowable. Rather, the following case studies focus on which stories mattered, which were displaced, and how well publicly shared narratives in the groups dovetail with doctors' private accounts of themselves. They give an entrée to the way that narratives, and the feeling they engender, are not simply discovered, but created and performed, allowing doctors to explain themselves to themselves and to others in plausible ways. As miniature social dramas, the stories told both shaped and reflected key social values within medicine, producing order out of the disorder of everyday experience.[24]

Scholars under-appreciate the different roles of emotion in the biopsychosocial model. In our case example, there is the emotional thought-feeling of the individual (the product of neurological activity). There is also a description of a prior emotion in an illness narrative. Additionally, there is the emotional content of the office visit itself. This last 'real time emotion' is often not recognized. These emotions are very strong cultural communications, each with culturally prescribed range of responses.[14, 17, 25] Doctors do not generally factor their own emotional experiences into the process of care, but expression of these emotions is often culturally proscribed and restricted. Despite this, emotions are recognized to mutually interact with each part of the bio-psycho-social-bio model.[24, 26, 27]

Healing is often referred to as being 'whole.' It is a small step to say that 'whole' is the 'whole story' of the individual self. Narrative works as a healing modality in the West because we tell the story of our self. The healer's role is to harmonize the individual's needs and the needs of the society. Healers regulate the relationship between the individual and society. Cross culturally, there are many ways to do this, but in Western thought, we need to control bodies and maintain individuality simultaneously. Doctors can do that by listening to stories and translating them into the language of technology and conversely translating technology into personal meaning. The individual has to have a sense of meaning – it doesn't have to be narrative – just meaning and harmony with society. In the West, we create individual meaning by telling our story to a socially authorized individual. You can't tell your life story to an institution – that institution has to be 'embodied' by a human. Thus both the individual and society have to be 'embodied.' That is the doctor–patient relationship. *By integrating narrative medicine and evidence based medicine and creating a co-constructed narrative, we have demonstrated an instantiated example of 'healing.'*

THE BODY POLITIC AND SOCIAL CONTROL OF THE HUMAN BODY
The 'disease model' of medicine arose in the 1700s when the power of the Catholic Church was waning and the Enlightenment put a greater emphasis on empirical observation.[28] Michele Foucault detailed the historical development

of medicine as an institution, describing the transition from the world view of the human body as sacred to the fledgling 'scientific' practice of medicine.[29] At this time, the first human dissections occurred. These dissections with their obvious empiricism – 'seeing is believing' – started to localize disease to specific organs. In other words, an obviously deformed internal organ on autopsy was correlated with the clinical signs and symptoms of the clinical history, physical exam, and clinical course of illness. Thus, there was a transition from a spiritual paradigm to a new medical paradigm based on diseased organs. Foucault referred to the development of stethoscopes and exam skills as the 'clinical gaze' where doctors try to see beneath the skin and 'visualize' the diseased organ. Who would have ever guessed that today's version of the clinical gaze is the 64-slice CT coronary angiograms (and beyond). The cognitive schemata of the 'clinical gaze' gave doctors the cultural authority to identify, diagnose and treat disease. Evidence based medicine is a perpetuation of the specialized knowledge and language to control 'bodies' through the use of social institutions.[30] This social control of bodies can be thought of as 'the social narrative.' It is a socially structured story of the way bodies should behave and be treated.

Concurrently with the development of the clinical gaze, doctors began working in 'the clinic,' a social institution. Thus they acquired not only cultural authority, but also social (institutional) authority. The cultural artifacts of this social transition are embedded in almost all institutions of Western medicine, structuring education and training, hospital departments, medical specialty certifications, as well as the cognitive artifacts of 'disease management' protocols. Unfortunately, this even extends to individual humans, as evidenced by our proclivity to refer to patients by their diseases, 'The case of heart failure in 243B.' This abstraction from a life lived to a disease is often dehumanizing. Michele Foucault goes on in a subsequent historical exploration of prisons to explicate how social institutions result in the 'control' of bodies.[31] Again, he cites multiple examples from military formations, prisons, and the industrialization process of how institutions 'control bodies' referred to as 'docile bodies.' Notice that docile invokes the lack of control of the individual and places total control within the social institution. In our case, the agent representing these social institutions has often been the doctor. The socialization process is so strong that we as physicians have developed cognitive structures that 'define reality' in terms of diseases. With such specialized knowledge, we speak with authority and define/control our patients with disease labels, prognoses, and available treatments.

Howard Brody, a noted physician and ethicist, gives many examples of this social, institutionalized power over the lives of our patients in his book, *The Healer's Power*.[32] Sharon Kaufman extends the argument by stating that within our highly technological, ICU hospital environment we even control the time of a person's death. The social institution of the medical Intensive Care Unit has 'progressed' to the point of being able to adjust the time of death – the ultimate power to define the reality of a human's existence.[33] These types of social controls over the body have been demonstrated in other settings. Again, these examples by other authors are specific examples of concepts developed by Foucault.[34, 35]

THE BODY POLITIC IN AMERICAN MEDICINE

The control of bodies described above seems at odds with the American values of Life, Liberty, and the Pursuit of Happiness, some of the core values in American culture. This set of values was a reaction or re-balancing to another system that describes the body politic – political economy. Political economy is a social theory that describes how power and money gravitate to the center while the periphery of the social system contributes resources to sustain the central (government, etc.). The American Revolution was a reaction to a system structured in this way: the British Empire. A closer look at the societal values that came out of the American Revolution demonstrates how each of these values is constrained and has inherent social conflicts. It is a series of checks and balances trying to manage the tension of centralized power and individualism. The commodification of health care is simply an example of these national and global economic trends described by the theory of political economy.[36] My theoretical sketch attempts to keep these large scale perspectives in mind while also addressing local culture and the individual.

Let us review the core American values and examine some of their inherent conflicts and constraints. *Life* today in many ways equates to access to health care. Health care reflects our deeply held belief in technology and American ingenuity – so powerful that we imagine that technology can extend life indefinitely. But that same technology becomes frightening if we lose our individuality and become 'dependent on machines.' Currently, the health care debate has been conflicted over this very issue – do we let market forces determine access to healthcare or is life (access to health care) a civil right? 'Big business' and 'big government' are threats to individualism. The ambiguity is structurally part of our political body. Does freedom of speech extend to telling my illness story to a doctor? Not really. All of these conflicting and contested values are part of the body politic. It is vital to understand that all of these values get played out in the exam room during a clinical encounter. *Recognizing these macro-level forces in the micro-level setting of the exam room gives us an understanding of how we might harmonize these multiple levels of analysis.*

The Social Practice of Healing Defined

When doctors listen to patients' stories, they merge the individual's narrative with the cultural power of the medical profession and produce a co-constructed narrative within the context of an institutionalized social framework, creating coherence between the 'inner experience' of the individual and the socially authorized version of the same story. This practice harmonizes two stories, creating personal meaning and reinforcing social norms.

Re-inventing the Wheel (of Medical Knowledge)

Although this chapter provides a theoretical outline from an anthropological perspective, it is entirely consistent with a medical perspective of healing as described by Kurt Stange, *et al.*[37] Although the following illustration uses quadrants (so typical of an epidemiological 2 x 2 table) with the columns of

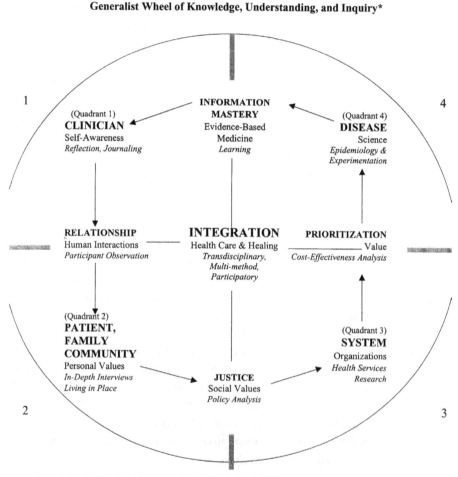

Generalist Wheel of Knowledge, Understanding, and Inquiry*

For each item, bold capitalized words on the first line signify the **"FOCUS OF KNOWLEDGE,"** normal text on the second line signifies the "Task of Understanding," and italicized words on the third line signify the *"Mode of Inquiry."*

Figure 13.1 Generalist Wheel of Knowledge, Understanding, and Inquiry
Reprinted with permission from the Society of Teachers of Family Medicine, www.stfm.org

inner versus outer reality and the rows of individual versus collective, resulting in what Stange, *et al.* described as 'I knowledge (quadrant 1),' 'we knowledge (quadrant 2),' and 'It knowledge' (quadrants 3 and 4). It should be noted that both the patient and the doctor live in the same society, so this could easily be collapsed into a triad of 'I knowledge,' 'we knowledge,' and 'it knowledge,' thereby approximating the triad – trinity (so typical of the symbolic anthropologist). 'I knowledge' is recognizable as the reflective physician and also as the Illness Story (the individual body). 'We knowledge' is the social interaction between the doctor and the patient (the social body). 'It knowledge' is recognizable as the body politic. This is a robust description of individual, social, and political realities that all factor into the practice of medicine. The next step in the science of healing practices is to explicate the 'observables' in each of these domains and establish the relationship between them; that would otherwise be called 'the healing relationship.'

Notice the centrality of integration and healing in this diagram. Notice also that disease, information mastery, doctor–patient relationships, self-reflective doctors, social institutions and values, as well as patient and family [stories] are all represented. If this knowledge is integrated, then it becomes a 'way of knowing' that is contingent, emergent, situated, and contextual. It is a doctor's way of knowing. It represents a call for doctors to be healers. It is time to take theory into research and practice.

REFERENCES

1   Scheper-Hughes N, Lock MM. The mindful body: a prolegomenon to future work in medical anthropology. *Medical Anthropology Quarterly*. 1987; 1: 6–41.
2   Ravnskov U. The fallacies of the lipid hypothesis. *Scand Cardiovasc J.* 2008; 42(4).
3   Mattingly C. Emergent narratives. In: Mattingly C, Garro LC (eds). *Narrative and the Cultural Construction of Illness and Healing*. Berkeley, CA: University of California Press; 2000: pp. 181–211.
4   Egnew TR. The meaning of healing: transcending suffering. *Annals of Family Medicine*. 2005; 3(3): 255–63.
5   Casson R. Schemata in cognitive anthropology. *Annual Review of Anthropology*. 1983; 12: 429–62.
6   Strauss C. Models and motives. In: D'Andrade R, Strauss C (eds). *Human Motives and Cultural Models*. Cambridge: Cambridge University Press; 1992.
7   D'Andrade RG. Schemas and motivation. In: D'Andrade R, Strauss C, op. cit.
8   Holland D. How cultural systems become desire: a case study of American romance. In: D'Andrade R, Strauss C, op. cit. pp. 31–89.
9   Mathews HF. The directive force of morality tales in a Mexican community In: D'Andrade R, Strauss C, op. cit. pp. 127–78.
10 Lutz C. Motivated models. In: D'Andrade R, Strauss C, op. cit. p. 181.
11 Strauss C. What makes Tony run? Schemas as motives reconsidered. In: D'Andrade R, Strauss C, op. cit. p. 191.

12 Romney AK, Moore CC. Toward a theory of culture as shared cognitive structures. *Ethos.* 1998; **26**(3): 314–37.

13 Wothman CM. Emotions: you can feel the difference. In: Hinton AL (ed). *Biocultural Approaches to the Emotions.* Cambridge: Cambridge University Press; 1999: p. 41.

14 Fessler DMT. Toward an understanding of the universality of second order emotions. In: Hinton AL, op. cit. p. 75.

15. Edgewater ID. Music hath charms ... : Fragments toward constructionist biocultural theory, with attention to the relationship of 'music' and 'emotion'. In: Hinton AL, op. cit. p. 153.

16 Lyon ML. Emotion and embodiment: the respiratory mediation of somatic and social processes. In: Hinton AL, op. cit. p. 182.

17 McNeil KE. Affecting experience: toward a biocultural model of human emotions. In: Hinton AL, op. cit. p. 215.

18 Laughlin CD, Throop J. Emotion: a view from biogenetic structuralism. In: Hinton AL, In: Hinton AL, op. cit. p. 329.

19 Meza J, Fahoome G. The development of an instrument for measuring healing. *Annals of Family Medicine.* 2008; **6**(4): 355–60.

20 Scott J, Cohen D, DiCicco-Bloom B, *et al.* Understanding healing relationships in primary care. *Annals of Family Medicine.* 2008; **6**(4): 315–22.

21 Ginsburg FD. *Contested Lives: the abortion debate in an American community.* Berkeley, CA: University of California Press; 1989.

22 Engel JD, Zarconi J, Pethtel LL, Missimi SA. *Narrative in Healthcare: healing patients, practitioners, profession and community.* Oxford: Radcliffe Publishing, Ltd; 2008.

23 Balint M. *The Doctor, His Patient and the Illness.* Edinburgh: Churchill Livingstone; 2000 [1957].

24 Pinder R, McKee A, Sackin P, *et al.* Talking about my patient: the Balint approach in GP education. *British Journal of General Practice.* 2006; Occasional Paper 87.

25 Worthman CM. Emotions: you can feel the difference. In: Hinton AL, op. cit., p. 41.

26 Balint M. *The Doctor, His Patient and the Illness.* Edinburgh: Churchill, Livingstone; 1957 [2000].

27 Moerman D. *Meaning, Medicine and the 'Placebo Effect'.* Cambridge: Cambridge University Press; 2002.

28 Artz FB. *The Enlightenment in France*: Kent OH: Kent State University Press; 1968.

29 Foucault M. *The Birth of the Clinic: an archeology of medical perception.* New York, NY: Vintage Books; 1973, 1994.

30 Bordieu P. The production and reproduction of legitimate language. In: Thompson JB, editor. *Language and Symbolic Power.* Cambridge, MA: Harvard University Press; 1991, p. 43.

31 Foucault M. *Discipline and Punish: the birth of the prison.* New York, NY: Vintage Books; 1995 [1977].

32 Brody H. *The Healer's Power.* New Haven, CT: Yale University Press; 1992.

33 Kaufman S. ... *And a Time to Die: how American hospitals shape the end of life.* Chicago, IL: University of Chicago Press; 2005.

34 Rhodes LA. *Total Confinement: madness and reason in the maximum security prison.* Berkeley, CA: University of California Press; 2004.

35 Scheper-Hughes N. *Death Without Weeping: the violence of everyday life in Brazil.* Berkeley, CA: University of California Press; 1992.

36 Singer M, Valentin F, Baer H, *et al.* Why does Jan Garcia have a drinking problem? The perspective of critical medical anthropology. *Medical Anthropology* 1992; **14**: 77–108.

37 Stange KC, Miller WL, McWhinney I. Developing the knowledge base of family practice. *Family Medicine.* 2001; **33**(4): 286–97.

CHAPTER 14

What is Healing and Who Needs it Anyway?

James P Meza

INTRODUCTION

Dan and I have described and demonstrated an example of two clinical encounters that I believe demonstrate the social practice of healing. Although we concentrated on learning methods in Part I and Part II, methodology alone does not help explain the more interesting questions of 'What is healing?', 'Who needs healing, anyway?', 'Why do we need healing now?', and 'Are today's doctors still healers?' These more interesting questions can be explored using the theory outlined in Chapter 13. In this chapter, I will simply expand on these questions and how they might begin to be understood using the theory proposed in the last chapter.

WHAT IS HEALING?

The word 'healing' evokes positive associations. It is a desired value in our society and indeed most others as well. Frequently, the word 'healing' is paired with the word 'power' making the term, 'healing power.' I believe that doctors have to acknowledge their power[1] and prevent abuse of that power in order to enter into healing relationships.

The unfortunate reality is that the word healing means many different things to many people. It is invoked by surgeons to characterize wound healing. Just check out a Medline search using the key word 'healing' and see how many thousand citations are related to surgical endeavors. Narrative theorists use it and compare it to psychoanalysis for a theoretical grounding. Psychologists pair the word 'healing' with 'trauma' and 'recovery.' Not even that captures the essence of the theoretical basis underlying the methods described in this book. On the other extreme, a nearby billboard emphasizes the word 'healing;' because of the positive attributes of the word, it is used in advertising campaigns to sell hospital services. Healing is like the five blind men describing an elephant – each determines it is something unrelated to the others' descriptions. It is for this very reason that senior scholars advise me to stop using the word.

Instead of discarding the word 'healing' because it is ambiguous, I have taken the alternate approach and tried to clarify exactly what I mean when I say 'healing.' Although there have been many attempts to describe what healing is and how to do it, most of the descriptions rely on a method only; unfortunately *a method without a theory is unscientific.* In this section of the book, I argue that healing is a *social practice* and explicate the theory behind the methods described throughout the rest of the book.

The evidence for healing being a social practice is substantial. In WHR Rivers' book, *Medicine, Magic, and Religion,* he states that 'mankind in general' believes the cause of disease to be from human agency, the action of a spiritual or supernatural being, or from a natural cause.[2] In this statement we have a hint of why societies need healers – the problem of disease and death. A modern version of this social dilemma embedded within the role of 'healer' comes from Egnew,[3] who states that healing is the ability to 'transcend suffering.' Other cross cultural studies reveal that healers share three characteristics: (1) they are invested with *social power,* often through specific training,[2][4] (2) a sufferer who seeks relief from the healer, and (3) a *healing relationship* that often involves words, acts, and rituals believed to benefit the sufferers emotions, attitudes, and behavior and ultimately 'restoring the victim's health and reestablishing or *strengthening his or her ties with the group.*' (italics added) In these initial descriptions, it becomes apparent that both the needs of the individual and the needs of society are being addressed. Disease and death threaten the integrity of both.

ARE DOCTORS HEALERS?

Medical schools do a good job of teaching about diseases and treatments, but curricula in healing are marginalized. This is a reflection of science and technology which are dominant values in American society. Whereas science and technology have an empiric basis in physics, there is no existent 'science of healing.' I'm suggesting healing needs to be explored within the realm of social science. Arthur Kleinman made the same observation and recommendation: we need to develop a medical social science[5] and 'narrative is a form of medical psychotherapy.'[6] Unless a theoretically based science of healing can be articulated and tested, the social functions of healing will remain mired in obscurity, overshadowed by technological advances. Doctors, after all, consider themselves 'scientists.' I agree with Kleinman that doctors also need to embrace the social sciences in order to be complete physicians.

The love of technology with an absence of medical social science has pushed us into our current 'crisis.' This crisis is articulated in the title of Bernard Lown's book, *The Lost Art of Healing.*[7] Lown details how doctors form relationships with technology and neglect the healing relationship with the patient. There are powerful psychological and social dynamics that are fueling this tendency.

First of all, disease, suffering, and death are messy and emotionally painful to deal with. Technology is trendy and cool. There are few medical school curricula to help medical students (or doctors) deal with the pathos of human existence. Although Balint work is designed for just this purpose, it is hard work. Before investing in such difficult activities, there has to be a perceived return on investment. I suggest that Balint work trains doctors to be healers.[8] Others who recognized this need formed the beginnings of the narrative medicine movement, best exemplified by Rita Charon's work with medical students and continued work with narrative evidenced based medicine.[9-14]

WHO NEEDS HEALING ANYWAY?

From a cross cultural perspective, I suggest that healers and healing rituals function at the interface of the individual and society and address the needs of both, resulting in the re-integration of a distressed individual back into the community, the creation of meaning for the individual and his/her experiences, and re-constitution of order and relationship within the larger group. Victor Turner defines the healing ritual in the following way:

> The healing rite in 'folk' or 'tribal' medicine is seen to be more than the typing and labeling of diseases and symptoms and the restoration of health. It is rather the mobilization of efficacy through symbolic action for restoring internal integrity to the patient and order to his community ... Here health represents a restoration of wholeness both to person and group; *mens sana in societate sana*.[15]

What I am suggesting is that Western medicine functions in exactly the same way. The interface between the person and the group in Western biomedicine is our symbolic system of what constitutes 'a body.' The concept of a body is a lot more complex than we can appreciate from the perspective of our dominant cultural ideology.

So who needs healing? Both the individual and society need healing. What is healing? It is both an individual and social process that allows both individuals and society to deal with the threat of disruption brought about by disease and death. Healing is not something that one does by oneself. If we conceptualize healing from the holistic viewpoint, recognizing that it is both an individual and social process mediated by a healing relationship, we can approach a better understanding and can hope to assimilate prior work into a theoretical model. Culture is an adaptive way to live in the world. Healing as a cultural construct begs the question of what and where is culture? Although not argued here, I take the stand that culture exists both within the individual and within the super-organic whole of society. Culture reproduces as humans reproduce; there is a constant ebb and flow of cultural material between the two.

REFERENCES

1 Brody H. *The Healer's Power*. New Haven, CT: Yale University Press; 1992.

2 Rivers W. *Medicine, Magic and Religion*. London: Routledge; 1924.

3 Egnew TR. The meaning of healing: transcending suffering. *Annals of Family Medicine*. 2005; 3(3): 255–63.

4 Frank JD, Frank JB. *Persuasion and Healing – A Comparative Study of Psychotherapy*. 3rd ed. Baltimore, MA: The Johns Hopkins University Press; 1991.

5 Kleinman A. *Patients and Healers in the Context of Culture*. Berkley, CA: University of California Press; 1980.

6 Kleinman A. *The Illness Narratives – Suffering, Healing, and the Human Condition*. New York, NY: Basic Books; 1988.

7 Lown B. *The Lost Art of Healing*. New York, NY: Ballantine Books; 1996.

8 Balint M. *The Doctor, His Patient and the Illness*. Edinburgh: Churchill Livingstone; 2000 [1957].

9 Charon R. Narrative medicine: form, function, and ethics. *Annals of Int Med*. J2001; 134(1): 83–7.

10 Hunter K, Charon R, Coulehan J. The study of literature in medical education. *Academic Medicine*. 1995; 70(9): 787–94.

11 Charon R. Literature and medicine: origins and destinies. *Academic Medicine*. 2000; 75(1): 23–7.

12 Charon R. Narrative medicine: attention, representation, affiliation. *Narrative*. 2005; 13(3).

13 DasGupta S, Charon R. Personal illness narratives: using reflective writing to teach empathy. *Academic Medicine*. 2004; 79(4): 351–6.

14 Charon R. Narrative medicine: a model for empathy, reflection, profession, and trust. *JAMA*. 2001; 286(15): 1897–1902.

15 Turner V. Symbolic Studies. *Annual Review of Anthropology*. 1975; 4: 145–61.

CHAPTER 15

Commodification of Health Care and the New Professionalism of Translational Practice

James P Meza

HEALING POWER

In medicine, the doctor and patient necessarily have vastly different socially constructed power – one is well, the other sick. One has specialized knowledge and the other is bewildered with a narrative dilemma.[1, 2] One has cultural authority and the other is vulnerable. Such differential power can of course be used or abused. The social contract that regulated this power became known as professionalism – the power was only to be used for the good of the patient. This chapter reviews some of the social changes that have made what we have previously known as professionalism obsolete and challenges all of us to understand the new dynamics of professional power.

An interesting part of the Hippocratic Oath is the pledge to 'keep inviolate' that which should not be revealed. Embedded right there in our guiding code of ethics is the structure of safety to tell stories – stories of good and evil, stories of confession, weakness, fears, worries, guilt, pain, suffering, sadness, and rage; stories with a narrative structure. Thus, the power of medicine is regulated by the ethics of the profession. Professionalism has historically been the regulatory force protecting the patient from abuse of the doctor's power. It is interesting to note that narrative theory is also well represented in the field of ethics.[3–5] A Google Scholar search using the words 'narrative' and 'ethics' returned 260 000 hits, and at least the first 100 were all relevant to health care (I did not look further).

The Social Transformation of American Medicine Continues

Paul Starr wrote an excellent history of how physicians became ascendant in terms of social prestige and power and the forces that are destabilizing that monopoly.[6] He made a clear distinction between social authority and cultural authority. This distinction will become important as we try to analyze the current social forces facing medicine today. One way to understand the long term change is to use the social theory called political economy. Very briefly, political economy theory predicts that power and resources are centripetal. Surveying American medicine, as more money and social resources have been channeled into the health care industry, power is moving first to regional centers and then to national centers.

Let us start at the beginning. At the turn of the century, doctors made house calls and attended the sick. They helped people understand how 'to be ill.' With penicillin and other technological advances, they added technological power to their social position and role. The process continued and soon not all the doctor's tools fit into the doctor's black bag. Hospitals were built to house the specialized services. These hospitals were run by physicians. Medicare money and increasing technology together made for a powerful combination. No one questioned the authority of the doctor to distribute these social resources. This power was regulated with a social contract – professionalism. However, as the resources intensified and CT scanners were introduced, followed by MRI scanners and then PET scanners, not every hospital could afford one. Hospitals merged into hospital systems and networks were built to send patients and resources to tertiary care hospitals. Power tended to shifted to the super specialized hospitals. Even these hospitals have begun to crumble under the financial strain of providing care, shifting power to more centralized corporations or governmental agencies.

Commodification of Healthcare

The United States is facing tremendous financial strains and health care is taking an ever increasing amount of societal resources. When healthcare is bought and sold, it loses its cultural and personal meaning. Bernard Lown describes this as 'the commodification of healthcare.' Commodification is a term that implies standardization and interchangeability in the marketplace. The concern is that healing relationships are not standardized and interchangeable. The previous ethic of professionalism, focused on the patient, is eroded by the commodification of healthcare,[7, 8] which introduces profit motives. Physicians are often distressed by power shifting to other social institutions not regulated by this moral grounding in professionalism. The interference of insurance companies or a market economy destabilizes the previous balance of power. We now have 'corporate medicine,' which has started to separate the cultural authority of the doctor as healer from the social authority of the institution of healthcare. This disruption is a threat to the practice of healing as it has been traditionally understood.

The shift in power initially enhanced physicians' social authority because they maintained control of community hospitals, but in most recent years, the social authority of doctors has declined. Health care institutions now make major decisions about resources, often using physicians for advertising purposes. The relative power of the physicians has peaked and is now competing with large economic enterprises. Although physicians retain tremendous cultural power, they often *perceive* these social changes as a relative deprivation. Doctors stripped of power can't do their doctoring; they can't perform their social function. After all, the role of the healer requires cultural and social authority to determine which ritual is required to restore health. On a more sobering note, I have seen the occasional physician get caught up in the market forces and profit motive. More frequently, I have seen doctors simply accept this new environment and adapt their practice to a new reality.

During President Eisenhower's farewell address to the nation on January 17, 1961 he commented on a momentous societal change, 'the conjunction of military establishment and a large arms industry is new in America.' He labeled this change the 'military-industrial complex.' He warned of abuse of misplaced power whose influence could be felt in the economic, political, and spiritual life of the nation. He advised that only an informed electorate could prevent such abuse.

In a similar way, the past 46 years since Medicare legislation was enacted, we have seen the development of a healthcare-industrial complex, with all the same benefits and hazards that President Eisenhower spoke of. This equally momentous societal change has been labeled by others as *the commodification of healthcare.*

ARE DOCTORS STILL HEALERS?

Social change has also handicapped the development of training a new generation of healers. Over his career, Bernard Lown bemoans the changes in how young doctors think (or order technological tests instead of thinking).[7] Today, large organizations embedded in a market economy with a profit motive directly affect the office consultation of a doctor and patient. The former social contract of professionalism is changing under the pressure of these social changes. As physicians no longer have power, there is no need to have professional constraints on behavior. Glossed with 'lifestyle choice' among young practitioners, this probably is a social calculation that values market forces and physicians as wage laborers above social needs of healing relationships. These changes have all taken their toll on maintaining professionalism as a part of the social regulation of power.[9-14] *You can sell a cure, but you can't sell healing.*

STORY TIME

I was recently observed (along with a group of other doctors) an undeniable breach of professionalism. As it turned out, the needs of the health care institution (a corporation) prevailed over the moral obligations of professionalism. I was upset that the profession of medicine failed to regulate physician behaviors. One of my closest colleagues told me, 'Jim, your problem is that you care too much. You need to realize that you are simply a wage laborer. You need to do your job and go home; otherwise you are simply causing your own suffering.' His words demonstrated to me how far apart the drift between social authority and cultural authority has become for doctors. I asked him, 'Are we still doctors or not?'

The point of the story is ... what is a doctor? ... are doctors healers? ... and who cares?

DOCTORS AND 'CORPORATE CITIZENSHIP'

Very few doctors are in solo practice. Of course we have duties to healthcare institutions – we are obligated to be good employees and institutional structure is absolutely necessary for effective health care delivery – we would do our patients a disservice not to respect that. In most instances I have always been able to see 'the big picture,' and using narrative, help my patients understand how health care institutions strive to improve the health of each patient. In this particular case, it was a sentinel event where the correct balance was disturbed. I believe as the political economy of healthcare evolves, doctors will increasingly be faced with challenges such as these. How well are we as doctors prepared to face these challenges? How well is society as a whole prepared to face these challenges? We explore that next.

Who Needs Healing? Doctors Do

In Chapter 13, I spoke about the need for healing individuals and society. If that is ever going to happen, doctors themselves need to be healed. The profession is under inordinate stress. In fact, it faces the very real possibility of losing its status as a profession. Embedded in the concept of a profession is having a specialized body of knowledge. In Chapter 10 we found that the pharmaceutical industry is writing the medical literature for us. (An example of the health-care-industrial complex.) Another aspect of a profession is self-regulation. As commodification increases, we seem to be losing that as well. Our obligations to the corporation are starting to overshadow our obligation to our colleagues and our patients. This relationship to a corporation is also drawing us away from our patients. Shannon Brownlee, in her book *Overtreated: why too much medicine is making us sicker and poorer*, wrote a compelling exposé of our current healthcare system.[15] Doctors figure prominently in a broken social system. She argues (I believe correctly) that doctors do not know or practice Evidence based medicine; doctors manage the uncertainty in clinical practice by recommending procedures that enhance their own wealth without perceiving the negative consequences and complications of these recommendations; and doctors are unduly influenced by pharmaceutical and medical device corporations. The system of financial rewards and power structures has created a monster that the medical profession has been unable to respond to appropriately.

Consider the following thought experiment. Currently doctors bill third party payers for their services. In order to do this, doctors are required to provide a diagnostic code. The entire medical record and audit system is designed around this fact. The billing process and re-imbursement is a part of the 'commodification complex.' What if doctors were required to provide the patient's narrative dilemma instead of, or in addition to the diagnosis? Imagine all the changes that would have to occur if we re-focused on the patients' concerns.

DOCTORS NEED TO BE HEALERS FIRST

I described social power shifting to corporate institutions. My personal example was when a physician administrator showed me a 'regression line' with four data points – the four doctors in our small practice. I was an outlier and therefore a 'bad doctor.' Inside I knew I was not a bad doctor, but I did not even know what a regression line was, so I could hardly defend myself. I went back to school and got a masters degree in health services administration simply to defend myself because I worked in a healthcare corporation that used business methods to manage me and patient care.

Doctors do feel a 'relative deprivation' from yesteryear when not that many people were telling them how to practice medicine. Healthcare today is different. Some doctors go back to school for an MBA. Unfortunately, this has a snowball effect because now doctors are thinking with the tools of business and the marketplace. As with all positive feedback loops, this results in hastening the commodification of healthcare. In order to regain cultural and social authority, doctors need to be healers, not businessmen. This change in mindset is not yet widely appreciated.

A Restoration Narrative for Western Healers

Doctor, heal thyself. So how do doctors heal themselves? I believe our best choice is a restoration narrative: doctors need to recover the 'doctor's way of knowing.' Jorgensen documented the social deprivation and stress on the Shoshone and Ute Indian societies.[16] Their land was taken away, their way of life was taken away, their economic survival was threatened. They experienced extreme deprivation from what they remember as a traditional way of life and they experienced deprivation compared to whites living on their land and in nearby towns. The stresses on the Shoshone came from outside the tribe – from a government that did not understand, care, or honor its commitments. It came from a government that favored business interests. In response to the extreme stress, they developed the Sun Dance to restore the 'Indian way of life' using 'Indian powers.' This social phenomenon is called a *restoration narrative*. The key point to remember about this restoration narrative was that it was to give power to the individual who participated, but also resulted in societal benefit by strengthening the Indian family and society. Other examples of social responses to perceived or relative deprivation include 'nativistic movements'[17] or 'revitalization movements.'[18] These are examples of how societies respond to extreme stresses.

The 'narrative medicine movement' and 'the practice of healing' are to doctors what the Sun Dance was to the Shoshone Indians. It is a way to restore the social and cultural authority of the doctor, having 'lost' the 'turf wars' of social authority. That same favoring of business over professional power is the relative deprivation that doctors are experiencing. Narrative medicine, evidence based medicine and the role of the 'healer' draw on traditional sources of power for physicians – specialized knowledge[19] and mediation between the individual's life experience and society.

Doctors need to restore 'the doctor's way of knowing' and to be able to reclaim 'the healing power' that derives from their traditional role of harmonizing the individual experiences of patients who suffer with the constraints of life as lived and the controls of society. The integration of narrative medicine and evidenced based medicine, as portrayed in this book, is an appropriate response to the uncertainties of clinical practice. It refocuses the efforts of the doctor back to the patient and lessens the impact of personal gain and institutional mandates.

The airline industry is often used as a model of 'safety' that health care needs to emulate. Perfecting and standardizing processes to result in safety is a typical business model approach to improving healthcare delivery. Although I acknowledge the benefits of such an approach, I also believe that the systematic intellectual errors and the lack of focus on the patient's experience are not yet part of the discourse in health care reform and safety. The social practice of healing offers added benefit to address these vexing problems. Reclaiming the cultural power of 'the social practice of healing' directly responds to many of the problems identified that chronicle what is wrong with medicine today. *Healing practices rather than professionalism is the counterbalance to commodification; this is what I call the new professionalism.*

It remains to be seen if the value of healing will be appreciated outside narrative medicine counter-culture movement within the medical profession. Although the Institute of Medicine stated that health care in the twenty-first century should be based on 'continuous healing relationships,'[20] the current fad is the Patient Centered Medical Home. It seems we are trying to create a healing relationship with an institution, not a real person. I am proposing that society's emphasis needs to shift back to the doctor–patient relationship. In a recent report, it appears that the government of the United Kingdom is shifting the National Health Service in that direction:

> In one of the biggest changes, the government said it plans to eliminate a layer of financial managers and ask doctors instead to decide how the bulk of the National Health Service's £105 billion annual budget should be spent.[21]

What guiding principles will doctors use to make such important societal decisions? At least narrative evidence based medicine can open the discussion of harm and benefit in a way that commodification of health care seems unable to do. Perhaps the logic of care will help set the correct balance between overtreating and undertreating. My own personal answer is that I want to be a better doctor; I want to be a better healer. I believe we should draw on the cultural authority embodied in the Hippocratic Oath: 'I do solemnly swear ... That I will share the knowledge and skills which I have received with my colleagues and with future generations of physicians ...' I think medical school curricula should guarantee we graduate doctors capable of entering into healing relationships with their patients. I believe that we should pursue a research agenda to support curricula such as these. The advantage of the theoretical outline described in Chapter 13 is that it forms a basis for the scientific study of healing practices. I would call such a program of education and research a restoration narrative for doctors.

TRANSLATIONAL PRACTICE, T3 IS ANOTHER NAME FOR HEALING

The Narrative Evidence Based Medicine Working Group at Columbia University has come to the same conclusion that we have. Narrative and evidence are co-constitutive of each other.[22] The National Institute of Health has laid out a translational research roadmap that emphasizes bench science to clinical application and clinical research to practice (T1 and T2).[23] The Narrative Evidence Based Medicine Working Group at Columbia University expands these definitions, recognizing translation 'begins at the point that practitioners have themselves elected to adopt and recommend strategies and interventions based on high-level evidence and guidelines ...and encompasses all aspects of care that converge on the practitioner-patient relationship and ultimately determine what therapies and choices patients actually make regarding their care.'[24]

Yes, times have changed, but like our patients, we still have an obligation to decide what to do next. This book describes a process of care that doctors can start practicing today. I encourage all of my colleagues to use *Translational Practice* with the next patient they see.

REFERENCES

1 Landro L. Finding a way to ask doctors tough questions. *Wall Street Journal*. March 4, 2009.

2 Frank AW. *The Wounded Storyteller: Body, Illness, and Ethics*. Chicago, IL: University of Chicago Press; 1995.

3 Jones AH. Narrative Based Medicine: narrative in medical ethics. *BMJ*. 1999; **318**: 253–6.

4 Hartzband P, Groopman J. Money and the changing culture of medicine. *New England Journal of Medicine*. 2009; **360**(2): 101–3.

5 Nicholas B, Gillett G. Doctors' stories, patients' stories: a narrative approach to teaching medical ethics. *Journal of Medical Ethics*. 1997; **23**(5): 295.

6 Starr P. *The Social Transformation of American Medicine: the rise of a sovereign profession and the making of a vast industry*. New York, NY: Basic Books; 1982.

7 Lown B. *The Lost Art of Healing*. New York, NY: Ballantine Books; 1996.

8 Lown B. The commodification of health care. *Physicians for a National Health Program Newsletter 2007* available at www.pnhp.org/publications/the_commodification_of_health_care.php (accessed December 10, 2010).

9 Morris RT, Sherlock BJ. Decline of ethics and the rise of cynicism in dental school. *Journal of Health and Social Behavior*. 1971; **12**(4): 290–9.

10 Pescosolido BA, Tuch SA, Martin JK. The profession of medicine and the public: examining Americans' changing confidence in physician authority from the beginning of the 'health care crisis' to the era of health care reform. *Journal of Health and Social Behavior*. 2001; **42**(1): 1–16.

11 Prechel H, Gupman A. Changing economic conditions and their effects on professional autonomy: an analysis of family practitioners and oncologists. *Sociological Forum*. 1995; **10**(2): 245–71.

12 Reeder LG. The patient-client as a consumer: some observations on the changing professional-client relationship. *Journal of Health and Social Behavior*. 1972; **13**(4): 406–12.

13 Reid AE. The development of work-related attitudes and behavior of professional recruits: a test of the functionalist argument. *Journal of Health and Social Behavior*. 1979; **20**(4): 338–51.

14 Ritzer G, Walczak D. Rationalization and the deprofessionalization of physicians. *Social Forces*. 1998; **67**(1): 1–22.

15 Brownlee S. *Overtreated: Why Too Much Medicine is Making Us Sicker and Poorer*. New York, NY: Bloomsbury US; 2007.

16 Jorgensen JG. *The Sun Dance Religion: Power for the Powerless*. Chicago, IL: University of Chicago Press; 1972.

17 Linton R. Nativistic movements. In: Lessa W, Vogt E (eds) *Reader in Comparative Religion: an anthropological approach*. 3rd ed. New York, NY: Harper & Row; 1972.

18 Wallace AFC. Revitalization movements. In: Lessa W, Vogt E, op. cit.

19 Bordieu P. The production and reproduction of legitimate language. In: Thompson JB (ed) *Language and Symbolic Power*. Cambridge, MA: Harvard University Press; 1991. p. 43.

20 *Crossing the Quality Chasm: a new health system for the 21st century*. Washington, DC: Institute of Medicine; 2001.

21 Whalen J. U.K. will revamp its health service. *Wall Street Journal*. July 13, 2010.

22 Charon R, Wyer P. Narrative evidence based medicine. *The Lancet.* 2008; **371**: 296–7.

23 Graham I, Tetroe J. Nomenclature in translational research. *JAMA;* **299**(18).

24 Goyal R, Charon R, Lekas, H, *et al.* 'A local habitation and a name': how narrative evidence-based medicine transforms the translational research paradigm. *Journal of Evaluation in Clinical Practice.* 2008; **14**(5): 732–41.

PART IV
Epilogue

CHAPTER 16

Epilogue

INTRODUCTION

Narratives have a beginning, middle, and an end. Human life has a beginning, middle and an end. Although we talk about healing and medical decision making, it is often with the implied assumption that we are solving problems. Death is not a problem to be solved, but a part of living that can add or detract from the meaning of that life. This is where we have found that the healing process described in this book demonstrates its real value. Stories do not really have an ending; they just get told and re-told. The end of one story is often the beginning of another.

> ### STORY TIME
>
> We had a patient who was 82 years old and had severe Chronic Obstructive Lung Disease, a repaired Abdominal Aortic Aneurysm, Hypertension, and many more chronic medical conditions. She continued to smoke, but since she couldn't afford to buy cigarettes, she rolled her own from loose tobacco and cigarette papers. Every time she came to the clinic, we would give her juice and crackers and she was never seen except when nibbling on something; she looked like one of those cute little mice, constantly nibbling. Despite that, her total body weight was only 87 pounds. Her family consisted of a son and daughter-in-law who lived 100 miles away. She was content, however, since she had a boyfriend in the assisted living facility across the street from our clinic. One of the major social outings was coming to the clinic and having the clinic staff hug and fuss over them (she always came with her boyfriend). After 15 years of tending to her chronic medical conditions and listening to life stories, she eventually developed Congestive Heart Failure and had several hospital admissions. I knew the end was drawing near. After one of the hospitalizations, her family drove into town and accompanied her to the clinic. We perceived that as a narrative moment and took time from a busy clinic to have an end-of-life discussion. We were all in the same room and heard the same story. Quite typically, the patient and family never filled out the paperwork for the Advanced Directive, but I recorded the conversation in my dictation from that visit. The next week, the patient was back in the Emergency Department.

Upon our arrival, she was sitting on the gurney, holding a sandwich between her thumb and forefinger with a look of absolute elegance. It did not matter that she couldn't breath and was in severe heart failure. We decided she needed transfer to the regional tertiary care hospital. The family was not pleased because it would only lengthen their drive to visit their loved one. Later that night, the patient had a cardiac arrest and was put on a ventilator. Miraculously after being resuscitated for 28 minutes, the patient was fully awake. When we visited, the Intensive Care Unit routine was in full swing – intubation, naso-gastric tube, arterial line, central venous catheter, Foley catheter, ECG monitoring pads and wires, wrist restraints, surgical tape, and all the rest. The son was distraught because he said he 'wasn't ready to let her die.' We struggled through 10 minutes of miming and attempts at writing to understand the patient's wishes – she wanted a sandwich. The sandwich became the metaphor for all future decision making in the ICU. It represented 'quality of life' that the patient spoke about during our end-of-life discussion. We had only to ascertain a few medical facts to integrate her medical status into her narrative. Decision making in this stressful, intensive place and time became simplified because we all knew the narrative context. If she was able to be weaned and enjoy a sandwich, then we planned a week of ICU support. If she developed a medical complication, she was to be terminally weaned and allowed to die gracefully, elegantly, and in the style that she always embodied. The blending of narrative and technology was coherent and effortless because we had all written the co-constructed narrative together before the life-story ended.

The point of the story is ... one of the highest impact moments in the healing process is at the end of the life-story; you can't tell the end of the story unless you know the beginning and the middle.

THE COST OF END OF LIFE CARE

With approximately one third of Medicare expenditures in the final year of life concentrated in the last month of life, mostly for life-sustaining care, it seems that the end of the story is quite expensive.[1] With the demographic imperative of the age distribution of the United States population, we can anticipate the next healthcare crisis and contested social narrative will involve the costs of end-of-life care. So here is the narrative twist in the story – perhaps those with social authority (healthcare institutions and government) will recognize that it is in their own best interest and the best interest of society to train doctors who know how to be in healing relationships. Healing is good medicine for everyone involved.

THE ZONE OF INDISTINCTION VIEWED AS *NARRATIVE FAILURE*

Sharon Kaufman wrote a superlative ethnography of dying in America (an ethnography is a detailed description of the cultural and experiential life as lived).[2] She talks extensively about what death was and has become in America. Many of her examples include Intensive Care Unit experiences. She makes it clear that the system constrains what is possible and why we in America are so bad at end-of-life care. In the extreme form, she describes the 'Zone of Indistinction', referring to bodies that are biologically functioning, but have no 'embodied self'. They are neither alive nor dead; these bodies are ventilator dependent and 'warehoused' in special hospitals with alternate re-imbursement rules. If you examine how such a situation was created, you find that doctors and patients, doctors and patient's families, and patients and patient's families all avoided talking, storytelling, and sharing enough information to be prepared to know what to do when the time of death arrives. This type of uncertainty results in overly aggressive care and creates the dilemma of being unable to tell if a person is still a person; we do not know how to create the story of the patient's end of life. *Amongst all the super high technology, we consider this to be another narrative failure.*

The New Professionalism

Shannon Brownlee mentions at least seven times in her book[3] that doctors do not know how to read medical literature, do not have the analytic skills to interpret evidence and says that medical schools do not teach these vital skills to future practitioners. That, combined with the lack of attentiveness to what the patient wants, the incentives to 'do more procedures', and the co-dependence of doctors to healthcare institutions increase costs and increases harm. Between Kaufman and Brownlee, we have a very clear picture of almost everything that is wrong with American medicine. We believe that one step that we can take right now is to start practicing a type of medicine that integrates narrative medicine and evidence based medicine – we encourage doctors to reclaim their role in society as 'healers'.

APPLICATION TO OUR CLINICAL SCENARIO

(10 years later)

Doctor: Jason, I'm glad you're here ... your mom is anxious to see you. She's made some decisions ...

Jason: How is she, doctor?

Doctor: She's stable and in good spirits. The car accident did a lot of internal damage; they had to remove most of her intestines during the first surgery and she knows that she will never live without depending on the IVs for all of her nutrition. She misses her chocolate cake ... I think you should go see her.

(After a time delay when Jason was alone with his mother)

Doctor: How did it go?

Jason: (Crying) I don't know. She asked me about the kids and Michelle and then asked how I was doing. It should have been the other way around. She's the one that needs help. We're all doing well. The last kid will be going off to school and ...
Silence ...
Sobbing ...
Silence ...

Jason: I'm just glad she got to see baby Shannon.
Silence
Silence
She told me she was so proud of me for getting my life together. I had to learn a lot of things the hard way, but when I think about it, she was always there. She forced me to make tough choices, but I'm glad I did.
Silence ...
She said something weird ... she called it 'my grandfather's blessing' ... I don't know what that meant. I don't understand. She told me she had one last lesson she wanted me to learn ... sobbing ... sobbing ... sobbing ...
Silence ...
She wants to go home with the IVs for two weeks so she can be surrounded by the ones she loves and have a chance to say good-bye without rushing anything. Then she wants the IV disconnected even though she knows she'll die in a matter of days. She said she wants to show me how to die gracefully so when my turn comes I know what to do. It's like she has this story all written out. I didn't know what to say.
I'm so scared ... I don't know if I can be as brave as she is, but she said she had such confidence in me.
You'll be there won't you?

Doctor: I've known your mother a long time ... we're pretty good friends. We've talked about her plan a lot. She truly understands what she wants and the consequences. I support her decisions. Of course I'll be there. I need to be able to say good-bye, too. There will be nurses to help and your Pastor will support you.
Jason, through your mother's eyes, I've watched you grow into a man. I have to say I'm proud of you too and I have confidence you can do this.

Jason: Thanks, doc ... Oh yeah ... she said she appreciated the way the two of you worked together so well.

Doctor: It was my pleasure. We'll talk again tomorrow. Take care, Jason.

NARRATIVE INTERPRETATION OF THE CLINICAL SCENARIO

This is the point when we encourage the reader to contemplate for themselves the meanings and personal reactions to the story – in order to practice narrative medicine, doctors need to be self-reflective. Now is a good time to practice.

LIFE IS CONTINGENT, EMERGENT, SITUATED, AND CONTEXTUAL

Life is contingent – we never know what types of surprises await us when we walk out the door or wake up in the morning. We plan, we dream, we hope; these are the *contingencies* of life.

Life is emergent. Think of pregnancy and all the possibilities in that new life. But then we watch our children grow up and they become exactly their own personality, making their own choices. They *emerge* into the world as their unique selves.

Life is situated. None of us got to choose our parents. It is just *the situation* into which we entered the world.

Life is contextual. Haven't you ever wondered what your life would have been like if you had been born in Africa, or Singapore? The rules we live by would have certainly been different because of the difference in the *context* of our life.

REFERENCES

1   Zhang B. Health care costs in the last week of life: associations with end-of-life conversations. *Archives of Internal Medicine.* 2009; **169**(5).
2   Kaufman S. *... And a Time to Die: how American hospitals shape the end of life.* Chicago, IL: University of Chicago Press; 2005.
3   Brownlee S. *Overtreated: why too much medicine is making us sicker and poorer.* New York, NY: Bloomsbury; 2007.

Afterword

The Wednesday night call caught me at a vulnerable moment. I was just beginning to read this book – and the Monday deadline for writing the Afterword was looming.

On the other end of the phone was the grandmother of two former young patients. I'd cared for them from birth before leaving my 19-year practice for a sabbatical and then for a new practice at a community health center. The younger brother now was a junior in high school. At 300 pounds, Zachery was a star lineman on his school football team. His grandmother had been raising Zack and his brother since their mother was killed in a tragic car accident nine years earlier. I could hear simultaneous concern and confusion in the grandmother's voice as she told me why she was calling.

In front of her were two conflicting reports and a DVD of scans from two respected major medical centers. Could her grandson continue to play football? She felt pressure from the coach and from her grandson. One doctor said no – the boy's spinal stenosis could result in paralysis from the next errant hit on the field. The other said yes – the risk was small enough that he could play, as he and his coach so desperately desired.

Could I help the grandmother somehow decide? The conflict from her siding with the conservative plan was tearing up the family.

I wish I'd had the benefit of this book before taking the grandmother's call. But while reading the book over the ensuing weekend, I found myself pulled back into her story, wondering how I might have reacted differently if I'd had its guidance. Meza and Passerman have given us a lens with which to see new events in ways that honor the past, are open to the unknown future, and more aware and mindful of the moment-to-moment.

Meza's and Passerman's text teaches us new techniques and reminds us of deeply known truths about healing. Their method integrates two fundamental and complementary ways of knowing. It shows us how to bring together stories and statistics, numbers and narratives. In this sharing, the authors open possibilities that move beyond knowing to understanding. In that understanding is the hope of wisdom.

The six 'As' of their method unite personal story and impersonal science. This integration brings with it the potential to restore wholeness to the person, value to our ailing health care system, and solidarity between the patient and his community. Flowing from personal narrative to general evidence and back again, the six As in this book join story and science.

Acquiring information is about identifying the nugget in the patient's story that is a unique opportunity for healing in this moment. Discovering the most helpful information today is about co-constructing narrative – drawing out the patient's 'narrative dilemma' in a way that frames a clinical question with true healing potential. This reflective bearing witness in itself can be healing – for both the teller and the listener. Healing – being whole and reconnected to meaning and community – can be facilitated just by the act of hearing someone's whole story.

Asking a clinically relevant question, in Meza and Passerman's method, is an explicitly collaborative boundary-spanning action. Translating the language of the patient's illness narrative into the language of clinical medicine requires diving below the surface of the story to find the source from which the question and the illness spring. This asking often involves swimming against the rip tides of time pressure to deliver the commodities of evidence based health care, in order to make sure the evidence and the care are relevant to the patient. Before following a stream of evidence, the authors ask us to deeply understand the patient's story to be sure we are in the right channel.

Accessing information to answer the clinically relevant question involves moving from the patient's world of individual lived experience to the researcher's world of systematic experience gained from studying many people. The clinician's role is that of guide, and Meza and Passerman show us how to use readily available free technology to minimize search work and maximize relevance and validity. I had thought I knew how to effectively use PubMed and Google, but the authors' approach is more effective and transparent and more open to use in furthering the patient's co-constructive narrative than my old approach.

Assessing the quality of the information is a new need of patients as they struggle with the overload of data and the paucity of relevance, understanding and wisdom that characterize the information age. The method of assessment in this book can help us as clinicians to effectively move from purveyors of doctor's orders to colleagues who help patients to use the best quality and most relevant information to advance their life story.

Applying the information to the clinical question is a branch point in the stream of the patient's narrative. Moving from dehumanized evidence to re-personalized information in the context of the patient's story has healing potential beyond what may be conveyed by numbers needed to treat. The technical aspects of this involve Bayes' Theorem, which tells us that what we believe beforehand affects how we interpret new information. When what we believe beforehand is informed by astutely asking the patient's story, and the new information is guided by carefully accessed and assessed information, the streams of narrative and evidence based medicine begin to merge to make health care both personalized and scientific – a science of the personal. This personalizing and grounding of health care one person and one problem at a time also is a passageway for healing a dysfunctional system and for making society more robust, resilient and connected.

Assisting the patient to make a decision in the Meza-Passerman method goes beyond an isolated cognitive choice. It involves situating information within the context of the patient's story so that it can be used to help a meaningful solution to emerge. This may involve multiple translations to find one that resonates with the patient's lived experience. Assisting goes way beyond science-supported recommendations. It is care that helps the patient to get on with his or her life.

A seventh 'A' – *abiding* – also is needed, and actually is implied in the final 'theory' chapters of the book. Relationship-centered health care requires patients and healers to stick together over time. Yet, as we have merged the two words of *health care* into the one word commodity of *healthcare*, we have turned the promising rush of technology and information into a swamp of depersonalized doing *to*, rather than abiding *with*. Meza and Passerman show us a different way. They call for a renewed social practice of healing to save us, our patients, and our country from having turned caring into commodity: 'Relationship centered care harmonizes two stories and brings the patient back into the community of empowered social actors, creating personal meaning and reinforcing social norms.'

Just as a fish is unaware of the water in which it swims, the experienced primary care clinician often is unaware of how vital the ongoing shared story – the relationship – is for our healing work. We see this when a student happens to see our patient, coming up with a new and sometimes helpful diagnosis. But when we follow up, the 'history' given to the student is totally different from the narrative we co-construct, as the story is retold as part of our ongoing conversation based on deep shared experience. A new view – starting a new shared story – sometimes can be very helpful in getting out of the rut of old streams of narrative. But it is the abiding story, the bringing together of rivulets of shared meaning over time that is desired by patients and needed by healers. It is this abiding story that unifies the cutting torrents of health care into a river of meaningful narrative that is connected to the Source, is a reservoir of hope, and a passage toward healing.

Zack's grandmother called me because her story of raising her grandson in a way that honored her deceased daughter was broken. The two healers whose expert evidence and advice she held in front of her had no abiding story with Zack or his departed mother. No matter how authoritative, these experts had a difficult time bridging the evidence of a scientific medical evaluation with the story of a young man and his family. My own narrative stream was incomplete

– blocked by my abandonment (an eighth A – the opposite of abiding). But the river of our relationship was deep enough to form a large reservoir that unites multiple streams: Zack and his medical condition; Zack as a football player and team member; Zack and his future life beyond football; Zack as part of a multigenerational family already experienced in loss from a rare event.

When the call came, I agreed to try to help. Looking back through the lens of this book, what I did was to *acquire* enough information to begin to understand the patient's concern. I *asked* the clinically relevant question: 'What is the likelihood of paralysis in a young football player with spinal stenosis?' Then, after hanging up, I *accessed* and *assessed* information from Google, PubMed, and a sports medicine colleague. I scheduled a home visit for the next evening after football practice to *apply* the information to Zack's grandmother's question and to *assist* them in making a decision.

Still not having read the book (distracted by my day job and by preparing for the family meeting), I called Zack's grandmother before departing for the home visit.

'I don't think you should bother coming over,' she said with a reflective, resigned tone.

Resisting my rescue fantasy, I listened as she reflected on how hard she'd worked to raise her grandsons as her daughter Jocelyn would have wanted. Together, we recalled how hard Zack had worked over the years to get schoolwork done despite his attention deficit disorder, and how playing sports had been such an important outlet for him. I brought up what I thought was the real issue – helping Zack to develop his identity and skills outside of football, since whether or not he played on this team this season, it was unlikely that football would be his life. Zack's grandmother was way ahead of me on this. She told me about all she had done over the years to draw out his other talents, including singing, and how she had saved up to take both boys to visit their uncle last summer. The uncle lives in another country, and the lesson was about the whole range of possibilities that life has to offer.

Her voice got even softer as she ventured further. Since the more experienced doctor had said the risk of paralysis was small and only a little above the risk of anyone else playing football; and since he and the coach had talked about tackling techniques that would minimize the risk; since Zack would soon be 18 and would then do what he wanted; and since Jocelyn probably would have wanted him to follow his dream, the grandmother was thinking about sitting down with Zack and talking about letting him play again.

As I recounted the positive effect that she'd had on the lives of these two boys, endorsed her decision, and gave a few contingencies, I realized that my patient for this encounter was not Zack. It was his grandmother.

Finally reading this book the following weekend helped me to make sense of the week's discussions with Zack's grandmother. This book named the acquiring, asking, accessing, assessing, applying, and assisting steps I'd taken. Organizational theorist Karl Weick uses the term 'sensemaking' for this process of giving meaning to experience. Making sense of the past enhances mindfulness in the present, and sets the stage for continued learning and growth.

On Sunday night I went back and used the Meza-Passerman method for accessing information using the specificity of Google Scholar and the sensitivity of PubMed. I found information of much greater relevance than my prior search or consultation with an expert had yielded. Knowing the actual rate of paralyzing injury in high school football, the increase in risk from spinal stenosis, and the (limited) predictive value of radiographic evidence might have changed the flow of my shared narrative with Zack's grandmother, although her changed decision to allow him to play football likely would have been the same.

But more transformative for me is to imagine future collaborative health care that uses the model in this book to bring both the head and the heart to healing. Recent Institute of Medicine reports call for more effective use of information technology and for basing health care on 'continuous healing relationships.' Linking narrative and evidence based medicine, as we are shown how to do in this book, is how this can be accomplished. Health care that is informed by high quality information made relevant by being embedded in co-created patient stories can generate a new narrative. That narrative is of a sustainable system that wisely uses resources for the enablement of the lives of people and their communities. By linking stories and science as taught in this book, we can build healing relationships, a new professionalism, and a high value health care system. Let us start with the next patient. The next story. The next relevant evidence. The next relationship. Let us make the integration of narrative and evidence based medicine the foundation of who we are as patients, healers, and a health care system.

Kurt C Stange, MD, PhD
Cleveland, Ohio

PART V
Appendices

Introduction to Appendices

Throughout the book, we talked about how we have come to use the process described simply as 'the way we practice medicine.' Using some of the terms we have described, what we have actually done is cognitively changed the way we practice medicine; it has become 'just the way we do it ...' We do not have to struggle to double think everything. It comes naturally and flows. In the office, we invite narratives when we greet the patient by saying, 'So, give me the update about what's happening with you ...' This implies that we know the previous episodes and are ready to listen to the patient's perception of their health status. We know enough to forgo questioning until we understand the patient's narrative dilemma. We facilitate the telling of the story. This is particularly important as health care is shifting to chronic disease management.

When teaching the process to learners, we always use actual cases that they are struggling with at the time. We follow the 'six As' format. It takes only slightly longer to review the process in a teaching setting. We have successfully used '20 minutes of unstructured listening time' to help learners listen and appreciate the narrative aspects of the process. Residents are expected to stop by a patient's room after rounds and just sit and listen. The rule is that they are not allowed to ask a question. (That is the difficult part, but the part that is most instructional.) The next day on rounds, they share what they heard and we apply it to the care of the patient that day. The resident fills out a 'procedure card' and the attending physician signs it just as they would sign a procedure card for a paracentesis or other invasive procedure.

Likewise, when faced with high impact clinical decisions, we understand that it is in the best interest of the patient to get every test that is needed, but avoid every unnecessary test. We model that behavior. Once when we were making rounds in the hospital, the resident said, 'We're planning to order a CT-Pulmonary Embolism Protocol ...' We just stood there silently, letting the awkward silence do all the talking until the resident finally said, 'I suppose you expect me to draw those lines on that thing with all the numbers ...' With bedside computers and interactive nomograms, clinical decision making is structured by a cognitive process that is adapted to the future practice of medicine.

In Parts I and II we went into great detail to explicate the important highlights of the process because we were writing in textbook style. Here in the Appendix, we simply want to demonstrate what we have already stated; this is the process we use to provide medical care. Imagine that this is simply the 'progress note' that would be entered into the medical record detailing why and how the process of care proceeded as it did. For learners, it is a good way for them to learn the scaffolding or structure of the process. We will not go into detailed explanations here in the Appendix. We only want to demonstrate that the process works. Hopefully the reader can 'fill in the blanks' of the cognitive processes of care. By making short sketches like these, learners understand how the process becomes interdependent. They learn what is inscribed on their diploma, 'Doctorate in the Art and Science of Medicine.' They learn what works and what doesn't. They learn to think with narrative and use evidence based medicine. They learn to become healers.

In the Preface we talked about Translational Practice and contrasted it with Translational Research. As mentioned above, consider the structure of a progress note changing from biomedical model to a translational practice model – our writing or case notes should also change the structure in which they are recorded in the chart. Consider these next two examples as just that. We also wrote about the science of the social practice of healing – in order to do that, we will also need a new literature base. This new type of literature would have to demonstrate how to make the transitions from narrative dilemmas to clinical questions and what research data was used, how it was found, and what it meant to the patient at that time. We would have to demonstrate how the quality of the data and how to put it into terms the patient could use effectively deal with uncertainty. These cases are examples. Perhaps some day we will have such a medical literature to use and study.

Appendix A

Acquire Appropriate Information to Understand the Patient's Concern.

Doctor:	Hi Mrs Cohen, what brings you into the urgent care today?
Patient:	Well, doctor, I am not feeling well. I am having some trouble breathing.
Doctor:	Silence
	Silence
	Silence
Patient:	I've never had this problem before. I'm always short of breath, whether I'm sitting in my chair, eating, or even taking a shower. I thought the warm mist from the shower would loosen this up and help me breath, but it doesn't matter. I can't walk, I can't go to work. I have been just miserable. I do have a cough, but I don't have any pain. I just can't breathe well.
Doctor:	That sounds miserable.
Patient:	Do you think that I have congestion?
Doctor:	Before we discuss that, what do you know about congestion?
Patient:	Well, I am afraid that I have congestion.
Doctor:	Silence
	Silence
	Silence
Patient:	John, my husband died of congestion. He went to the hospital because he couldn't breath, just like me, and they told him that his heart wasn't beating very strong. Six months later, he died. It was very sad. Even with the oxygen he was gasping for air. They had to give him medicine to help with the gasping.
	See, John and I lived very similar lives. We both smoked, we both had high blood pressure but since we don't have a lot of money, we could not see the doctor regularly. We could not afford our medicine, so, we couldn't take it. Even when we went to the doctor, they would get mad and say that we had to take our medicine or we would die. They were right about John. He did die. Now it's my turn.
Doctor:	Let me check to make sure I understand what you're sharing with me ... you think you have 'congestion' and it's so bad that you are going to die from it.
Patient:	That's right.

Doctor: What does 'congestion' mean to you?

Patient: That's when the water comes out of your lungs ... I never really understood what that had to do with the heart, but that's what John's doctors told me.

Doctor: The job of the heart is to pump the blood out of the lungs and into the body. If the heart muscle is weak, then the blood backs up in the lungs. The blood cells are too big to get into the tiny air sacs of the lungs, but the clear straw fluid they float in does get in there and fills the air sacs with fluid. That's what people mean when they say 'water' in the lungs. It's like trying to breathe after you inhaled water, like partially drowning. I think you're using the word 'congestion' for something we call 'congestive heart failure' – a weak heart muscle with build up of fluid in the lungs.

Patient: Do I have that?

Doctor: Let me examine your lungs ...
The good news is that I don't think that you have congestion. Your lungs do not sound like congestion. Actually, I hear wheezing. Did you ever have asthma?

Patient: I had asthma as a kid. I am 48 now, so, that was 35 years ago since I had a problem with it. I am glad that you don't think that I have congestion. The medical student that was just in here told me he just did a rotation ... is that what you call it? ... in the Emergency Department and he said I could have a test called ... wait a minute, I wrote it down ... (patient rummages in her purse) called BNP and that would tell me if I have congestion. I really want that test today.

Doctor: There is a test, called BNP. Before we order it, let's first discuss whether it would be helpful for you. Before we get started, let me see if I have your concern correct: you want to know if you have fluid backing up in your lungs, called congestion, or congestive heart failure ... is that right?

Patient: That's right. I think that test will answer my question.

Ask an appropriate clinical question

The patient is looking for a test that can help her with the diagnosis for congestive heart failure. We have to include her understanding of BNP and 'congestion.' In order for us to be able to help her with this disease diagnosis, we need to find the sensitivity and specificity to calculate the likelihood ratio.

What is the sensitivity and specificity of BNP for the diagnosis of congestive heart failure?

Access information to answer the question

The Google Scholar search terms, which are directly from the clinical question, are as follows: sensitivity, specificity, BNP, congestive, heart, failure.

The Google Scholar search page is:

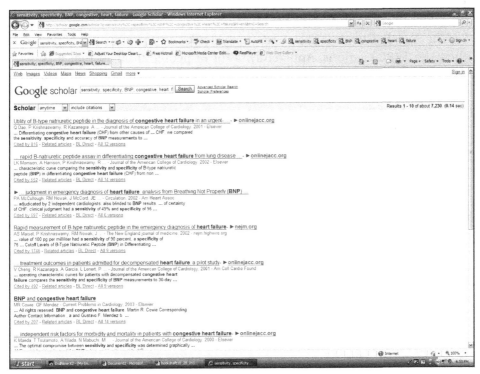

Figure A.1 Google Scholar Search.

The first Google Scholar summary is promising; however, after following the link to the abstract, there were 250 patients who were predominately male, and 94% who presented to a Veterans Affairs center. The fact that it is a Veterans Affairs center explains the sex distribution. Since our patient is a woman, she does not quite fit in with this patient population. Additionally, the military background of all of these patients does not match our patient's background. Military veterans have a different pattern of chronic disease burdens. For these reasons, we should look for another article.

The second Google Scholar summary also looks promising. However, after following the link to the abstract, there are only 321 patients. They all presented to the emergency room for dyspnea. The abstract also stated, 'Patients with CHF ($n = 134$) had BNP levels of 758.5 ± 798 pg/ml, significantly higher than the group of patients with a final diagnosis of pulmonary disease ($n = 85$) whose BNP was 61 ± 10 pg/ml.' Our clinical question is 'What is the sensitivity and specificity of BNP for the diagnosis of congestive heart failure?' not does our patient have congestive heart failure or a pulmonary disease as the cause of her dyspnea? Essentially, our patient wants to know if she has congestive heart failure or not. Let us look at the third Google Scholar summary.

The third Google Scholar summary states that it is an analysis from the Breathing Not Properly trial. We are looking for original research, so we will move onto the fourth Google Scholar summary.

The fourth Google Scholar summary looks very promising. Notice how there are 1786 citations. Apparently, a lot of people thought that it was relevant as well. After following the link to the abstract, there are 1586 patients in this study. They presented to the ER for acute dyspnea and they used the BNP to determine if the patients had congestive heart failure or not. After searching the rest of the page and the next page, there were not any articles that appeared more relevant to the fourth Google Scholar abstract. I think that we found our article.

Before we move on with the fourth article, let us check for more recent articles by setting the Google Advanced Scholar Search dates to 2008–2009, the last two years, and use the same search terms as above, BNP congestive heart failure sensitivity specificity.

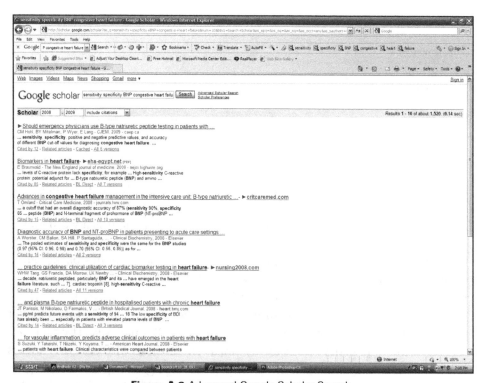

Figure A.2 Advanced Google Scholar Search.

The first two Google Scholar summaries are editorials, not original research. We are interested in original research. The third Google Scholar summary is studying the prohormone NT-proBNP. Our institution cannot perform this test rapidly enough for clinical application. Thus, this article is not relevant to our search. The fourth article compares BNP to NT-proBNP, again, not relevant to our patient.

At this point, we can proceed confidently to the next step as we have the most relevant article of the subject matter.

We are going to locate the article in PubMed and search by 'related citations.'

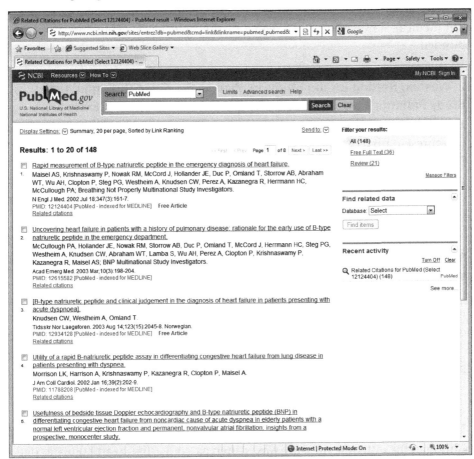

Figure A.3

The most noteworthy study is the 'Breathing Not Properly' Study (catchy title). After reviewing several of the papers, none is better than our original choice, so we're going to proceed.

Assess the validity of the information

1. Was There an Independent 'Blind Comparison' with a 'Gold Standard'?

The gold standard for the diagnosis of congestive heart failure is clinical judgment. Chest X-ray and echocardiogram aid in the diagnosis, but they lack a high degree of sensitivity and specificity. For example, if a patient has clinical

CHF and a normal 2D-echo, then by definition, they have diastolic failure. In this study, the clinical judgment of the two independent cardiologists was used as the gold standard and BNP was compared to their assessment. The cardiologists were able to make the diagnosis with all of the information, such as, the chest X-ray, echocardiogram, symptoms, and treatment course.

The article also states that the cardiologist 'independently reviewed the medical stay without knowledge of the BNP levels.' Thus, the study was blinded.

2. Was the Setting for the Study, as Well as the Filter Through Which Study Patients Passed, Adequately Described? (Inclusion/Exclusion)

The inclusion and exclusion criteria were adequately described and seem to be representative of our patient, as the patients presented to the Emergency Department with dyspnea. The only difference is that a potential bias is that one might imagine sicker patients go to the Emergency Department and less ill patients present to the clinic. Nonetheless, this is about as good of a match as we hope to find, so we will accept it.

3. Did the Patient Sample Include an Appropriate Spectrum of Patients to Whom the Diagnostic Test will be Applied in Clinical Practice?

In other words, has the diagnostic test been evaluated in a patient sample that included an appropriate spectrum of mild and severe, treated and untreated, disease, plus individuals with different but commonly confused disorders?

Table A.1 details a robust spectrum of patients with varying degrees of symptoms and baseline illness.

4. Have the Reproducibility of the Test Result and its Interpretation Been Determined?

Although the outcome measure was written as 'congestive heart failure as determined by two cardiologists' reviewing all the clinical information, the actual data of these clinical assessments were not provided. Instead, they reported out sub-group analyses and did regression analyses to determine (presumably) who has CHF and who did not. The reality is we do not know what they did because they did not tell us.

5. Have the Tactics for Carrying Out the Test Been Described in Sufficient Detail to Permit Their Exact Replication?

The methods were sufficiently described, but the results were not reported in a format that we would have preferred. We have to accept some assumptions they made when writing the research manuscript.

Apply the information to the patient's problem

In order to calculate the likelihood ratios, we need the sensitivity and specificity. Table A.1, below, summarizes the results found in the study. Most of the literature uses the cutoff of 100 for BNP being positive or negative; if the BNP is greater than 100, then the test is positive for congestive heart failure and if the BNP is less than 100, then the patient does not have congestive heart failure. The authors provided different cutoffs, demonstrating how that affects the test characteristics. The different cutoffs will have different test characteristics. Since much of the literature uses a cutoff of 100, we will use that cutoff.

Table A1. Summary of results from study. These values can be found on Table 3 of the article. (*New England Journal of Medicine.* 2002; **347**(3))

BNP	Sensitivity	Specificity
50	97	62
80	93	74
100	90	76
125	87	79

In order to calculate the likelihood ratio for a positive test, we will use the following equation:

$$\text{LR}(+ \text{ test}) = \frac{\text{Sensitivity}}{1 - \text{Specificity}}$$

$$\text{LR}(+) = \frac{\text{Sensitivity}}{1 - \text{Specificity}} = \frac{.9}{1 - .76} = 3.75$$

In order to calculate the likelihood ratio for a negative test, we will use the following equation:

$$\text{LR}(- \text{ test}) = \frac{1 - \text{Sensitivity}}{\text{Specificity}}$$

$$\text{LR}(-) = \frac{1 - \text{Sensitivity}}{\text{Specificity}} = \frac{1 - .9}{.76} = .13$$

In order to use the likelihood ratios, we first need to determine the patient's pre-test probability. This patient is a middle aged woman with a history of tobacco use, worsening shortness of breath, and a long history of what can assume to be poorly controlled hypertension. She has no paroxysmal nocturnal dyspnea or orthopnea. There hasn't been prior angina or myocardial infarction. The good news is that on exam, she has wheezing, not crackles, no JVD, and no leg edema. The JVD and lower extremity edema correlate to right heart failure, and her symptoms correlate to left heart failure. Many times, though, right and left heart failure are seen together as the most common cause of right heart failure is left heart failure. The chest X-ray has not been done yet, but would likely be part of her evaluation. At this point, we feel that her pre-test probability for congestive heart failure is 10%.

In Figure A.4, the application of the above numbers if the test is positive is seen below:

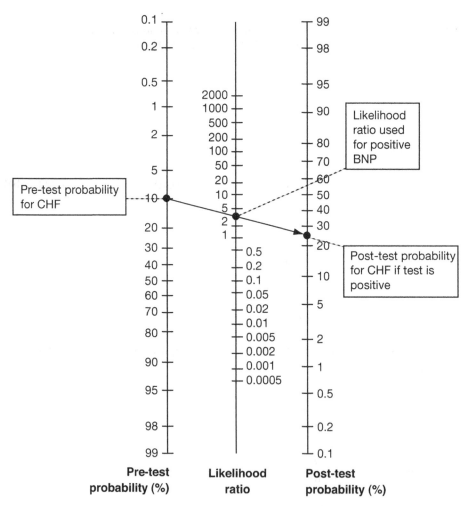

Figure A.4 Nomogram for a Positive BNP.

In Figure A.5, the application of the above numbers if the test is negative is seen below:

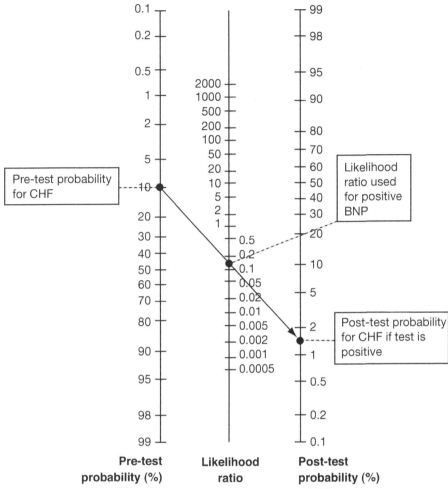

Figure A.5 Nomogram for a Negative BNP.

If the test is positive, then the patient has a 25% chance of having congestive heart failure; if the test is negative, then the patient has a 1.5% chance of having congestive heart failure.

Assist the patient to make a decision

Doctor: Mrs Cohen, after looking at some of the research, it seems as though if we order that test the medical student told you about, it would only be helpful if the test was negative. If the test is positive, we won't be able to tell you anything more about 'congestion' than we already know. I'd like to hear something about your expectation of what this test could do.

Patient: I'm afraid of congestion. How do you check to see if I really have it?

Doctor: Well, the way the research article was performed gives us a good idea how we should do it for you. They collected information about the physical exam, chest X-ray findings, echocardiogram tests and that type of thing. The diagnosis of congestion was then made by the clinical impression of the doctors. I know that's hard to believe in our world of technology, but this is one of those cases where a careful history and physical together with simple testing is more accurate that the test described in the research study used to test for congestion.

Patient: Do you mean I won't know?

Doctor: When we were talking, it seemed as though you equated 'congestion' with dying ... is that true?

Patient: Yes ...

Doctor: I told you that the best test is the doctor's clinical opinion ... I think your trouble breathing is from asthma ... if we treat you for that and later do a different test to verify that you do have asthma, will you feel confident enough that you don't have congestion?

Patient: I'm confused.

Doctor: I'm sorry to have confused you. What part of it do you want me to explain again?

Patient: Did you say that the test won't tell me if I have congestion?

Doctor: That's true. The best test to determine that you do have congestion is a history and physical exam. The only thing the test is capable of is telling you that your small chance of congestion is even smaller. The problem with ordering the test is that I think it is just as likely to confuse things and cause you more worry. I'm comfortable with the diagnosis we have now without running the risk of ordering a test that might confuse us and cause you to have more testing that has as much potential to cause harm as to help you.

Patient: So the best thing is for me to trust your opinion?

Doctor: Do you trust me?

Patient: Well, the doctors that took care of my husband didn't even bother to talk to me ... and I was too afraid to ask a question. I wish there was a test to prove I have congestion, but if you tell me this test the medical student told me about can't do that, then I guess I don't want it. Promise me you'll check me closely and tell me if you have any suspicion I'm getting congestion.

Doctor: I promise. I want to see you again in two weeks.

Appendix B

Acquire Appropriate Information to Understand the Patient's Concern.

Doctor:	Good morning Mr and Mrs Engle, how are you doing today?
Patient's wife:	I am concerned about my husband. He has not been doing very well. I think that the dementia is getting worse. As you know, he doesn't talk much anymore. He has recently been sitting around a lot. He just sits and watches TV. Two days ago, I noticed that he had swelling in his right leg. It seems to hurt him –I sometimes hear him moaning. He moans louder when you touch the leg.
Doctor:	What have you been doing for the leg?
Patient's wife:	I was worried, so I took him to the ER Sunday. They did some tests and told me he has a blood clot. Here, I have the papers with me.
Doctor:	That's scary.
Patient's wife:	Yes it is. I know that people can die from blood clots.
Doctor:	Is he being treated for this?
Patient's wife:	They gave him this pill (warfarin) and this shot (low molecular weight heparin) that I have to give him twice daily. I haven't given him the shot yet. Don't people stay in the hospital for a blood clot?
Doctor:	They used to admit people to the hospital for blood clots. Since the shot was invented, we can treat people at home.
Patient's wife:	I tell you, they just don't want people to be in the hospital anymore. I think they are just being cheap.
Doctor:	Pause Pause Pause
Patient's wife:	I want the best for my Steve. I am not ready for him to die. Is this shot any good?
Doctor:	Let's find out how good the shot is.

Ask an appropriate clinical question

Since the patient is concerned about a treatment modality and wonders whether her husband should be in a hospital (for unfractionated heparin drip), we can develop a PICO question as follows:

P = Patient Population = Deep vein thrombosis
I = Intervention = Low molecular weight heparin
C = Control therapy = Unfractionated heparin
O = Outcome = Mortality

Does low molecular weight heparin, when compared to unfractionated heparin, reduce mortality in deep vein thrombosis?

Access information to answer the question

The Google Scholar search terms, which are directly from the clinical question, are as follows

The Google Scholar search page is: low, molecular, weight, heparin, deep, vein, thrombosis, mortality

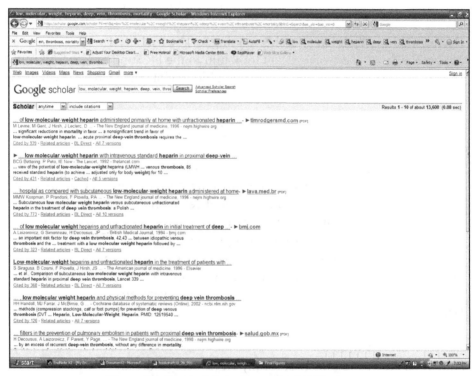

Figure B.1 Google Scholar Search for DVT Treatment.

The first Google Scholar summary looked relevant as it compared outpatient low molecular weight heparin to hospitalized unfractionated heparin for the treatment of DVT. However, after following the link, the article's endpoint was recurrent thromboembolism, not mortality. Our patient is interested in mortality reduction.

The second Google Scholar summary also looks appropriate. We followed the link to the article's abstract, and found the article was also looking for recurrent thromboembolism and bleeding risk. Again, mortality was not an endpoint.

The third Google Scholar summary, like the first two, initially looks relevant. Also like the first, after following the link we learned that the endpoint was not relevant to our patients concern. The endpoint was recurrent thromboembolism, bleeding, quality of life, and cost.

The fourth Google Scholar summary also looked relevant. After following the link to the abstract, we learned that this was a meta-analysis of 16 studies. One of the endpoints is mortality. The article was published in 1994. We are interested if more relevant, more current information is available. We will keep this in mind and continue looking.

Looking down the screen, the sixth Google Scholar summary is a Cochrane Systematic Review. The Cochrane Collaboration is one of the foremost authorities in evidence based medicine. They review all of the information for a given subject in a high degree of detail. The fact that there is a Cochrane review of this subject matter, our search can stop here. Cochrane is the most authoritative source of evidence. We have found our article, the Cochrane Review.[1]

In real life application of this process, we would use the Cochrane Review to help our patient make a decision. But, for illustration of this process and to carry onto the next step, we have randomly selected 'Fixed-dose, Body Weight independent Subcutaneous LMW Heparin versus Adjusted Dose Unfractionated Intravenous Heparin in the Initial Treatment of Proximal Venous Thrombosis' an article that was used in the Cochrane Review. We will use this article for the remainder of the discussion.

Assess the validity of the information

1. Was the assignment of patients to treatments really randomized?
Yes. It states it in the Study Design section.

2. Were all clinically relevant outcomes reported?
The primary outcome measure according to the authors is a DOE – the Marter score on repeat venography. Who cares? The secondary outcomes are the relevant ones. It was a composite outcome, but they go on to report death separately, so this is an appropriate outcome measure.

3. Were the study patients recognizably similar to your own?
No. This was a selected group of patients from a venous embolism service from an inpatient setting – our patient is from the office.

4. Were both clinical and statistical significance considered?
Statistically, there was no difference with regard to mortality.

5. Is the therapeutic maneuver feasible in your practice?
Yes, we use low molecular weight heparin routinely.

6. Were all the patients who entered the study accounted for at its inclusion?
Yes, the numbers all add up.

7. Were patients analyzed in the groups to which they were randomized?
Yes, an intention to treat analysis was used.

8. Were all patients, health workers, and study personnel blinded?
No. This is very important. However, is it possible with these medications? With the unfractionated heparin, the patient gets a PTT test every four to six hours in addition to an IV drip. The LMWH are boluses injected into the skin daily. A possible solution to this problem would be to give a placebo drip or placebo injection and then draw a PTT every six hours on every patient regardless. The physician would not be blinded as they would have access to the lab results. In really well designed studies, they have two sets of physicians so that the lab results can still be blinded – you can titrate placebo IV drips and preserve blinding for the treating physicians. Having an unblinded study critically weakens the study. This article focuses on the fact that the radiologist read the repeat venogram. However, who really cares if the clot is smaller? We are more interested in the secondary outcomes for which the treating health care professionals were not blinded. Neither were the patients. This can still be biased from the lack of blinding – who decides if bleeding is significant or not? Who decides whether or not to repeat a work-up for recurrent disease? So, the lack of blinding is a problem with this study.

9. Aside from the experimental intervention, were the groups treated equally?
No. Care for experimental and control groups can differ in a number of ways besides the test therapy, and differences in care other than that under study can weaken distort the results. If one group received closer follow-up, events might be more likely to be reported, and patients may be treated more intensively with non-study therapies.

Apply the information to the patient's problem
We are going to first calculate the number needed to treat (NNT) for mortality reduction for the individual article reviewed and then compare it to the Cochrane Systemic Review.

Individual Article's Number Needed to Treat

Table B.1 summarizes the mortality results for the individual study. There are three categories of death – death at initial treatment, death within the first six months (the study length), and total mortality. Our patient is interested in total mortality – is he going to live or die. 'N' stands for the total number of patients in each group; (%) indicates that the number in parenthesis is the percentage of patients in that group with the measured outcome. In other words, (4.5) means that 4.5% of the patients in the unfractionated heparin group had died by the six months follow-up.

Table B.1. Summary of Results for the Individual Study.

	LMWH N = 265 (%)	Unfractionated heparin N = 273 (%)
Death upon initial treatment	0	3 (1.1)
Death by 6 months follow-up	6 (2.3)	12 (4.5)
Total death	6 (2.3)	15 (5.5)

Harenberg J, Schmidt J, Koppenhagen K, *et al.* Fixed-dose, body weight-independent subcutaneous LMW heparin versus adjusted dose unfractionated intravenous heparin in the initial treatment of proximal venous thrombosis. *Thromb Haemost.* 2000; **83**: 652–6.

We can calculate the NNT with the following equation:

$$NNT = \frac{1}{arr}$$

The equation to calculate the absolute risk reduction (arr) is:

$$arr = \frac{\text{Patients in the control group with the measured event}}{\text{Total number of patients in control group}} - \frac{\text{Patients in the treatment group with the measured event}}{\text{Total number of patients in treatment group}}$$

Using the numbers from the first equation above:

$$arr = \frac{15}{273} - \frac{6}{265}$$

arr = .055 – .023

arr = .032

Plugging the absolute risk reduction of .032 into the number needed to treat equation:

$$NNT = \frac{1}{.032}$$

$$NNT = 31$$

Thus, for every 31 patients that are treated with low molecular weight heparin instead of unfractionated heparin; one of their lives is saved. However, this number needed to treat is for a poor quality study. Let us see what happens when we use the Cochrane Review's data.

Cochrane Review's Number Needed to Treat

The following excerpt is from the Cochrane Review's abstract:

> Nine studies ($n=4451$) examined proximal thrombosis; 2192 participants treated with LMWH and 2259 with UFH. Subgroup analysis showed statistically signifi- cant reductions favouring LMWH in thrombotic complications and major haem- orrhage. By the end of follow up, 80 (3.6%) participants treated with LMWH had thrombotic complications, compared with 143 (6.3%) treated with UFH (OR 0.57; 95% CI 0.44 to 0.75). Major haemorrhage occurred in 18 (1.0%) partici- pants treated with LMWH, compared with 37 (2.1%) treated with UFH (OR 0.50; 95% CI 0.29 to 0.85). Nine studies ($n = 4157$) showed a statistically significant reduction favouring LMWH with respect to mortality. By the end of follow up, 3.3% (70/2094) of participants treated with LMWH had died, compared with 5.3% (110/2063) of participants treated with UFH (OR 0.62; 95% CI 0.46 to 0.84).[1]

Again, our patient is interested in mortality. In the last sentence, they state that 70 of 2094 patients treated with low molecular weight heparin died compared with 110 of 2063 patients treated with unfractionated heparin. Let's use these numbers to calculate the absolute risk reduction as seen below:

$$arr = \frac{110}{2063} - \frac{70}{2094}$$

$$arr = .053 - .033$$

$$arr = .02$$

We can then calculate the number needed to treat:

$$NNT = \frac{1}{.02}$$

$$NNT = 50$$

Thus, we would have to treat 50 patients with low molecular weight heparin instead of unfractionated heparin for the treatment of a DVT to save one of their lives. This is quite a bit higher than the individual study that we reviewed. Which one should we use to discuss with out patient? Cochrane Review is more accurate than any individual study, thus we will use a number needed to treat of 50 in our patient discussion.

Assist the patient to make a decision

Patient's wife: So is it OK if I just give him these shots?

Doctor: Actually, it's better if you use the shots … the research shows that fewer patients die with using the shots compared to IV drips in the hospital.

Patient's wife: I would never have imagined that. Thanks for checking it out for me, doctor.

REFERENCE

1 Van Dongen CJ, van den Belt AG, Prins M, *et al.* Fixed dose subcutaneous low molecular weight heparins versus adjusted dose unfractionated heparin for venous thromboembolism (Review). *Cochrane Library.* 2008(4).

The Hippocratic Oath

'I do solemnly swear by that which I hold most sacred:

That I will be loyal to the profession of medicine and just and generous to its members;

That I will share the knowledge and skills which I have received with my colleagues and with future generations of physicians;

That I will lead my life and practice my art in uprightness and honor;

That into whatsoever house I shall enter, it shall be for the good of the sick to the utmost of my power; holding myself aloof from wrong, from corruption, from the tempting of others to vice;

That I will exercise my art solely for the good of my patients, and will give no drug, perform no operation for a criminal purpose, even if solicited, far less suggest it;

That whatsoever I shall see or hear of the lives of patients which is not fitting to be spoken, I will keep inviolably secret;

These things I do promise and in proportion as I am faithful to this my oath may happiness and good repute be ever mine – the opposite if I shall be forsworn.'

Index